Developing Your Identity as a Professional Counselor

Standards, Settings, and Specialties

Sylvia C. Nassar-McMillan
North Carolina State University

Spencer G. Niles
Pennsylvania State University

BROOKS/COLE
CENGAGE Learning™

Australia • Brazil • Japan • Korea • Mexico • Singapore • Spain • United Kingdom • United States

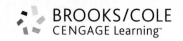
BROOKS/COLE
CENGAGE Learning

Developing Your Identity as a Professional Counselor: Standards, Settings, and Specialties
Sylvia C. Nassar-McMillan and Spencer G. Niles

Acquisitions Editor: Seth Dobrin

Assistant Editor: Nicholas Albert

Editorial Assistant: Rachel McDonald

Media Editor: Dennis Fitzgerald

Senior Marketing Manager: Trent Whatcott

Marketing Assistant: Darlene Macanan

Marketing Communications Manager: Tami Strang

Content Project Manager: Rita Jaramillo

Creative Director: Rob Hugel

Senior Art Director: Jennifer Wahi

Print Buyer: Paula Vang

Rights Acquisitions Account Manager, Text: Katie Huha

Rights Acquisitions Account Manager, Image: Leitha Ethridge-Sims

Production Service: Pre-PressPMG

Copy Editor: Gail Fay

Cover Designer: William Stanton

Cover Image: SuperStock

Compositor: Pre-PressPMG

For product information and technology assistance, contact us at **Cengage Learning Customer & Sales Support, 1-800-354-9706.**

For permission to use material from this text or product, submit all requests online at **www.cengage.com/permissions.** Further permissions questions can be e-mailed to **permissionrequest@cengage.com.**

Library of Congress Control Number: 2009943635

Student Edition:

ISBN-13: 978-0-618-47492-9

ISBN-10: 0-618-47492-7

Brooks/Cole
20 Davis Drive
Belmont, CA 94002-3098
USA

Cengage Learning is a leading provider of customized learning solutions with office locations around the globe, including Singapore, the United Kingdom, Australia, Mexico, Brazil, and Japan. Locate your local office at **www.cengage.com/global.**

Cengage Learning products are represented in Canada by Nelson Education, Ltd.

To learn more about Brooks/Cole, visit **www.cengage.com/ brookscole**

Purchase any of our products at your local college store or at our preferred online store **www.CengageBrain.com.**

Printed in the United States of America
1 2 3 4 5 6 7 14 13 12 11 10

BRIEF CONTENTS

DETAILED CONTENTS

PREFACE

The main purpose of this text is to provide current, state-of-the art information regarding the counseling profession. To achieve this purpose, we assembled leaders in the profession to serve as chapter authors. Thus, each chapter of this book is authored by persons who are intimately familiar with the respective topics addressed. They each have substantial professional experience, not simply as counselor educators and statespersons within the profession, but also as counseling practitioners. They draw upon their collective experiences to share their wisdom and insights regarding their chapter topics.

A second, but equally important, purpose of this text is to inspire readers as they develop their identities as professional counselors and learn about counseling standards, settings, and specialties. We seek to engage the reader in each of the topics we address in this book. The chapter authors provide personal statements and include material from a "day in the life" of practitioners working in the primary counseling settings and specialty areas. The authors provide real and accurate information regarding what it is like to work as a professional counselor in the 21st century.

At the onset of this project, we quickly determined that it would be challenging at best for one or two authors to write from an expert's perspective on every topic that should be addressed in an introduction to counseling book. One or two people could not possibly possess a deep level of expertise across such a wide range of topics. Even though one could argue that a deep level of expertise may not be required for a book that introduces readers to the counseling profession, we strongly disagree. Consider this question for yourself. If you were to attend a lecture regarding any particular topic included in this book, would you rather the lecturer be a generalist who perhaps has never worked in the area that she or he is writing about, or would you prefer that the lecturer be a person who has specialized in the topic she or he is discussing? Which lecturer do you think may have a deeper under-standing of the challenges, issues, opportunities, and benefits of working in the area about which she or he is discussing? We think the answers to these questions are obvious. We also think that using the "expert" approach to developing this book results in an excellent resource that readers can rely upon for learning the essential information related to becoming a professional counselor.

To achieve these purposes, we provide important pedagogical informa-tion in each chapter. Each chapter begins with important learning objectives that provide an overview to the key material presented in the chapter. Chapter authors also provide "thought questions" to guide readers in reflecting upon important chapter points. Authors also provide a window into what it is like to be a professional counselor working within a specific counseling specialty or setting. Through the "day in the life" sharing of what counselors actually experience in their work, authors provide you with more of an experiential moment as you read about what it might actually be like working as a profes-sional counselor. Special topics and further considerations are also included in the chapters. Summary points and suggestions for additional resources help to reinforce and extend learning about chapter content.

To help instructors adapt the book to their courses, we provide ancillary materials that include PowerPoints, sample tests, and related pedagogical fea-tures. Collectively we sincerely hope that this book becomes a valued resource for students and instructors. We are proud of the contributions that have been made by each chapter author. We are grateful for their willingness to share their vast experience, knowledge, and insights regarding professional counseling. We hope that this book helps readers develop their professional identities and inspires them to become the best professional counselors that they can possibly become. We also hope that readers acquire a deep sense of pride in the rich traditions that characterize a profession that is dedicated to helping others live more fulfilling, satisfied, and productive lives.

ACKNOWLEDGEMENTS

In addition to the important contributions of the chapter authors, the editors are deeply grateful to Mary Falcon for her skilled and professional editorial assistance and guidance. In her typical exemplary fashion, Mary has helped raise the quality of the book significantly. We also acknowledge the helpful feedback provided by the reviewers. Finally, we are grateful to the support provided by Seth Dobrin throughout the development and the completion of this project.

ABOUT THE AUTHORS

RICK BRUHN is a professor of counselor education at Sam Houston State University. He also has a private practice in marital and family therapy in Huntsville, Texas, along with his wife, Sara. Dr. Bruhn's career as a university instructor started in 1984. Since then he has taught a wide range of counseling and marriage and family therapy (MFT) courses at three universities, at the undergraduate, master's, and doctoral levels. His current favorites are Techniques of MFT, Theories of MFT, and Supervised Practice of Counseling (master's and doctoral levels). Dr. Bruhn is a Licensed Professional Counselor-Supervisor, and a Licensed Marriage and Family Therapist-Supervisor in Texas. He also is a member of the American Counseling Association, the American Association for Marriage and Family Therapy (Clinical Member and Approved Supervisor), and the American Society of Clinical Hypnosis. Dr. Bruhn's Ed.D. in counseling and guidance is from East Texas State University and his M.S.Ed. (school psychology) is from University of Wisconsin–Stout.

JOLYNN CARNEY, Ph.D., is an associate professor of counselor education at Penn State University. She is a Licensed Professional Clinical Counselor who has experience working in community mental health agencies, private practice, and schools. She has been a trustee on a number of boards of directors that service at-risk youth, has served on state counseling boards, works closely with local school districts, and is a recipient of several service awards from professional groups. Dr. Carney is the current president elect of Chi Sigma Iota International and has served as regional chapter facilitator for the North Atlantic region. Dr. Carney's research and publishing focuses on intervention/prevention aspects of youth violence and adolescent suicide. Scholarly work also includes wellness programming and counseling techniques. A significant focus is on the psychophysiological influence of chronic bullying on youth. She currently serves on editorial boards of nationally recognized counseling journals, publishes, and does local, regional, and national trainings/ workshops.

AMY CHEUNG received a bachelor of arts in psychology from the University of Maryland, Baltimore County. She attended Loyola College in Maryland and attained a master's of education in school counseling. She has been employed with the American Psychological Association and the Carroll County Public School System.

DENNIS ENGELS, Ph.D., LPC, MCC, NCCC, has been Regents Professor in the Counseling Program at University of North Texas, Denton, since 1976. He is also a past president of the Texas Counseling Association; past president and a charter fellow of the National Career Development Association; editor emeritus of *Counseling and Values*, journal of the Association for Spiritual, Ethical, and Religious Values in Counseling; past chair of the American Counseling Association Council of Journal Editors; and former secretary and newsletter editor for the Association for Counselor Education and Supervision. Dr. Engels spent 30 years on editorial boards of the *Journal of Counseling and Development, Counselor Education and Supervision*, and *Career Development Quarterly*. He has extensive experience with accreditation, has been published in over 100 professional publications, and has prepared hundreds of presentations. Consultant with public and private sector organizations and agencies. Dr. Engels teaches and/or supervises courses in career counseling, ethics, life-career development, and internship. His research and scholarly interests center on career development, decision making, ethics, human resource development, multipotentiality, organizational and disciplinary history, and strategic and operational planning.

DELINI M. FERNANDO, Ph.D., LPC, NCC, has been assistant professor in the Counseling Program at the University of North Texas, Denton, since 2006. Dr. Fernando teaches the master's and doctoral group counseling courses and coordinates master's internships. She supervises interns on the community/ agency, school, and college/university tracks. She also supervises doctoral student group leaders and doctoral student supervisors. She has presented at numerous state, regional, and national conferences, as well as published in major counseling journals. Dr. Fernando's research and scholarly interests center on group work, counselor supervision, multicultural and social justice issues in counseling, and international disaster counseling. She has experience in a variety of counseling settings including agency, school, international disaster groups, and private practice.

LINDA H. FOSTER is the vice president for professional practice at the National Board for Certified Counselors (NBCC). Dr. Foster is a Licensed Professional Counselor, Supervising Counselor, National Certified Counselor, and National Certified School Counselor. She served on the NBCC Board of Directors for five years and previously worked with NBCC on a standards revision and test development committees. Dr. Foster was a school counselor for over 10 years and held a tenure track position as a counselor educator. She has published several book chapters and journal articles primarily in the area of professional practice and assessment.

PERRY C. FRANCIS, Ph.D., is a professor of counseling and the coordinator of counseling for the College of Education Clinical Suite at Eastern Michigan University (EMU). The clinic is a training facility for advanced level graduate counseling students where they see clients from the community and student body of EMU. He is a member of the American College Counseling Association and has served on the leadership team as a board member-at-large and as the president. Dr. Francis has authored articles and book chapters on several subjects and has presented on common and not so common ethical issues in supervision and college counseling, as well as suicide assessment and prevention at conferences in the United States and Canada. Dr. Francis earned his degree in counselor education at the University of Northern Colorado (UNC). Before completing his degree, Dr. Francis was a Lutheran parish pastor and a campus pastor. He also served as an interim staff psychologist at the UNC Counseling Center.

GARBETTE MONTIE GARRAWAY is an assistant professor in the Department of Counseling and Addiction Studies at the University of Detroit Mercy in Michigan. He received his master's degree in counseling psychology from the University of British Columbia, Canada, and his doctorate in counselor education and supervision from Penn State University. He worked for 14 years as a high school teacher and elementary school counselor and was the coordinator of the School Counseling Program at Oakland University in Michigan. Dr. Garraway has made several international, national, and regional presentations on the counseling process and issues in multicultural counseling and has coauthored a textbook on career planning.

JANE GOODMAN is professor emerita, counseling, at Oakland University in Rochester, Michigan. She is a past president of the American Counseling Association (ACA) and the National Career Development Association (NCDA). Professor Emerita Goodman is the author of several books and many book chapters and journal articles, mostly in the area of adult career development and adult transitions. She is a fellow of ACA and NCDA and received the Eminent Career Award from NCDA. Professor Emerita Goodman is a frequent presenter at local, national, and international conferences. Most recently she led an ACA People to People delegation to China and Tibet and made a series of presentations in Peru on behalf of NCDA. She is the mother or stepmother of seven and grandmother of eight amazing children and young adults.

CHARLES F. GRESSARD is an associate professor in the Counselor Education Program at the College of William & Mary. He has worked in the counseling profession for close to 40 years, and he has been a counselor educator for 30 years. He has specialized in addictions counseling from the beginning of his career, and he currently coordinates the Addiction Counseling emphasis in community counseling at William & Mary. Dr. Gressard also has interests in ethics, international issues, and credentialing. He has served on the Virginia Board of Counseling; the Virginia Impaired Professionals Committee; the American Counseling Association Ethics Committee; the National Board for Certified Counselors (NBCC) Addictions Academy; the NBCC Board of Directors, which he chaired in 2004; and the 2009 CACREP (Council for Accreditation of Counseling and Related Educational Programs) Standards Revision Committee. He is currently a member of the CACREP Board of Directors. In 2008, Dr. Gressard received Chi Sigma Iota's Thomas J. Sweeney National Professional Leadership Award.

RICHARD J. HAZLER, Ph.D., is professor of counselor education at Penn State University. He earned his Ph.D. at the University of Idaho and has been a faculty member for 30 years. Other professional work includes being an elementary school teacher and counselor in schools, prison, military, and private practice. Dr. Hazler's national and international reputation extends to holding editorial board positions on major journals; writing articles, books, and book chapters on counseling and humanistic-oriented approaches; and being a regular speaker on counseling issues. His early and continuing research on school violence and bullying has received particular notice. A sample of books include *Helping in the Hallways: Expanding Your Influence Potential*, 2nd edition (2008); *The Emerging Professional Counselor: Student Dreams to Professional Realities*, 2nd edition (2003); *The Therapeutic Environment: Core Conditions for Facilitating Therapy* (2001); and *Breaking the Cycle of Violence: Interventions for Bullying and Victimization* (1996).

EDWIN L. HERR, Distinguished Professor Emeritus of Education and emeritus associate dean, College of Education, Penn State University, received his Ed.D. in guidance and counseling from Teachers College, Columbia University. He served as the first director of the Bureau of Guidance Services in the Pennsylvania Department of Education and has served as a visiting professor in many universities in Europe, Asia, Africa, and North America. The author of more than 300 journal articles and invited book chapters and 34 books and monographs, Dr. Herr has served as president of the American Counseling Association, National Career Development Association, Association for Counselor Education and Supervision, and Chi Sigma Iota. He also served on the Board of Directors of the International Association for Educational and Vocational Guidance and the International Round Table for the Advancement of Counseling. He is an Overseas Fellow of the National Institute for Careers Education and Counseling, England, a member of the Executive Committee of the International Centre for Career Development and Public Policy, as well as a fellow of numerous professional societies including the American Psychological Association.

BRANDON HUNT is a professor of counselor education at Penn State University. Prior to becoming faculty she worked as a rehabilitation counselor serving clients with mental illness as well as clients with alcohol and other drug concerns. Her current research interests include counselor professional identity and assessing counselor attitudes toward their clients. Dr. Hunt has served on three national counseling boards (National Board for Certified Counselors, Council for Accreditation of Counseling and Related Educational Programs, ARCA) and is the associate editor for qualitative research for the *Journal of Counseling & Development*. She has a strong commitment to teaching and advising undergraduate and graduate students and has a history of mentoring new faculty.

CAROLYN W. KERN, Ph.D., LPC, NCC, is an associate professor in the Counseling Program at the University of North Texas. She is also a past president of the American College Counseling Association and an American Counseling Association Governing Council Member. She also served several years as an editorial board member for the *Journal of College Counseling*. Dr. Kern teaches doctoral counseling supervision, counseling skills based courses, practicum, internship, college student development, counseling adolescents and school counseling. Her research and grant interest includes suicide intervention and prevention and developing resiliency. She has presented at numerous state, regional, and national conferences as well as published a number of articles and book chapters. Dr. Kern also coordinated supervision of students in internship. She has experience in a variety of counseling settings, including agency, school, and college counseling centers.

SONG LEE, Ph.D., is an assistant professor at California State University, Fresno, in the Department of Counseling, Special Education, and Rehabilitation. She received her master's degree in counseling, with a concentration in marriage and family therapy, and the Pupil Personnel Services Credential in School Counseling from California State University, Fresno. Dr. Lee earned her Ph.D. in counselor education from North Carolina State University. Dr. Lee's clinical experiences include providing counseling services to diverse groups of children, family, and couples. Dr. Lee's primary research interests include identity development of marginalized populations in general and of the Southeast Asian population specifically, and multicultural issues relating to the provision of counseling services. She has presented at international, national, state, and regional conferences on topics relating to identity development, the Hmong population, multicultural counseling issues, and culturally and linguistically appropriate interventions. Dr. Lee also co-hosts a radio show for the Hmong elderly population.

ELIZABETH MELLIN, Ph.D., LPC, is an assistant professor of counselor education at Penn State University. Prior to joining Penn State University as an assistant professor in 2006, Dr. Mellin was a child and adolescent counselor, clinical supervisor, and grant writer for a large, public community mental health program in Atlanta, Georgia. She is a nationally published author on issues related to promoting mental health among children and adolescents. Dr. Mellin's research and scholarly interests are specifically focused on the contribution of interprofessional and cross-system collaboration to improving outcomes valued by schools, families, and communities. In addition to her appointment as an assistant professor at Penn State University, Dr. Mellin is also an invited member of the Mental Health-Education Integration Consortium, which is a national group of scholars and practitioners focused on research, training, and policy related to the mental health professional development of educators and all other school personnel as well as the preparation of mental health professionals for working within educational environments.

SYLVIA NASSAR-MCMILLAN, Ph.D., is an associate professor and program coordinator for counselor education at North Carolina State University. Over the past 20 years, her research, service, and practice foci have included counselor training and supervision and intersections of career, gender, and multicultural issues. She is the current associate editor of multicultural issues for the *Journal of Counseling & Development*; a member of the Census Information Center Advisory Board to the Arab American Institute and the North Carolina Board for Licensed Professional Counselors; and a former board member of the National Board for Certified Counselors. Dr. Nassar-McMillan has authored or coauthored over 50 publications and 75 presentations. Among her awards are the Association for Counselor Education and Supervision's Publication in Counselor Education and Supervision Award (2008), the UNCG Department of Counseling and Educational Development Alumni Excellence Award (2006), the North Carolina Counseling Association Research and Professional Writing Award (2006), and the American Counseling Association Best Practices Award (2003).

JUDITH A. NELSON is an assistant professor in the Educational Leadership and Counseling Department at Sam Houston State University in Huntsville, Texas. She is a Licensed Professional Counselor, a Licensed Marriage and Family Therapist, and a Certified School Counselor. Dr. Nelson is the president of the Texas Counseling Association for the 2009–2010 term, and she was the recipient of the Texas Counseling Association Professional Writing Award in 2008. Before working in higher education, she was a school counselor and worked in a small private practice. Dr. Nelson currently teaches Theories of Marriage and Family Therapy and Counseling for Sexual Concerns. Her research interests include family systems and school systems working together; counseling in alternative schools; organizational cultural competence; and the notion of commitment in marriage.

MARY NICHTER, Ph.D., is an associate professor of counselor education at Sam Houston State University in Huntsville, Texas. She is a Licensed Professional Counselor and Supervisor, Licensed Marriage and Family Therapist, and a Certified School Counselor. Dr. Nichter has been a counselor educator for 10 years. Dr. Nichter has eight years of clinical practice working as a marriage and family therapist in private practice, hospitals, and at a clinic for pain stress and depression. She is also the editor of an online counseling journal, *Profession Issues in Counseling*. Dr. Nichter's research interest includes theoretical orientation of beginning counselors, identifying student impairment, and supervision.

SPENCER NILES, Ed.D., is professor and department head for the Department of Counselor Education, Counseling Psychology, and Rehabilitation Services at Penn State University. He is the recipient of the National Career Development Association's (NCDA) Eminent Career Award (2007), a NCDA Fellow (2002), an American Counseling Association (ACA) Fellow (2007), ACA's David Brooks Distinguished Mentor Award (2003), the ACA Extended Research Award (2004), and the University of British Columbia Noted Scholar Award (2001). Currently, he is the editor of the *Journal of Counseling & Development* and has authored or coauthored approximately 100 publications and delivered over 90 presentations on career development theory and practice. Dr. Niles is an honorary member of the Japanese Career Development Association (2003) and the Italian Association for Educational and Vocational Guidance (2005).

JERRY TRUSTY is a professor in the Department of Counselor Education, Counseling Psychology, and Rehabilitation Services at Penn State University. He is coordinator of the Secondary School Counseling Program. He is the current editor of *Career Development Quarterly*, the journal of the National Career Development Association. Dr. Trusty has worked as a middle school and high school counselor, a school-dropout prevention coordinator, and a counselor educator. His research and scholarly work has focused on school-dropout prevention, adolescents' educational and career development, parents' influences on adolescents, and opportunity gaps in schools. In his recent published research, he investigated the effects of students' experiences and behaviors in high school on college graduation versus nongraduation. Jerry currently works with the Pennsylvania Transforming School Counseling Initiative. This initiative involves training school counselors to lead and advocate for effective school policies and practices.

RICHARD E. WATTS, Ph.D., is professor and director of the Center for Research and Doctoral Studies in Counselor Education at Sam Houston State University in Huntsville, Texas. He received his Ph.D. in counseling from the University of North Texas in 1994. Watts is the author of over 100 professional publications and has received numerous awards for his scholarship and service to the counseling profession. He is also the editor of *Counseling and Values*, the professional journal of the Association for Spiritual, Ethical, and Religious Values in Counseling, a division of the American Counseling Association. His scholarship interests include Adlerian, cognitive, and constructivist approaches to individual and couple and family counseling; counselor supervision and counselor efficacy; ethical and legal issues; play therapy; and religious and spiritual issues in counseling.

KEITH B. WILSON, Ph.D., CRC, ABDA, NCC, LPC, is a professor of counselor education and rehabilitation education at Penn State University, University Park,

Pennsylvania. Dr. Wilson has 25 years of service in higher education and teaches graduate and undergraduate courses in counselor education and rehabilitation services. He is the author of the book chapter "Skin Color and Latinos With Disabilities: Expanding What We Know About Colorism in the United States" (2008) and editor of the book *Expanding What We Know Through Research About the African Diaspora* (2009). His current research project, "Phenotype Discrimination: The Experiences of Black and White Latinos With Disabilities in the United States," examines phenotype discrimination among Black and White Latinos with disabilities and people with nonvisible disabilities not only in the United States, but globally as well. Dr. Wilson served as program chair for rehabilitation services for four years. Additionally, from 2006–2008 he served as director the African Research Center. He has delivered innumerable workshops and seminars to programs like Upward Bound, SORP, and McNair as a presenter, social and research mentor. These programs are in place to facilitate college and/or graduate school success for students from underrepresented populations. He has been the proprietor of Counseling, Consultation and Psychotherapy Services in State College, Pennsylvania, for the past seven years.

INTRODUCTION FOR THE STUDENT

As you've already learned from the Preface, we believe that this book represents both the current standards of the counseling profession, as well cutting-edge issues in the field. Actual chapter topics are aligned with the standards of the Council for the Accreditation of Counseling and Related Educational Programs by which your counselor education program may be accredited. We have divided the book up into four parts: Foundations of Professional Counseling, Professional Counseling Settings, Professional Counseling Specialties, and Developing a Personal and Professional Counselor Identity.

In Part I (Foundations), Chapter 1 (Theoretical and Historical Foundations of the Counseling Profession) will introduce you to the history of the counseling profession from both theoretical and practical perspectives. Chapter 2 (The Counseling Profession Today) will take over from there by bringing you up to date on what the counseling profession looks like today. Chapter 3 (The Counselor's Roles and Functions) will describe the roles that today's counselors play, as well as the counseling services they provide in those roles. Chapter 4 (Ethical and Legal Standards in Counseling) discusses the important ethical and legal issues that are critical for today's counselors to address in the scope of their work. Chapter 5 (Counseling With Diverse Clients) brings into focus the diversity of demographic factors in today's world, with a particular emphasis on counseling implications within the United States. In Chapter 6 (Using Assessment in Counseling), you will be introduced to the role of various types of assessment in counseling. Finally, Chapter 7 (The Role of Research in Counseling) discusses the role that research plays within an array of counseling contexts.

Parts II (Professional Counseling Settings) and III (Professional Counseling Specialties) will provide a more in-depth look at the actual work that professional counselors do, examining a broad spectrum of settings in which they may be employed as well as specialized training and interests that may be pursued to better serve the needs of particular groups of clients. Chapters 8 (Counseling in School Settings), 9 (Mental Health Counseling in Community Settings), and 10 (Student Affairs and Counseling in College Settings) detail both general information about professional counseling within those settings, such as credentialing and types of facilities, as well as special topics within and future considerations for those settings. Chapters 11 (Career Counseling), 12 (Substance Abuse Counseling), 13 (Rehabilitation Counseling), and 14 (Couple and Family Counseling) explain the more specialized orientations and considerations necessary when focusing on a specific client group or issue, such as special knowledge, information, or training needed, as well as, again, future considerations in these areas of professional counseling. Within Parts II and III, you will find many "Day in the Life Of" stories to illustrate professional counselor scenarios presented.

Finally, in Part IV (Developing a Personal and Professional Counselor Identity), we invite you to take a look within yourself to begin to identify your own journey. In Chapter 15 (Considering the Counselor as a Person), we will engage you in exploring aspects of yourself as a person that are relevant to yourself as a beginning counselor, or even as someone just becoming interested in the field. Chapter 16 (Developing and Maintaining a Professional Identity) will provide a historical perspective of various aspects of the professionalization of counselors and the counseling profession, as well as help you begin to set goals for your own professional career. Chapter 17 (Integrating Technology and Counseling) provides a glimpse at future considerations necessary for all professional counselors in today's technological world.

We hope that these chapters will engage you on a rich and exciting journey of professional counseling! Our intent in shaping the content, particularly the learning activities, is to stimulate your imaginations to enter this world, perhaps placing yourself within a specific setting or specialty of interest, perhaps focusing on a particular client issue or aspect of counseling. Wherever your journey takes you, we hope it will have been enriched by the material we have provided. We believe that, should you decide to pursue the counseling profession, your personal and professional journey will ultimately lead to better service delivery to clients and, thus, the betterment of society, and we are pleased to be a part of it!

PART 1

Foundations of Professional Counseling

CHAPTER 1

Theoretical and Historical Foundations of the Counseling Profession

LEARNING OBJECTIVES

After reading this chapter, you should be able to

- describe the short history of counseling as an organized body of techniques, interventions, and professional evolution that essentially arose in the 19th century and had its major advance in the 20th century;

- discuss the long view of scholars through 2,000 years of history who studied "mental health issues" and the persons who served and guided others;

- understand the origins of modern psychology, and its split from philosophy, as a base for understanding human behavior, grouping such behavior, and attaching these groupings to methods that may be used to "treat" mental disorders and other psychological problems;

- describe the rise of the terms *guidance* and *counseling* as the operative words for interventions in human behavior and the contextual factors that stimulated such interventions;

- understand the importance of federal policy and legislation in shaping the provision and definition of counseling in the 20th century;

- identify theories of counseling in the 20th century that grew in number and in emphasis; and

- discuss trends in counseling.

CHAPTER OUTLINE

INTRODUCTION

In this chapter, the history of counseling is discussed in two major ways: (1) in a short view, focusing on the "recent" events affecting the rise of a counseling profession in the last 150 years or so; and (2) in a long view, tracing the roots of counseling back to the time of Aristotle and other major philosophers and teachers of several hundred years ago who slowly but surely built the foundations for what we now conceive of as counseling. This long view of the evolution of counseling has many antecedents and many shifts in emphasis. In an oversimplified way, counseling originates in attempts to understand human behavior and in an evolution from philosophy to psychology to scientific methods used to test the conceptual and theoretical perspectives developing century after century.

Until the short view began some 150 or so years ago, scholars were focused on what could be called mental health issues, psychological matters, the etiology of individual differences, the impact on individual behavior of the external conditions and contexts in which people lived, and other important issues that gave insight into various explanations of human behavior.

During the Middle Ages, a remarkable set of theories were created to increase the understanding of mind-body relationships, the formation of personality and character, the stimuli to human growth and behavior, and the elements that cause individuals to be alike or different. These theories were refined and combined, and sometimes rejected, but they often were the forerunners of contemporary theories of behavior. As such, these scholars provided important propositions about human behavior, the influences upon it, and how it might be reinforced and changed. Inevitably, the latter began giving greater emphasis to the development of interventions or treatments and to research and experimentation.

As the short view of the history of counseling began in the late 1800s and the early 1900s, the terms *guidance* and, subsequently, *counseling* started being used as summary terms for the interventions in human behavior that were being developed. Many of these interventions were applied in schools, while others were provided for adults in community centers and settlement houses.

This chapter discusses in some detail the professionalization of counseling that occurred during the 20th century and has continued during the 21st century. This short view of counseling discusses

- a variety of contextual variables that have been instrumental in defining both the content and the processes of counseling;
- the visionaries who brought creativity to the development of assessments and other tools to help people with their decision-making;
- the public policies that reinforced the importance of guidance and counseling to achieve a variety of national goals;
- the rise of organizations (e.g., the American Counseling Association and its divisions) that increased the professional identity of counselors;
- the credentialing of counselors; and
- the accreditation of counselor preparation programs.

The chapter concludes with a discussion of some of the major trends in counseling. As such, it speculates about the future of counseling at the same time it is expanding its history.

RECENT EVENTS IN THE RISE OF THE COUNSELING PROFESSION

The history of counseling is both short and long. It is about a process and those who provide that process. Such comments are likely to be confusing, although they are each accurate observations. To say that the history of counseling is short is to suggest that as an organized body of techniques or interventions, or indeed a profession, counseling arose in the late 1800s and has evolved, been refined, and changed throughout the 20th century. Now in the first decade of the 21st century, counseling continues to be responsive to new theoretical concepts, new populations to serve, and new procedures.

During the 20th century, a counseling profession emerged; multiple theories were created to describe human behavior and the interventions that might affect change in adjustment issues, decisions to be made, or actions to be taken to solve individual dilemmas; and support for the importance of counseling evolved from an initially philosophical base to an empirical or scientific base providing support for counseling outcomes, the predictable outcomes of counseling. On balance, much of the 20th century was devoted to (1) creating a scientific base for counseling; (2) establishing the separate identity of counselors within the helping professions; (3) creating an infrastructure of counselor educators, preparation standards, program accreditation (Council for Accreditation of Counseling and Related Educational Programs), individual credentialing (National Board of Certified Counselors, state licensure) mechanisms, and ethical guidelines; (4) seeking legislation, statutory sanctions, and support for counselor licensure and for other forms of recognition of counseling as a profession; and, more recently, (5) spreading counseling across the world, strengthening its quality, and tailoring it to different cultural traditions.

These recent events and processes are essentially the legacy that counselors in training and professional counselors can claim as the building blocks of their profession and of the theory, knowledge, and evidence-based interventions encompassed by the term *counseling*.

THEORETICAL FOUNDATIONS OF COUNSELING

Also of significance, however, is the longer view of the history of counseling. That, too, is part of the important legacy that counselors can claim. Depending upon how one defines *counseling*, it is possible to argue that from at least the time of Aristotle, societies have had persons emerge who served and guided others as they dealt with crises or decision conflicts in their lives (Dumont & Carson, 1995; Miller, 1961; Williamson, 1965). In various places around the world and at different times in history, such "helpers" of others were students of what would now be called decision-making, psychological, or mental health issues. These persons in their time might have been known as sages, wizards, shamans, priests, physicians, mythological healers, or exorcisers, or by other labels that suggested that they had special powers that separated them from "ordinary people." Thus, in the distant past one could argue that the conceptual frames of reference for counseling were widely focused on mysticism, supernaturalism, mythology, astrology, and philosophy. Indeed, techniques such as phrenology and palmistry, among others, were employed in counseling as late as the early 20th century. These practices were still being written about and used in the 1930s as possible counseling methods (Jones, 1934).

Aside from such perspectives, however, there were major scholars contemplating and investigating what contemporary counselors would recognize as mental health issues far into antiquity. In a cumulative way their insights have become important elements of the conceptual legacy that has evolved over centuries. Many scholars, more than 2,000 years ago, shed mysticism, evil spirits, and related supernatural causes in their writings as the explanation for mental health problems and began to seek more common and observable factors. For example, Hippocrates argued that epilepsy was not due to demonic possession but to natural causes; Plato argued that mental disorders were partly somatic, partly moral, and partly divine in origin. Other physicians and scholars of the time argued for naturalistic causes of mental conditions, feeblemindedness, hysteria, dementia, madness, and insanity (Bromberg, 1963).

Early Scholars of Human Behavior

By the 17th and 18th centuries, considerable progress had been made in understanding and grouping mental disorders, although less so in determining interventions and other therapies. Such understanding occurred long before psychology became independent of philosophy in the late 1800s and before psychology came to fruition as a separate discipline, an experimental science, and one of the major disciplines undergirding the content and processes of counseling. Many of the views of important scholars in the 1600s and 1700s can be aligned with the field of philosophy. For example, René Descartes, sometimes called the father of modern psychology, was, in the 1600s, the first to make "a sharp distinction between mind and body and believed the mind may affect the body and the body the mind" (Keller, 1937, p. 49). John Locke, a noted British philosopher of the 1600s, provided the notion that the mind at birth is initially a blank sheet (tabula rasa) on which experience writes and the environment shapes one's ideas and behaviors. At the very least, Locke's work can be seen as the precursor of behaviorism and its related theories of counseling. The counterpoint to Locke's perspectives on how human behavior occurs and, therefore, what needs to be changed or modified by counseling is the work of Gottfried Wilhelm Leibniz, also a philosopher of the 1600s, who provided a different view of how individual personality is formed. In a classic essay in 1696 entitled "Observations on Locke's 'Essay on Human Understanding'" (Leibniz, 1890, pp. 94–99), Leibniz argued that human beings can be thought of as having the power to transcend physical and environmental forces through acts of will and volition and inherent appropriate striving. Thus, human beings are not simply captives of their environments but rather persons who can choose and act upon their choices as qualities of self-insight. Leibniz's view can be seen as an early precursor of humanistic or existential theories of man (Allport, 1962).

Many philosophical perspectives on human behavior and its variations stem from the insights of Locke and Leibniz, and these two streams of thought have in later centuries influenced perspectives on how humankind grows and changes and how these processes can be learned, relearned, modified, or otherwise changed. Central to such perspectives are philosophical issues; for example, Are human beings basically rational or irrational? How can different assumptions about the psychological make up of individuals suggest interventions that are aligned with such assumptions? Allport (1962), among others, suggested that variations in assumptions about human growth and development have led to interventions that emerge from such philosophical assumptions.

Allport (1962) cited three examples. If a human being is perceived to be a *reactive being*, as defined by Locke's assumptions about the tabula rasa—the power of one's environment on how one learns to behave and react to one's environment—then the counselor is more likely to use an intervention that deals directly with behavior modification, extinction of responses to certain cues, and learning or relearning of new behaviors. If a human being is seen as a *reactive being in depth* in which—as Sigmund Freud and several of his contemporaries believed—repression, regression, reaction formation, and other factors are involved, then a counselor might use interventions such as depth psychology, psychoanalysis, and a focus on psychodynamics. If, as Leibniz argued, humans are considered *beings-in-the-process of becoming* the counselor is more likely to use interventions that emphasize humanistic, existential, self-insight, client-centered, or constructivist approaches as advocated by Carl Rogers and others.

Allport's perspectives on these three philosophical models of human growth and behavior are helpful toward understanding major ways by which human beings can be classified, but they also emphasize that the philosophical and psychological emphases of scholars in the 17th, 18th, and 19th centuries were on the nature of human behavior, how individual differences could be identified and grouped, what individual differences had to do with the type of work that was pursued, and the complexity of contextual and hereditary factors that influenced group and individual behavior—rather than on counseling interventions.

Theories of Human Behavior Became More Scientific

It is also true that the 17th, 18th, and 19th centuries had many notable thinkers and, increasingly, researchers who provided important propositions about human behavior, the influences upon it, and how it might be reinforced or changed. Although we do not have time to deal with these theorists in depth, it is nevertheless useful to mention some of the influential voices dealing with mental health issues and psychological matters. They include Charles Darwin, who conceptualized evolution as a process of survival of the fittest and postulated that the human being's mind is only different in degree, not in kind, from the animal's and is an evolutionary outgrowth from a lower form. Many scholars of human behavior in the 19th and early 20th centuries valued Darwin's concepts as helping to explain individual differences.

Other scholars of note in the 19th century include Gustav Fechner, a German mathematician and physicist who has been widely identified as the father of quantitative or experimental psychology and psychophysics as he pursued quantitative studies of mental life as related to the stimuli found in the physical world; Wilhelm Wundt, who published the classic book *The Outlines of Physiological Psychology* in 1883, established the first psychological laboratory in the world in 1879, inaugurated the first scientific journal for the publication of psychological research in 1881, and provided the first view of "systematic" psychology and its methods of investigation including introspection and observation; and Edward Titchener, a student of Wundt who established and directed the new laboratory of psychology at Cornell University and instituted it as the standard for scholarship and research in psychology in North America for some 35 years between the late 1800s and the early decades of the 1900s. Titchener gave substance, structure, and definition to the emerging field of psychology. He contrasted the conceptual view of experience by other disciplines with that of psychology. In his view, psychology is the science of the mind, describable in terms of observed fact; a distinction between mind and body; and the importance of the nervous system, introspection, and classes of mental elements (e.g., sensations, images, and affections or feelings) that differ in quality, intensity, duration, vividness, perceptions, context, and the sensory and imaging processes that occur.

Following close on the heels of Titchener's structural approach to psychology, several American scholars at the University of Chicago—including John Dewey, the noted philosopher and educator; James R. Angell, former president of Yale; and Harvey Carr, senior psychologist at Chicago—opposed structuralism because of their interest in what the mind is for rather than what it is; in short they were interested in the *function* of the mind rather than its *structure*. They were seen as representing the Darwinian biological approach to psychology rather than its physiological tradition. These scholars were devotees of Darwin's views of mental evolution and the survival of the fittest. Their question was, What is the role of the mind in helping humans in their struggle for existence?

In addition, the small group of scholars from the University of Chicago cited as the originators of functionalism were also influenced by William James, who was a physiologist, philosopher, teacher, writer, and psychologist. James did not believe in using apparatus and techniques to study the mind. He saw the mind as personal, continuous, changing, and selective, and he took a Darwinian view that the mind had evolved to "steer" the nervous system that had become too complex to regulate itself. In this functionalist view the context of psychology was mental activity or psychophysical activity. This view contended that there was interaction between mental activity and the reactions of the physical organism. In general, then, the goals of the functionalists were to discover (1) how mental activity occurs, (2) what it does, and (3) why it occurs. These questions were seen as part of the relationship between an organism and its environment. Such perspectives yielded two major concepts that guided the functionalists' tasks of discovery about psychological matters: the *reflex arc* and *adaptive behavior*. The *reflex arc* suggests that humans and animals react to sensory stimuli or environmental influences even though the reactions are not learned and are involuntary. In essence, there is no physical reaction without a sensory stimulus; in the presence of such a stimulus some physical reaction will occur. The second major concept of the functionalist is that of *adaptive behavior*, which includes "a motivating stimulus, a sensory situation, and a response that alters that situation in a way that satisfies the motivating condition" (Carr quoted in Keller, 1937, pp. 48–49). In this view, a motive is always a stimulus, including both external and internal motives such as hunger, thirst, and pain. A motive is, in general, considered to be similar to terms that other psychologists use, such as "need," "urge," or "drive." The sensory situation can describe a whole range of stimuli present in a large environment although the individual may respond to only one dominant stimulus in that environment. Functionalism, among other contributions to the evolution of psychology, broadened the scope of psychological issues and included increasingly diverse material from many sources.

Before functionalism became fully established in the evolving definition of psychology, behaviorism gained significant credibility under the leadership and advocacy of John B. Watson. Although there were many other scholars whose work was embedded in a behavioral frame of reference, a legacy of John Locke's theoretical work a century or two earlier, Watson brought to his conceptions of behaviorism a significant background in experimental animal research and study in functionalism. Indeed, his first book dealt primarily with animal behavior. Some five years later Watson wrote a book, *Psychology from the Standpoint of a Behaviorist* (1919), focused on research on human beings. Watson's prolific writings were devoted to his effort to make psychology an experimental science, purely objective, and part of natural science. The central problem in turning psychology into a science, as he viewed it, was to make psychology focus on prediction and control of behavior. Within such a goal, one issue is what cause or stimulus gives rise to a response; the other is predicting the response likely to occur in a given situation. Watson was not interested in data that could not be objectively verified or defined clearly. He took his cues from the larger world of science, where he found in other disciplines methods that were objective and that could be reproduced by other scientists. The world of science led him to be concerned about experimental conditions, the use of small groups of selected subjects, and the primary application of introspection by the psychologist as the investigative method. To a large degree Watson was concerned that much research in psychology was continuing to employ philosophical speculation as a research tool rather than seeking the objective science that he sought. To study stimuli and responses, Watson suggested that objective observation could involve many specific methods, testing, studies of unconditioned and conditioned reflexes, observations with and without experimental controls, and verbal reports, among other possibilities.

Watson hoped that as questions of stimulus and response were answered in his laboratories, his efforts to make psychology an exact science would also yield insights that offered expert advice on many human problems and spheres of activity. In this context he valued both applied and basic research and the experimental problems that could be addressed in either approach. Among his many studies, Watson collected large amounts of data from studying newborn infants as they developed that gave important insights into unlearned and learned responses in children and subsequently adults. For example, Watson found that there were three patterns of emotional responses that arose early in infancy: rage, fear, and love. He also found that many of the emotional responses late in life were conditioned. Thus, according to Watson, many of the individual fears and failures in adulthood have their origins in infancy and early childhood, and are applications of the early response patterns associated with fear, rage, and love. As suggested previously, he believed that an individual's personality is a product of a large number of unlearned responses that have undergone particular types of conditioning. Such processes in adults, however, typically become obscure in their origins because of the overlay of habits and emotions. Watson's work almost inevitably turned to questions about whether emotional patterns can be implanted or conditioned and, in addition, whether such patterns can be unconditioned or unlearned. As such, he pioneered experimental techniques such as extinction and transfer of reactions to stimuli other than the original stimulus. Although he did not propose particular counseling techniques, Watson advocated that practitioners in psychology should use what is known about psychological issues to advise parents, educators, and policy makers; help individuals to organize their life activities; and help society grow in its knowledge and control of the individual.

The Evolution of the *Diagnostic and Statistical Manual of Mental Disorders*

The major scholars cited here laid a base for using the understandings being developed about human behavior, grouping such behavior, and attaching such groupings to methods or techniques that may "treat" persons suffering from mental disorders or other psychological impediments. One of the major outcomes that evolved from this growing knowledge base was the development of the predecessors to the *Diagnostic and Statistical Manual of Mental Disorders* (DSM; American Psychiatric Association, 1980), which has become a major tool of counselors; indeed, some people would say it is the "Bible" of psychological and mental disorders.

As such, the creation of the *DSM* began with the 1840 census and the development of a body of statistical data about the frequency of different types of mental illness in the United States. At the time, there were some seven categories of mental illnesses differentiated by scholars, including mania, melancholia, monomania, paresis, dementia, dipsomania, and epilepsy. According to the American Psychiatric Association's Web site, by 1917 several groups were involved in the planning of uniform statistics across mental hospitals and the development of "nationally acceptable psychiatric nomenclature" that would be incorporated in the American Medical Association's Standard Classified Nomenclature of Disease, used primarily to diagnose inpatients with severe psychiatric and neurological disorders. The organizations that were central to these processes included the National Commission on Mental Hygiene, the Bureau of the Census, and the American Medico-Psychological Association, which in 1921 became the Committee on Statistics of the American Psychiatric Association. The organizations particularly involved in this early development of psychiatric language and its classification were the New York Academy of Medicine, the American Medical Association, and the American Psychiatric Association. This nomenclature continued to enlarge in the post–World War II period under the stimulus of the U.S. Army and the Veterans Administration's concerns about the psychophysiological, personality, and acute disorders experienced by many servicemen and veterans. At essentially the same time, the World Health Organization published the sixth edition of the *International Classification of Diseases*, with a section on mental disorders for the first time. This information included 10 categories describing psychoses and psychoneuroses and 7 categories of character, behavior, and intelligence.

The first version of the *DSM* was published in 1952 (*DSM-I*) and was followed by increasingly refined subsequent editions, *DSM-II, DSM-III, DSM-IV*, and *DSM-IV-TR*. The current structure of the *DSM-IV* (American Psychiatric Association, 1994) and *DSM-IV-TR* is based on a categorical classification system; the categories are prototypes of disorders and are assessed by five domains, or axes, by which counselors or other clinical specialists can better understand the patients' illness and the potential treatment that might be effective, as well as providing help to third-party payers trying to understand the patient's needs. The five axes assess five dimensions of behavior:

- Axis I: Clinical Syndrome. This assessment is usually thought of as the diagnosis.
- Axis II: Development and Personality Disorders. These are disorders that are typically evident in childhood, for example, autism.
- Axis III: This domain discusses physical conditions which may be important factors in Axis I and II disorders.
- Axis IV: This axis has to do with severity of psychological stressors that have an impact on a person's life.
- Axis V: This domain discusses the "highest level of functioning" in the present and during the past year to help the counselor understand how the four axes are affecting the person.

Obviously, the *DSM* is not a "cookbook"; clinicians who use or intend to use the *DSM* need to be trained to understand the comprehensive content of this important tool.

In sum, then,

> the DSM-IV like its earlier editions, provides assistance to counselors in organizing their diagnoses and assessments of clients around a multiaxial system that classifies five types of information. The DSM-IV as well as the earlier interactions of the DSM have been of significant assistance in helping counselors understand the complexity of mental disorders, their assessment of the variety of factors that interact to influence or to stimulate the course and severity of mental disorders. Many of these factors lie outside the individual, in a range of psychosocial factors that may trigger problems or predispose individuals to being at risk. (Herr, 1999, p. 179)

THE RISE OF GUIDANCE AND THE EMERGENCE OF COUNSELING

There is much more to say about each of the theorists identified in the previous section, as well as the evolution of the *DSM* as one example of a tool that originated in the ongoing scholarship of many researchers and theorists over centuries. However, these brief vignettes suggest the beginning of the conceptual perspectives that underpinned the context in which counseling began to be advocated, although the term *counseling* itself was not used until the first decade of the 20th century and with increasing frequency until the 1930s forward. As work on psychological issues and mental health were splitting off from philosophy in the late 1800s and moving forward in their descriptions and explanations of the nature of humankind, persons from many disciplines—physics, physiology, philosophy, mathematics, medicine, education, social reform, engineering, and law—continued to make major contributions to research and experimentation, often in laboratories in Europe and in the United States, focused on examining individual differences, personality types, and so forth.

Counseling Takes Root in the Guidance Profession

By the end of the 19th and the beginning of the 20th centuries, the term *guidance* had become the operative word for interventions in human behavior, often subsuming the term *counseling* as one aspect of the guidance process. Perhaps more important, a variety of contextual factors began to create the need for "counseling" of young people and adults (Herr, Cramer, & Niles, 2004). Some scholars and practitioners began to advance the importance of working directly with children in schools or with adults needing "guidance" in making wise decisions about their life options or, more specifically, jobs. Early attempts at guidance began to focus on schools as important venues to help students learn content that complemented and reinforced academic subject matter. Among the important educators who first conceived of guidance as a systematic and integral part of the school curriculum were George Merrill, who in 1895 developed the first vocational guidance program in San Francisco; Eli W. Weaver, a high school principal in Brooklyn, who authored *Choosing a Career*; and Jesse B. Davis, principal of a high school in Grand Rapids, Michigan (Herr, 2003). Davis believed that all students should receive moral and vocational guidance, and he believed in inserting into academic classes—for example, English composition—activities to develop a conception of self as a social being in a future occupation and thus the appreciation of duty and obligation toward others, business associates, neighbors, and the law (Davis, 1914, p. 17). Davis, like other contemporary thinkers of the time, began to lay the foundation for what would become school counseling and a vocabulary for counseling that used the term *guidance* to subsume counseling and other interventions that in the second half of the 20th century became seen as part of the counseling process. The term *guidance*, however, had amazing staying power. Frequently being used as a term parallel to or inclusive of the term *counseling*, particularly in school counseling, the term *guidance* was accepted as an appropriate representation of what many counselors did, although many counselors and theorists were dismayed and disagreed that the term *guidance* described what they did in their profession. The latter believed that the term was too narrow and conveyed a directive, expert-subordinate (counselor-client) relationship in which test scores and occupational or other information were essential content, rather than a collaborative, nurturing relationship between counselor and client.

Part of the problem with the term *guidance* is that it was used many different ways and with many nuances. In some contexts, guidance was seen as a process, sometimes as a set of services or a program; sometimes guidance services were seen as part of the broader term *personnel services*, which was often used at the collegiate level to include such entities as health services, housing services, financial assistance, and so on. In other perspectives guidance was treated as an intervention in its own right, often parallel to or the same as counseling. However the term was used, scholars continued to argue that the focus of guidance or counseling is upon the individual and his or her plans, decisions, and development. Thus, while in its early years guidance arose primarily in the schools, it was not synonymous with such terms as *education* or *curriculum* or *instruction* or *discipline*. While counseling may be a part of each of these, it was and is seen as distinctive in its function. Miller (1961), a guidance specialist in the U.S. Office of Education, defined the major elements of guidance as it was understood at the time and summarized the basic meaning of the term as follows:

> Guidance seeks to aid the individual to develop according to his [*sic*] own emerging life pattern and expectancies by achieving a maximum self-realization in harmony with his own values and the values of the culture in which he [*sic*] will probably live. (pp. 450–451)

Miller goes on to suggest that

> the appropriate area of functioning of guidance lies between primary concern with subjective states on the one hand and primary concern with external social conditions on the other.... Guidance operates in the zone in which the individual's own unique world of perceptions interacts with the external order of events in his [*sic*] life context. It is here that the choice points and problems arise which are the distinctive concern of guidance. (p. 450)

With this perspective, one could in many ways substitute the term *counseling* for the term *guidance* and the implications, content, and process would essentially substitute one for the other. Viewing guidance through the lens that Miller provides apparently sustained the use of the term *guidance* over a longer period than one might predict.

The Growing Professionalization of Counseling

Indeed, from its beginning in 1952 until 1983, the largest organization of counselors in the world, the American Personnel and Guidance Association, highlighted the term *guidance* in its title, its organizational documents, and its representation of its members. Finally, in 1983, the title of the organization was changed to the American Association for Counseling and Development and in 1992 to the American Counseling Association, eliminating an emphasis on the term *guidance*.

In a larger sense, the name changes in 1983 and 1992 reflected the sense of professionalism of and identity with counseling that had been growing in the decades from 1960 onward. It also reflected the reality that guidance and counseling were no longer creatures primarily of schools but were being comprehensively applied across populations and settings. Such identity shifts rapidly spawned related accreditation processes that evaluated counselor education programs and accredited those that met specified criteria. These shifts also generated a rise in credentialing of individual counselors, through certification, licensure, or other recognition that affirmed through tests and interviews that they met the experience and training criteria necessary to function as a competent, independent practitioner.

Although we have jumped from early in the 20th century to essentially the last third of the century, before going back to the earlier history, it is important to point out other aspects of the evolution from guidance to counseling. This evolution included the transition from a person taking a few random courses to become a counselor to an increasingly sophisticated infrastructure to support the professionalization of counseling—accredited training, specific course requirements, and supervised practicum and internships; defined competencies to practice as a counselor; comprehensive statements of ethics undergirding counselor practice; and a nationwide core of counselor educators committed to the training of professional counselors—all complemented by a growing array of theoretical perspectives and empirical research. These advances in the constructs and practices of counseling were essentially responsive to external forces as well as internal dynamics in the counseling profession.

By the second half of the 20th century, legislation related to who could provide counseling and for what purposes also often focused on third-party payment, which meant that the payment of client fees to counselors in independent practice was provided by insurance plans and processes other than the client. These third-party payers wanted to be sure of the credentials of counselors and other mental health professionals. Thus, before licensed professional counselors became a reality, counseling and clinical psychologists, clinical social workers, and psychiatric nurses became providers of counseling and reinforced their competency through accreditation of preparation programs, licensure of providers, continuing education requirements, ethical guidelines, and related aspects that supported the quality of their profession and their readiness to receive third-party payment.

Counselors, before the 1960s or so, were primarily creatures of organizations, rather than independent practitioners, and often took the names of the settings in which they worked to identify themselves: for example, school counselors, rehabilitation counselors, employment service counselors, mental health counselors, college counselors, and so on. As such, with relatively few exceptions, counselors worked in institutions and agencies rather than in independent practice. However, in the 1970s and beyond there was an acceleration of mental health professionals in psychology, social work, and nursing moving into independent practice rather than continuing to be organization based. This meant that professional counselors needed to be able to distinguish themselves from the other mental health professionals and they needed to be able to identify effectively the characteristics of their professional competition for clients and third-party payments. As suggested previously, part of this accelerated movement away from institutional bases was occasioned by legislation that provided incentives to engage in independent practice. The Community Mental Health Act (1963) and the Social Security Act and its amendments (1935), among other factors, provided such motivation.

CONTEXTUAL VARIABLES IN THE 20TH CENTURY

But, as important as these points of growing professional identity are, a larger perspective is that counseling and its providers have historically been responsive to the social contexts that exist at a given time. Indeed, sometimes counseling has been called a sociopolitical process because it has so frequently been included in state or federal legislation identifying counseling as a major instrument to achieve particular goals at a given point in time. In this sense, the content and processes of counseling (or guidance), and to a large degree counseling specialties, have been shaped by national policy and legislative formulations, funding, and action since the early decades of the 20th century. Support for counseling (or guidance) as a stand-alone or independent focus of policy formulation has occurred, but more often such support for counseling or guidance occurs in conjunction with other intervention processes. Thus, counseling has frequently been seen as adding value; having utilitarian contributions to multidimensional programs related to such goals as facilitating equality of access to education and training opportunities; creating human capital; rehabilitating those on the margins of society; and helping persons find self-esteem, self-efficacy, purpose, and productivity in their life planning and adjustment.

Contextual variables affecting the provision and definition of counseling have been formed not only by policy and legislation but also by the congruence of theoretical perspectives and the state of the larger society at any given time. In gross terms, this perspective suggests that the urgency of counseling and expectations for its outcomes vary from decade to decade. Examples in which counseling was identified as making an important contribution include social reform and the integration of large immigrant populations in the late 1800s and early 1900s; the rise of individualism and the growing understanding of individual differences in the first decades of the 1900s; the concern for the handicapped and mentally ill (including the war wounded) in the 1920s; the economic exigencies and need to match persons with available employment opportunities during the Great Depression of the 1930s; national defense in the 1940s; the space race in the 1950s; social justice, desegregation, and the democratization of opportunities in the 1960s; the concerns for equity for special needs population in a climate of economic austerity in the 1970s; the transformation from an industrial to an information-based economy and the rise of the global economy in the 1980s and 1990s; and terrorism, intolerance, and posttraumatic stress disorder in the first decade of the 21st century (Herr, 1991).

Assessment Emerging

As a function of the national need to classify thousands of military personnel for roles in the First World War, the military borrowed from the laboratory work ongoing in Europe and the United States on measurement of individual traits, and used the first large-scale testing programs, called the Alpha and Beta tests, to identify the mental abilities of recruits. When World War I was finished, the Alpha and Beta Tests were revised to be used in the civilian sector to classify applicants for jobs and for use in some schools as part of the school counseling programs. At the time, the emphases in counseling and assessment were on the content of choice, attempts to understand and measure individual differences in performance, and efforts to predict who would be successful in what tasks. General aptitude and interest assessments were finding their stride. Such uses of measurement were also spawning other measures that laid the foundation for the use of tests in counseling. For example, at the nation's first applied psychology department at Carnegie Tech (now Carnegie Mellon University), developed by Walter Van Dyck Bingham, there was also an Education Research Department directed by a young assistant professor named E. K. Strong, who worked with several other young measurement experts to develop a 400-item vocational interest test. In 1923, Strong accepted an appointment to Stanford University, where he improved the interest measure that he and his colleagues had been working on at Carnegie Tech, published the measure in 1927 as the Interest Analysis Blank, the predecessor of the contemporary Strong Interest Inventory (Miller, 1961; Super & Crites, 1962).

Public Policy and Counseling

Throughout these decades in the 20th century, legislation including counseling was often instituted to emphasize a particular counseling specialty that gave promise of being able to provide support and empower particular populations. As only a few examples of such phenomena, one could cite such legislation as the Wagner-Peyser Act during the Great Depression, which supported the nationwide system of employment counselors as a free public service to employers and workers throughout the nation; the Rehabilitation Act amendments (1973), which provided counseling across the nation for persons with disabilities; the Carl D. Perkins Vocational and Applied Technology Act (1985), the largest source of funding for career guidance in the schools; the National Defense Education Act (1958), which vastly increased the elementary and secondary school counseling population, created the conditions for K–12 comprehensive guidance programs, institutionalized school counseling, provided year-long training institutes, provided tests and other resources to schools, and financially supported the hiring of elementary and secondary school counselors; and the Community Mental Health Center Act of 1963, which essentially ended the placement of mentally ill patients in state hospitals and asylums, established community mental health agencies, and stimulated the employment of counselors outside of educational settings.

The major point to be made here is that social, economic, and political changes affect individuals, sometimes directly and sometimes indirectly. And they affect the expectations of counseling held by policy makers, administrators, third-party payers, theorists, and so forth. Given the social and economic issues for which counselors have been included in legislation and policy, counselors have often been seen as change agents. The reality is that neither clients nor counselors exist in a vacuum. They adjust their images and learn new techniques as they respond to the contextual factors that press upon them in new and challenging ways. Thus, it is important to view changes and trends in counseling through contextual lenses that operate at a given time and that give insight into the persons and events that shape counseling. So it was in the pre-counseling period.

The End of the Pre-Counseling Period

At the end of the 19th century and the beginning of the 20th century, another visionary—Frank Parsons—emerged as the architect of vocational guidance and/or vocational counseling, using the term *counseling* for one of the first times in the United States. Although the focus was on vocational choice and employment, the term *counseling* in this context triggered other specialties in the ensuing decades for which counseling was the process but the content was educational choice, family relationships, rehabilitation, mental health, and so forth. As these specialties emerged, the application of counseling to a wider spectrum of problems and of persons for whom counseling was helpful continued to grow.

Specific Contextual Factors Affecting Counseling

To return to the development of vocational counseling in the late 1800s and early 1900s: Several of the contextual and implementation factors cited previously evolved and continued to be important as counseling was becoming established and growing in its application to individual problems. First, it is noteworthy that vocational counseling was directly associated with major shifts from a national economy that was, in general, agriculturally based to an economy that was increasingly industrial in its occupational structure. The Industrial Revolution that had begun in Europe was spilling over to the United States, promoting manufacturing throughout the northeastern part of the United States and rapidly moving westward to Detroit, Chicago, and other major cities. As the Industrial Revolution became part of the American identity, urbanization and occupational diversity increased as did national concerns about helping people distribute their energies and talents across a burgeoning industrial structure. This required mechanisms to identify and distribute information about job opportunities and work settings. By the late 19th and early 20th centuries, particularly in urban areas, such information was so differentiated and comprehensive that families or neighborhoods could no longer serve as the prime sources of such information or be knowledgeable about the vast array of jobs that were being developed and implemented. Other more formal mechanisms, including rudimentary forms of counseling and advice-giving, began to emerge in schools, in settlement houses, and in community centers.

A major factor in the rise of vocational counseling in the late 1800s and the early 1900s in the United States was the large waves of immigrants coming from nations with poor economic opportunities to seek new lives and options; a parallel phenomenon was occurring as people in the United States were migrating from rural to urban areas, spurred by the urbanization of jobs, particularly in the concentrations of manufacturing plants in major cities making steel, furniture, automobiles, and other large capital goods. Many, indeed most, of these immigrants from abroad and from within the United States moved into inner cities, where living conditions were crowded, dirty, and difficult.

It was inevitable that in the midst of such transitions in the occupational structure and the social services available to both native-born citizens and the tens of thousands of immigrants, questions of social reform would become major political issues. These took many forms, but included such emphases as appropriate education for children and effective placement of adults into a rapidly changing occupational structure; effective methods of helping immigrants to distribute themselves across the range of available occupations; how to bridge the gap between schooling and the realities of the adult world, with many critics arguing that schools were too "bookish," too college oriented, and had insufficient vocational education; how to address changing family structures, diminished extended kinship systems, opposition to child labor, and shifts in child rearing practices that were emerging in relation to migration and the consuming force of the industrial revolution; and concerns that workers, immigrants and domestic, needed to be seen as persons of dignity with a right to determine their own life plans, rather than be chattels of employers, as property to be consumed and cast aside.

THEORIES OF COUNSELING

The sum of the issues discussed so far is that counseling, theories of counseling, and other interventions emerged, in many instances, in response to specific social, political, and economic forces. In periods of social change, as was true in the latter quarter of the 19th century and the first quarter of the 20th century, people who advocate what needs to be done to convert ideas about counseling or other processes into action are critical.

The Parsons Model of Vocational Counseling

Frank Parsons was such a person. A social worker, engineer, and attorney, Parsons had long been involved in social reform. He was also a thinker who provided a major tripartite concept of vocational counseling. Published posthumously in 1909, Parson's book *Choosing a Vocation* was instrumental in providing this three-step plan that became the basis of vocational guidance for the first 50 years of the 20th century and beyond. Parsons did not call his tripartite model a counseling model, but rather a process of *true reasoning* that included

> first, a clear understanding of yourself, aptitudes, interests, resources, limitations, and other qualities. Second, a knowledge of the requirements and conditions of success, advantages and disadvantages, compensation, opportunities, and prospects in different lines of work. Third, *true reasoning* on the relations of these two groups of facts. (Parsons, 1909, p. 5)

We do well to remind ourselves that Parsons authored the concept of true reasoning, the conceptual frame of reference for vocational counseling, without the benefits of a body of career development theory, a repertoire of tests to use, or an *Occupational Outlook Handbook* to which to refer. Instead, he created his own information and assessments—self-reports, checklists, lists of occupations that welcomed men and women—as well as other primitive tools by which to help his clients with their job search. In the early 1900s, Parsons and other conceptual geniuses of the time worked diligently to find simple and straightforward ways to evaluate clients and to use this information in their counseling.

The professional literature frequently speaks about Parsons' model as defining what is now known as a trait-and-factor, directive, or actuarial approach to vocational counseling or to counseling in general. While such a premise is accurate, Parsons' model also outlined important areas for which assessment is required if vocational or career counseling is to be successful. Each of his three steps toward *true reasoning*, the process of making a decision, has stimulated the development of particular assessment emphases. For example, the first step of his tripartite model has led to emphasis on the importance of understanding individual differences; which traits are stable, consistent, and predictive of human behavior in training, performance, or other contexts; and how these traits can be measured. The second step has stimulated job analyses and, indeed, educational analyses of the differences in occupational and educational content and, therefore, the individual traits required to be successful in different settings and how these data can be reflected in the dependent or criterion measures used. The third step has led, in the last half of the 20th century, to efforts to assess decision-making skills, career maturity, and career adaptability, or the status of the client's ability to deal with the *process of choice* as well as to identify and choose the *content of choice*.

Parsons' model and the related interventions he created were first used in the community, in settlement houses, and in other places where individuals seeking work and assistance with obtaining relevant information and interaction could meet with a social worker or vocational guidance practitioner versed in matching persons and jobs. But, early in the 20th century, Parsons' tripartite model found its way into the schools, where it converged with emerging approaches to prepare students with educational guidance, personal guidance, and testing through structural programs in classrooms or provided by teachers assigned to supply such information and individual guidance about getting along with others, codes of individual behavior, job search skills, and related content (Parsons, 1909). This convergence of possible interventions designed to promote vocational, educational, and personal guidance began to define a model for school counseling as a specialty area and it emphasized a developmental rather than treatment model. But alternative models of counseling were emerging rapidly in other areas of clinical practice and counseling.

Early 20th-Century Models of Counseling

By virtually any criteria used, the first several decades of the 20th century were extremely fertile in their contributions to the provision of philosophical, psychological, measurement, and conceptual ideas as the underpinnings of counseling and, indeed, other helping professions and mental health specialties. In addition to the contributions of such important visionaries as Parsons, Strong, and their various colleagues was the ongoing work of such towering figures as Sigmund Freud. By the time Freud's work became prominent, mental illness was no longer conceptualized or treated as demon possession or witchcraft but was beginning to be understood as deserving humane treatment. Psychiatry was in the early stages of becoming a clinical field and humanitarianism was being seen as a psychotherapeutic approach (Bromberg, 1963, p. 740). The "moral treatment" as it was called replaced purges, bleedings, restraints, and rigid confinement of the insane and those with other mental problems. Researchers and theorists had begun to identify mental illnesses as the result of nervous system infections or exhaustion, the pressure of emotional strain, and distorted beliefs about the life history of patients. Rather than being restrained and confined in asylums, mentally ill persons started receiving help from newly emerging therapies that treated patients with respect. Included were hypnosis, rest cures, electrical stimulation, and increasing attention to dynamic psychotherapy and the focus of the unconscious mind on various nervous and dissociative symptoms described by Freud and his various colleagues. In rapid sequence, other factors associated with mental illness were emerging and affecting the provision of counseling and psychotherapy. Of particular concern were the importance of infant rejection and deprivation, psychosexual factors, and the significance of symbolism in how persons construed their personal realities, their psychological defenses, and the effects of their thinking on the frequent neurotic symptoms that resulted.

During these early decades of the 20th century, psychoanalysis and depth psychotherapy emerged, leaving their residue of knowledge about the factors affecting human behavior on the content and processes of counseling. During this period several contending streams of theory and therapy began to arise. One branch involved the psychoanalytic techniques that originated with Freud and were carried forth by his many colleagues. Fundamental to such perspectives were the use of therapy to uncover psychosexual issues in early childhood, unconscious drives and feelings, and the conflicting energies and powers of the id, ego, and superego.

A second important stream of theory and therapy was focused on social factors, social pressures, and social relationships. Such major theorists as Alfred Adler, Harry Stack Sullivan, Karen Horney, and Carl Jung, among others, believed that social factors were as significant causes of neuroses as the repressed individual's instinctual drives described in the work of Freud and his associates. Among the implications for counseling and therapy that arose from a social factor, rather than an unconscious drive, perspective were less passive behavior by the counselor, greater flexibility in the content of counseling, an emphasis on brief therapy rather than long-term depth analysis, much less attention to analyzing early psychological experiences of the client, and a focus on present behavior.

One of the results of the changing perspectives on therapy that occurred in the 1930s and 1940s was the use of group therapy in psychiatry and increasingly in counseling. Although the history of group therapy deserves a chapter in its own right, suffice it to say that as with individual therapy, there were several types of group therapy that responded to the theoretical perspective of the counselor and the setting in which it was conducted. These therapy types included activity and analytical group therapy; encounter group therapy; psychodrama, nondirective, or client-centered group therapy; eclectic group therapy; and, as was discussed briefly earlier, instructional group work. These are all different types/categories of group therapy. Throughout the 20th century, group therapy in its various emphases has grown in its application in and out of counseling, including its use in Alcoholics Anonymous, Gamblers Anonymous, relapse prevention, and support groups for those who have lost loved ones or are going through transitions in their lives.

The Evolution of Theory in the Second Half of the 20th Century

One of the characteristics of counseling through much of the first half of the 20th century was the influence of the medical model on how counseling was conducted. Many of the researchers who focused on human behavior and on mental illness during the 17th, 18th, 19th, and early 20th centuries were physicians or worked in medical settings. It would be natural for them to adopt the approach to working with clients that prevailed within medicine. That model portrayed the counselor as the expert and the client as the subordinate. In such a view, the counselor was the person in the counseling relationship who used batteries of tests (personality, interest, aptitude, etc.) to classify the problems; the psychological characteristics; and the individual's personality traits, interests, and aptitudes, as this information was relevant to the client's presenting problem. Following the use of such tests, including self-report information, the counselor then interpreted the results obtained and prescribed a set of interventions that would presumably help the client solve the dilemmas he or she brought to the counselor. Such a model of counseling or psychotherapy essentially paralleled the method used by physicians to interact with patients having physical problems.

One could argue that the medical model is more focused on the content of the interaction between physician or counselor and client than on the process. However, in the first of his major books, Carl Rogers (1942), the architect of nondirective or client-centered therapy, raised significant questions about how traditional views of counseling and psychotherapy were being seen. In Rogers' view counseling should not be based on psychometrics, testing, or imposing external information on clients. Instead, Rogers applied the postulates of existential or individual psychology to counseling, contending that tests and information should not be the content of counseling or be the major tools of counselors; the major content of counseling should be on the internal perceptual or phenomenal field of the client. Thus, the client should be an active part of the counseling dyad, a collaborator with the counselor in determining what types of external information, if any, would be relevant to the concerns brought to the counselor, rather than being an inactive recipient of information that may or may not be relevant to the client. In addition to his view of the content of the client's perspectives vis-à-vis the internal perceptual field, Rogers also spoke about the essential ingredients of the counseling process, known as the essential and necessary conditions for a therapeutic relationship, as including empathic understanding, unconditional positive regard, and congruence (Rogers, 1957): conditions that the counselor provides for the client.

It is worth noting here that Rogers' important perspectives on counseling or therapy initially occurred during World War II. Because of the needs of the military as well as many people at home concerned about their loved ones and the outcomes of the war, counseling services began to be available to more people; clinical psychologists, who prior to the war were test givers for psychiatrists, were pressed into service during the war as therapists, and counseling subsequently became a distinctive profession. In addition to Rogers' major theoretical impact, other changes were occurring. The social context of change and freedom following World War II did not lend itself to the rigidity and the medical model of counselor as expert that was an explicit part of directive counseling. Although psychoanalysis was helping to popularize individuals' search for meaning in the magazines, movies, and plays of the 1940s, 1950s, and 1960s, it simply took too long and was too expensive for wide application. It also was true that other theorists were emerging who rejected Freud's concepts and the practice of psychoanalysis.

There were many such persons who made important contributions to the direction and processes of counseling that went far beyond the scientific impact, if not the popular impact, of psychoanalysis. These individuals included Albert Ellis and his creation of rational emotive therapy; Victor Frankl and his perspectives on existential therapy or logotherapy; and Carl Rogers' client-centered, nondirective, humanistic psychology. Such theorists and theories were among the originators of major shifts in the counseling paradigms that shaped the counseling approaches that dominated and refined counseling in the last half of the 20th century. Rogers' theory, in particular, broke the hold on counseling as a directive process telling clients what to do. Instead, Rogers generated a model that emphasized the need to have the client operate within his or her phenomenological field in which all of his or her counseling content of importance resided. In this sense, the client was in charge of the perceptions of his experiences that guided his or her behavior and decided what to share; thus, the counselor was not the expert about what was important in the counseling relationship, the client was. It also meant that it was not necessary in counseling to revisit the early years of the client's life and reassess each of the perceptions that he or she developed at that time. Rather, the assumption was that the residual of those early experiences, if important, would be present in current behavior. In such cases, Rogers portrayed the client and the counselor as co-equals, both participating actively in discussing the concepts and perceptions of the client, with the counselor providing the necessary conditions for a therapeutic relationship.

As the 20th century progressed, increasing attention was given to the counseling process itself, specifically, the working alliance between clients and counselors. New counseling approaches emerged and an array of tools and techniques became part of the repertoire of counselors (including new assessments that allowed counselors to translate theory into practice from the work of such theorists as Donald Super, John Holland, and John Krumboltz, among others). Also of growing interest was the use of technology and computers as adjuncts to the counseling process; the specification of competencies that counselors should possess, whatever the counseling theory they espoused; the approval of counselor education programs to prepare counselors to be competent in the use of the competencies expected of them; and the credentialing (approval) of programs to prepare counselors and of the policies or state statutes that provide licensure or certification of counselors who have met the standards required of competent counselors.

Throughout the 20th century, new counseling theories and approaches continued to be spawned. These approaches were often responses to government policies or to the characteristics of the social contexts of the time. New metaphors or descriptive adjectives were often used to characterize these emphases: solution-focused brief therapy, crisis counseling, narrative therapy, strength-based theories, constructivist theories, and wellness. These theories varied in their intent. Many of them focused more on building client's strengths and potential than on their problems per se. Some theories focused on addressing an immediate problem rather than a comprehensive approach to all of the problems a client might be experiencing. In some cases, the emphasis was on the client's search for meaning or spiritual growth. In still other cases, the emphasis was on the promotion of wellness as a way of transcending problems.

A major counseling approach, for which there are many theoretical frames of reference, is family counseling. Family counseling has grown in importance and availability throughout much of the 20th century. As such it has made many contributions to counseling at large. For example, originally clients who were experiencing "family problems" were seen by the counselor alone, assuming that if parents were included in the counseling process, the client of focus would be reluctant to discuss the issues that brought him or her to counseling. However, as the century continued, group counseling and systems theory were also growing in prominence. Indeed, counseling theorists began to talk of families as systems to which all family members contributed roles and behavior. Family members, then, were interdependent, frequently presenting particular patterns of behavior that perpetuated family behavior and needed to be seen in a collective rather than simply an individual sense, thereby embracing the counseling of families as a unit.

Counseling Theories Today

As new counseling theories emerged during the latter decades of the 20th century, Rogers' perspectives on the counseling relationship, particularly his analysis of the necessary and sufficient conditions of a therapeutic relationship between counselors and clients, was debated as to the sufficiency of the conditions he proposed. Even so, however, as the last half of the 20th century witnessed a large outpouring of counseling theories and interventions, Rogers' concepts related to necessary conditions of a therapeutic relationship continued to be integrated into other counseling theories that may not share specific aspects of his premise.

In any case, it is fair to argue that as we identified the range of insights into human behavior and interventions in it that have grown during the past several centuries, there is a continuing stream of interdisciplinary perspectives that have shaped our current counseling theories. Different observers have classified these theories in various ways, but we will simply cite them here, since many will be dealt with in depth in the remainder of this book. For example, C. H. Patterson (1966) classified the major theories of counseling into rational learning theory; psychoanalysis; perceptual-phenomenological approaches; and existential psychotherapy. Shertzer and Stone (1974) classified counseling theories as those that are cognitively oriented (including trait and factor, rational emotive, eclectic, reciprocal inhibition, behavioral) and affectively oriented (including psychoanalytic, client-centered, existential, gestalt). More recently, Smith, Glass, and Miller (1980, p. 32) organized therapies by effect size. In order, their findings of the effectiveness of the major counseling approaches were ranked as follows:

1. Cognitive (reality therapy, rational emotive, transactional analysis),
2. Cognitive-behavioral,

3. Behavioral (systematic desensitization, implosion, behavior modification),
4. Dynamic (psychodynamic, hypnotherapy, Adlerian, other),
5. Humanistic (client-centered, Gestalt), and
6. Developmental (vocational-personal, other).

Such effect sizes are similar to findings from other studies. In general, these studies suggest that cognitive and cognitive-behavioral approaches to counseling yield the highest effect sizes, and therefore are more effective than verbal therapies or developmental approaches. However, it is also worth noting that while specific classes of therapies tend to be more effective in general than other therapies, it is also true that some approaches are more effective or equally effective for particular presenting problems and for particular client populations.

An overarching question still related to the efficacy (the effect size) of a particular approach to counseling or to psychotherapy is, What are the differences between counseling approaches and the specific ingredients that contribute to these differences? This question is as yet incompletely answered. However, a second question is also relevant: What is the impact of the counselor/therapist on the effect sizes? The answer provided by Wampold (2001) in a classic study of meta-models of effect sizes of different approaches to psychotherapy and contextual factors (therapist characteristics) is that the quality of the therapist is a critical factor in effect size, and while there is little to document the major ingredients separating approaches in psychotherapy, it is recommended that the client be helped to choose the counseling approach that is most compatible with his or her characteristics and that the counselor feels competent to provide. Thus, data reported by Wampold indicates "that the particular treatment that the therapist delivers does not affect outcomes, ... but yet the therapist delivering the treatment is absolutely crucial" (p. 202).

It is important to continue to acknowledge that counseling theories are not static; they are dynamic. They tend to grow in number and emphasis, even though new theories tend to be accommodated within the classification of theories cited previously. What does occur, however, is that theories and interventions tend to emerge in response to particular contextual factors, such as their multicultural efficacy, the costs of counseling that require less long and complex counseling processes, and events that push for particular types of counseling designed to address some emergent and important contemporary issue, for example, dealing with trauma, crisis, or posttraumatic stress disorder.

Although the fit between theory and context is never absolute and typically is a function of the historical time during which it is constructed, theory tends to respond to external realities relevant to a particular counseling approach. Thus, in terms of limits on the number of counselors available and the lack of capacity to engage in long-term counseling, brief therapy, time-limited therapies, and solution-focused therapies have been formulated to emphasize the most immediate problem a counselee has and try to find a solution for it, rather than conducting a comprehensive analysis of all of the areas of the client's life that counseling might help. In such a circumstance, the number of counseling sessions is likely to be reduced in number and cost; in general, the emphasis in newer counseling theories is on counselees' competence, related strengths, and possibilities rather than their deficits, weaknesses, and limitations. In such counseling, as is also true in crisis intervention or brief therapy, there is a focus on concreteness, on helping the counselee perceive the immediate situation as accurately as possible; assisting him or her in analyzing the meaning of the events at issue, the events' possible outcomes, and the resources available to help the client; and assisting the counselee to manage the feelings and emotions that the crisis has stimulated as openly and comprehensively as possible.

Other recent emphases in theory-building are variously labeled as narrative therapy and social constructivism. Neither of these methods is alien to other counseling approaches such as cognitive approaches. Rather, these methods provide an alternative frame of reference within which counselors can function, or, perhaps more important, they tend to make explicit what in other counseling theories may be implicit. For example, cognitive approaches to counseling are concerned with how clients perceive cues, process information, construct their belief systems, and create rational or irrational systems of self-talk ("I'm a loser," "I can't do that," "Nobody likes me," " I have no friends," etc.). But embedded in those elements of cognitive counseling is a concern for how individuals create meaning for themselves. Constructivist approaches to counseling suggest that people are meaning makers; rather than receive information or knowledge in pure form directly from their environment, the external world, they construct meaning out of their life experiences. Narrative therapy would suggest that such meaning is apparent in the narratives, stories, metaphors, and scripts that people construct to describe themselves and to use as a guide to how they play out their life stories and their behavior. These stories can cause one to be "stuck" in certain behavioral patterns and belief systems, or they can be freeing and liberating.

From either a constructivist or narrative perspective, human beings are not seen as passive recipients of information or universally similar to others who share a common reality. Thus, the emphases for counselors in using these counseling approaches is less on fixing and controlling a client's behaviors and much more on helping the client to deal with his or her efforts in meaning-making and analyzing client narratives to identify themes in a client's life and to help him or her sharpen, reconstruct, and alter or rescript these narrative themes as the individual comes to terms with the sense of meaning sought in his or her life (Herr, 1999, p. 240).

Time and space do not permit a further examination of the events, personalities, contextual factors, vocabulary, or theories that have shaped the history of counseling and the profession that has evolved from that history. There continue to be important additions to all of the dynamic factors that have been part of the rise of professional counseling in the United States and around the world. Economic, political, and social events change the lives of individuals, new insights into human behavior emerge, and new interventions are created to test or apply the related theories. Legislation and policy continue to define counseling as a sociopolitical instrument to help persons deal with employment, education, marginalization, discrimination, grief, loss, or crises; counseling theorists, researchers, and practitioners respond in ethical and comprehensive ways. And thus the cycle of professional counseling continues to build upon its history and continuously brings its knowledge, techniques, and ethics into contemporary contexts.

Active Learning Exercise **1.1**

Consider yourself a statesperson representing counseling in a school, a university, or a workplace, you have been asked to give a speech on the history of counseling, its issues, its trends. What would you say? You have 15 minutes for this presentation. What would you emphasize?

TRENDS IN COUNSELING

To end this overview of the history of counseling, several trends will be identified that represent future challenges for counseling and for counselors.

The Uniqueness of Counselors

Counseling theorists, counseling organizations, and other observers continuously seek themes that unify counselors and their profession (Herr, 1999; Paisley & Borders, 1995). Questions have long been raised about whom the primary constituents of counselors should be: "normal" populations of children, youth, and adults wrestling with decisions among multiple options? Persons with chronic and significant emotional and psychological problems? Persons on the margins of society who need to be assisted to learn behaviors and skills that assist them to be integrated into the main stream of society? Persons of minority status who have not had access to education, occupation, or social opportunities or counseling and who need insight, support, and strategies to master such circumstances? Persons who want to optimize their behavior and move toward wellness in their lives? Persons who have had an addictive disorder and now want help to break such restraints? Persons coping with transitions, with crisis, with loss in their lives? Persons who feel adrift, trying to find meaning in their life and spirituality?

It is likely that, if examined, most mission statements would contend that counselors distinguish themselves from other professions by emphasizing optimal human development for primarily "normal" persons across the life span. That answer is certainly correct at a philosophical level, but the reality is that counselors work in many settings and with many populations who need significant help to become healthy, interpersonally effective, and productive. Indeed, many counselors have clients who represent all of the persons depicted earlier. The question in such a reality is, What are the themes that unify counselors rather than separate them?

One hopeful sign clarifying the themes of the school counseling profession and its priority contributions to the school setting is found in the

National Standards for School Counseling Programs developed over several years and adopted by the American School Counseling Association (ASCA, 1997). The National Standards for School Counseling Programs are developed around three major areas: academic development, career development, and personal/social development. These standards and the associated student competencies, implementation materials, and evaluation instruments available from the ASCA have affirmed that whatever specific model of school counseling is implemented, there is a series of outcomes (knowledge, attitudes, and skills) that should result from every school counseling program, that can be measured, and that are central to the mission of the school. Since at least the 1970s, a variety of foundations, government programs, cities, and states throughout the United States have created standards or, in some cases, thematic structures within which school counselors could find identity and offer clearly defined processes and outcomes of significance to student development and to the missions of schools. Such standards will continue to be refined and advocated in the years ahead, but in the present and the recent past, they have provided important tools and concepts to advance the professionalization of the school counseling profession.

Beyond standards for school counseling programs, there is an array of standards, guidelines, and of competency requirements applied to career counselors and to counselors with specialties other than school counseling. Examples of the sources of such information include such diverse organizations as the National Career Development Association, the National Board of Certified Counselors, Chi Sigma Iota, the Council for the Accreditation of Counseling and Related Educational Programs, the American Mental Health Counselors Association, and the Association for Counselor Education and Supervision. The perspectives of these organizations on counselor roles and their uniqueness from those of other mental health providers, while perhaps unintentional in their purpose, continue to provide significant insight into the themes that unify counselors and their profession.

The Interaction of Behavior, Intervention, and Context

There is a growing awareness that clients and the content of counseling are shaped by events and contextual factors external to clients. In large measure, how the client processes, interprets, and acts upon these external events becomes the content of counseling (Herr, 1999). Human development does not occur in a vacuum; it interacts with environmental influences within which an individual negotiates an identity, aspirations, and meaning (Rosen, 1996). This growing awareness raises questions regarding how contextual factors the person experiences impact the effectiveness of counseling approaches. What approaches are most effective in addressing such individual-environment transactions? Is the preparation of counselors too fully focused on intrapsychic theories rather than on contextual factors, within the client's environments?

Evidence-Based Practices

With the plethora of presenting problems that clients bring to counselors, there is a continuing need to match counseling interventions to problems for which the interventions have been effective, reliable, and efficient as demonstrated by research. Essentially, this is the focus of what has become known as evidence-based, empirically supported, or results-based approaches to identifying preferred or best practices in counseling for specific purposes (Frank & Frank, 1991; Marotta & Watts, 2007; Wampold, 2001).

Group Processes

Although many counselors are most comfortable with and prefer one-to-one counseling, there are a growing number of psychoeducational group models that allow counselors to work with multiple clients simultaneously, either for treatment or prevention of problems. These programs include a large array of foci: for example, career education, personal constructs, role relationships, deliberate psychological education, stress management, test-taking and studying skills, anxiety or anger management, job-search strategies, parent effectiveness training, assertive training, social skills development, and communication skills. Many of these programs are targeted on children and youth; others on adults in different settings. These planned and structured learning approaches differ in their content, but they typically involve teaching of pro-social or career skills, homework and practice, the use of audiovisual materials, and simulations or similar approaches. While these programs have typically demonstrated significant learning for clients (Truneckova & Viney, 2007), they have rarely been evaluated against individual counseling focused on the same content. In any case, many counselors have an important role as program planners of group interventions, which are likely to expand in the future (Herr, Heitzman, & Rayman, 2006).

Cybercounseling and the Use of Advanced Technology

The use of advanced technology as an adjunct to counseling continues to expand; so does the vocabulary related to counseling by technology. One such important and recent term is *cybercounseling*. Maples and Ham (2008) quote the definition of cybercounseling that has been promulgated by the National Board for Certified Counselors: "The practice of professional counseling and information delivery that occurs when client(s) and counselors are in separate or remote locations and utilize electronic means to communicate over the Internet" (p. 178). While an important and useful definition, it fails to mention the many uses of advanced technology that support the process of counseling with clients as well as with other administrative and support roles.

Some uses of computers and related technologies help with the scheduling of clients, billing, word processing, record keeping, and other administrative processes. Such uses of technology save counselors time or make the counseling practice or program more efficient. In other cases, advanced technology is more directly used as part of the counseling process. (Herr, Heitzmann, & Rayman, 2006).

Computers, the Internet, and other communications devices provide the opportunity to work with clients at a distance through e-mails, chat rooms, video conferencing, and related processes (Sampson, Kolodinsky, & Grenno, 1997). Advanced technology also provides information about *DSM* classifications of mental disorders, their etiology, and the preferred practices, which can serve counselors as a quick reference library. To a growing degree, computers can be used to score tests and assessments and interpret the results. They can interact with clients as the latter take tests or as they explore information about jobs or other options. Computers can also provide total programs of career development, typically conceived as a series of modules that will help clients test their interests, abilities, and educational achievements; explore and practice decision-making skills and strategies; examine career and personal options; match their aspirations and characteristics to the options available to them; learn about job search methods; and identify other salient information relevant to their needs. Such uses of advanced technology in counseling increasingly require the counselor to be sufficiently computer literate to choose the software and databases that will be appropriate to the client groups and likely content with which they will work.

The Growing Need for the Promotion of Counseling

In most settings where counseling programs exist, the principal mission of the larger institution is not counseling. Thus, in most instances, counseling is not a stand-alone program. It is intertwined with the goals of the larger organization (Herr, Heitzmann, & Rayman, 2006). In the cases of schools or universities, the primary mission is education and development. In corporations it is to provide quality products or services, and if counseling is available, the corporation's mission is to increase the purposefulness and productivity of employees who receive counseling in-house or through employee assistance programs. In other governmental settings, the availability of counseling is, again, akin to the reasons for counseling in corporations or elsewhere—help troubled employees to function more effectively, serve as a referral source for employees and their families, help employees use their educational benefits wisely, help employees understand the career pathways through an organization, and prepare employees for advancement to supervisory and management roles.

If counseling programs are to be incorporated in organizations that are not primarily about counseling, then counselors and counselor administrators must increasingly advocate for and promote the utility of counseling in the particular organization at issue; in essence, they must demonstrate the *added value* that counseling can provide in support of the organization's mission, the health and well-being of its employees, and the improvement of employee readiness for work tasks and for advancement. In essence, then, counselors in virtually any organization must help to articulate how the goals of the counseling program can be seen as relevant to the strategic plans of the larger organization (Herr, Heitzmann, & Rayman, 2006).

The Increasing Use of Triage Approaches

In every public and private sector that incorporates counselors and counseling programs into its organization, there are resource limitations to be dealt with. Therefore, policy makers and administrators want to know how to provide counseling services in the most economical way.

In essence, a triage approach is similar to the diagnosis of patients in medicine to determine how much and what kind of physician help they need. In the case of counseling, clients are usually divided at intake into three or more groups based upon their likely need for individual counseling rather than other types of non- or limited counselor interventions. Using career settings as an example, a first group of clients may be assigned to self-directed activities (e.g., exploring the content of interest stations to identify possible jobs, reading available resources about jobs, interacting with a computer program designed to provide relevant information about specific jobs that they are seeking); a second group of clients may be evaluated as needing something more than self-directed activities but not intense individual counseling. In such cases, they may be assigned to a support group to discuss job search methods and/or engage in assessments and role play of various career emphases. The third group may be evaluated as requiring several sessions of intense individual counseling. These clients may be seriously indecisive or unable to find and use information independent of a counselor's support. In this three-group scenario, the counselor may only need to get heavily involved with the third group, although he or she may spend a brief time orienting the persons in Groups 1 or 2 and then turn the clients over to a technician, so that the bulk of the counselor's time is committed to the clients in Group 3. Such a triage approach can be used within any counseling program in schools, universities, government, or corporate settings to conserve counselor's time for clients in most need of individual help while also serving many other clients whose needs can be met using less expensive processes such as the Internet or specific information resources.

Prevention, Behavioral Optimization, and Wellness

The classic perspectives on the purposes of counseling are (1) treatment/remediation of relational or transition problems of career and life crises or (2) helping to develop attitudes, knowledge, and skills through which clients can acquire the behaviors necessary in the future to prevent problems or crises (Herr, 1999). In the first approach counseling tends to be triggered by immediate problems or crises; in the second approach counseling is seen as preventive, strength-building, and educative rather than focused on repairing deficits or other major problems. Increasingly, however, there is a third purpose of counseling that is not solely focused on overcoming negative environmental and family situations, poor personal intrapsychic images, or the development of particular skills. Terms like *optimization of behavior, renewal, spirituality,* and *wellness* are all finding their way into the vocabulary of counseling. While overlapping with the second purpose of counseling—development— the third purpose focuses on helping clients aspire to personal excellence, to making their behavior the most effective it can be, to seek meaning in life or a commitment to their spirituality, to live a healthy lifestyle, and to be resilient. In general, such an approach in its various configurations focuses on client strengths that help them absorb negative life experiences; bounce back from adversity; be resilient, self-confident, and optimistic; and be able to take control of their life. Such a mind-set is essentially a counselor strategy of promoting continuous individual self-renewal (Myers & Diener, 1997). Such an approach is in contrast to being reactive to or oppressed by negative life experiences that then become triggers for depression, unhappiness, or inability to function effectively.

Cost-Benefit Analyses

Implicit, if not explicit, in several of the trends cited in this chapter, is a concern for conserving the time of counselors so that it can be applied to clients for whom the need is the greatest. But also implicit in such concerns is the overall effect of counseling programs. One major issue is how much does it cost to staff and equip a counseling program, what are the likely results, and what is the economic value of counseling? Such questions have frequently been addressed in rehabilitation counseling and in addictions counseling but much less frequently in counseling in general. However, it is not unusual to hear policy makers or administrators ask, "What do I get, if I invest in counseling?" Is counseling an added cost or an added value? When counseling is included in legislation, there is often a *presumptive benefit* that the results of counseling with clients will yield *less* incarceration, crime, addictive behavior, and unemployment and *more* reintegration of clients into the work force, productivity, effective interpersonal skills, and deliberative and informed decision-making. Each of these results is expected to yield cost-benefit ratios that demonstrate that the economic returns to clients or to society exceed the costs of providing counseling. Unfortunately, the empirical tests, the analyses for many of these cost-benefit ratios, have not yet been done. In the future, it is likely that such demonstrations of the added value of counseling in many settings will include cost-benefit analyses as resources available for human services become more limited and their access becomes more competitive (Herr, 2001; Herr, Cramer, & Niles, 2004; Whiston & Brecheisen, 2002).

Multicultural Approaches

There is little doubt that demography, the population profile of the United States or of specific regions within the Untied States, is becoming more multicultural. Immigration into the United States now occurs at a rate approximately the same as that which occurred during the late 1800s and the early 1900s. The difference is that the nations of origin for immigrants have changed since the major immigrations to the United States 100 or more years ago. At that time, many, if not most, immigrants were from Europe; now they are from Asia, Mexico, and Central and South America. In any case, cultural diversity and pluralism in traditions and beliefs is a reality among clients seeking counseling.

As sensitivity to the importance of the changing demography of the U.S. population has grown, so have other concepts. In a special issue of the *Journal of Counseling & Development* focused on multicultural counseling, the guest editors, Michael D'Andrea and Elizabeth Foster Heckman (2008), made clear that multicultural issues are not only matters of race, ethnicity, or cultural traditions. They are also about social justice issues, and the multicultural/social justice counseling movement is linked to several other movements such as feminism, psychological liberation, empowerment, advocacy, and ethical professional practices and training endeavors. Implicit in such linkages is also the reality that many persons who come from different cultural traditions or from minority groups also suffer from being marginalized and devalued by the larger society. Thus, they are persons for whom social justice has often not been provided.

As a result, counselors will increasingly need to be trained in more comprehensive ways than currently exist to be able to reflect in counseling the cultural traditions that motivate clients, whether newly arrived or who are first or second generation. In these cases, continuous study of the characteristics of the cultural groups from which the clients of a particular counselor come is a minimum need; in many more cases than now exist more counselors will need to be bilingual or multilingual to work with clients who are not English speakers or who are not fluent in English. In some cases, counselors and clients will need interpreters to ensure that the subtleties of language and culture of clients will be understood. Counselors will need to be fully competent to implement the multicultural competencies that now exist and to learn the care-giving approaches that define relationships between clients and counselors in various cultures (for example, how much and what kind of interaction with a client's family should a counselor have if the results of counseling are to be acceptable within that cultural context). Counselors will need to know how to provide respect for the cultural history of the client and monitor any communications obstacles that may arise. They will need to learn skills by which to help multicultural clients deal with and react to being marginalized and devalued by the larger society. While much of importance has been achieved in increased sensitivity to the significance of culture and ethnicity in the relationship between counselors and clients, there is much yet to be achieved to provide counselors who are educated in and capable of addressing the needs of immigrant populations and those who live in families who are straddling majority and minority cultures.

Active Learning Exercise **1.2**

You are speaking to a board of directors who want to know why they should continue to support counseling in this organization. They want to know what they should expect to get from their investment in counseling. What has the history of counseling demonstrated that you think the board members should know about? What trends do you think are of particular interest to the board of directors?

CONCLUSION

Given the trends in counseling just discussed, it is clear that the history of counseling is not complete. Indeed, every day extends the history of counseling while at the same time adding speculation about the future.

In this chapter, we have discussed the antecedents to contemporary theories and practices, as well as to the professionalization of counseling. We have acknowledged that throughout history, people have emerged who serve and guide others as they deal with crises or decision conflicts in their lives. Increasingly, over the centuries, knowledge bases have been created to add to our understanding of human behavior and its disorders and how different behavioral problems can be changed, strengthened, or eliminated.

Discussed in this chapter have been both the "long view" and the "short view" of counseling. The intent has been to describe how historical content about counseling changes as scholars and thinkers find new ways to discuss mental health issues and how to respond to them. However, in the short view, the emphasis has been on the professionalization of counseling, the contextual variables that have shaped and given support to counseling, the collective impact of organizations that have represented counselors and their value to the larger society, the accountability mechanisms (e.g., counselor licensure or certification; accreditation of counselor education programs; ethical codes) that identify standards of professional behavior by counselor, and the major issues, or trends, in counseling that need to be studied and incorporated into counseling.

CHAPTER REVIEW

1. The long view of the history of counseling focuses on the major scholars who have provided insight into human behavior, mental health, and mental illnesses. Many of these theories have been refined and become the "seedbeds" for contemporary theories.

2. The short view of the history of counseling has spanned approximately the last 150 years, the period when counseling has emerged as a significant process supported by public policy and by the initiatives that resulted in the professionalization of counseling.

3. This chapter has discussed the shifts from philosophy to empirical, scientific approaches to human behavior and interventions matched with groups of persons who share similar symptoms and mental disorders. This is the basis for the growing focus on evidence-based, empirically supported, results-based approaches, or best practices.

4. As the importance of counselors and counseling has grown, new trends have emerged to increase what counselors need to know about and address. Included are such matters as the use of advanced technology in counseling, the promotion of counseling, multicultural/social justice approaches, cost-benefit analyses, and so on.

REVIEW QUESTIONS

1. How have the terms related to counseling changed over time?
2. What are the differences between a *long view* and a *short view* of counseling?
3. How have the classifications of persons with mental illness changed over time?
4. How would you differentiate between *guidance* and *counseling*?
5. Identify and briefly discuss five of the major scholars who offered major theories of human behavior.

ADDITIONAL RESOURCES

- http://nbcc.org/
- http://www.person-centered-counseling.com/carl_rogers.htm
- http://www.counseling.org/Counselors/TP/PodcastsHome/CT2.aspx
- http://www.simplyhired.com/a/jobtrends/trend/q-Counseling

REFERENCES

Allport, G. W. (1962, Fall). Psychological models for guidance, *Harvard Educational Review, 32*(4), 373–381.

American Psychiatric Association. (1980). *Diagnostic and statistical manual of mental disorders* (3rd ed.). Washington, D.C.: Author.

American Psychiatric Association. (1994). *Diagnostic and statistical manual of mental disorders* (4th ed.). Washington, D.C.: Author.

American School Counselor Association. (1997). *The national standards for school counseling programs.* Alexandria, VA: Author.

Bromberg, W. (1963). History of treatment of mental disorders. In A. Deutsch & H. Fishman (Eds.), *The encyclopedia of mental health*, Vol. 3 (pp. 737–746). New York: Franklin Watts.

D'Andrea, M., & Heckman, E. F. (2008). Contributing to the ongoing evolution of the multicultural counseling movement: An introduction to the special issue [Special issue]. *Journal of Counseling and Development, 86*(3), 258–259.

Davis, J. (1914). *Vocational and moral guidance.* Boston: Ginn.

Dumont, F., & Carson, A. (1995). Precursors of vocational psychology in ancient civilizations. *Journal of Counseling and Development, 73*, 371–378.

Frank, J. D., & Frank, J. B. (1991). *Persuasion and healing: A comparative study of psychotherapy* (3rd ed.). Baltimore, MD: Johns Hopkins University Press.

Herr, E. L. (1991). Multiple agendas in a changing society: Policy challenges confronting career guidance in the USA. *British Journal of Guidance and Counseling, 19*(3), 267–282.

Herr, E. L. (1999). *Counseling in a dynamic society. Contexts and practices for the 21st century.* Alexandria, VA: American Counseling Association.

Herr, E. L. (2001). Career development and its practice: A historical perspective. *The Career Development Quarterly, 49*(3), 196–211.

Herr, E. L. (2003). Historical roots and future issues. In B. T. Erford (Ed.), *Transforming the school counseling profession* (pp. 21–38). Upper Saddle River, NJ: Merrill Prentice Hall.

Herr, E. L., Cramer, S. H., & Niles, S. G. (2004). *Career counseling and counseling through the life-span systematic approaches.* Boston: Allyn and Bacon.

Herr, E. L., Heitzmann, D. E., & Rayman, J. R. (2006). *The professional counselor as administrator: Perspectives on leadership and management in counseling services.* Mahwah, NJ: Lawrence Erlbaum Associates.

Jones, A. J. (1934). *Principles of guidance* (2nd ed.). New York: McGraw-Hill.

Keller, F. S. (1937). *The definition of psychology. An introduction to psychological systems.* New York: Appleton Century-Grofts.

Leibniz, G. W. (1890). Observations on Locke's "Essay on Human Understanding" [Originally published in 1696]. In G. M. Duncan (Ed.), *The Philosophical Works of Leibniz* (pp. 94–99). New Haven, CT: Tuttle, Morehouse, and Taylor.

Maples, M. F., & Ham S. (2008). Cybercounseling in the United States and South Korea: Implications for counseling college students of the millennial generation and the networked generation. *Journal of Counseling and Development, 86*(2),178–183.

Marotta, S. A., & Watts, R. E. (2007). An introduction to the best practices section in the *Journal of Counseling and Development. Journal of Counseling and Development, 85*(4), 491–503.

Miller, C. H. (1961). *Foundations of guidance.* New York: Harper & Brothers.

Myers, D. G., & Diener, E. (1997). The science of happiness. *The Futurist, 31*(5), 1–7.

Paisley, P. O., & Borders, L. D. (1995). School counseling: An evolving specialty. *Journal of Counseling and Development, 74*(2), 150–152.

Parsons, F. (1909). *Choosing a vocation.* Boston: Houghton Mifflin.

Patterson, C. H. (1966). *Theories of counseling and psychotherapy.* New York: Harper.

Rogers, C. R. (1942). *Counseling and psychotherapy: Newer concepts in practice.* Boston: Houghton Mifflin.

Rogers, C. R. (1957). The necessary and sufficient conditions of therapeutic personality change. *Journal of Consulting Psychology, 21*, 95–103.

Rosen, H. (1996). Meaning-making narratives: Foundations for constructivist and social constructionist psychotherapies. In H. Rosen & K. T. Kuehlwein (Eds.), *Constructing realities: Meaning-making perspectives for psychotherapy* (pp. 3–54). San Francisco, CA: Jossey-Bass.

Sampson, J. P., Kolodinsky, R. W., & Greeno, B. P. (1997). Counseling on the information highway: Future possibilities and potential problems. *Journal of Counseling and Development, 75*(3), 203–212.

Shertzer, B., & Stone, S. C. (1974). *Fundamentals of counseling* (2nd ed.). Boston: Houghton Mifflin.

Smith, M. L., Glass, G. V., & Miller, T. I. (1980). *The benefits of psychology*. Baltimore, MD: Johns Hopkins University Press.

Super, D. E., & Crites, J. O. (1962). *Appraising vocational fitness* (Rev. ed.). New York: Harper & Row.

Truneckova, D., & Viney, L.L. (2007). Evaluating personal construct group work with troubled adolescents. *Journal of Counseling & Development, 85*, 450–460.

Wampold, B. E. (2001). *The great psychotherapy debate: Models, methods, and findings*. Mahwah, NJ: Lawrence Erlbaum Associates.

Watson, J. B. (1919). *Psychology, from the standpoint of a behaviorist*. Philadelphia: J. B. Lippincott.

Whiston, S. C., & Brecheisen, B. K. (2002). Annual review: Practice and research in career counseling and development: 2001. *The Career Development Quarterly 51*, 98–154.

Williamson, E. G. (1965). *Vocational counseling: Some historical, philosophical, and theoretical perspectives*. New York: McGraw-Hill.

CHAPTER 2

The Counseling Profession Today

LEARNING OBJECTIVES

After reading this chapter, you should be able to

- discuss the major distinctions among counseling, psychiatry, psychology, and social work;
- list the areas of specialization within the professional counseling field;
- describe the various practice settings for counselors;
- explain counselor certification and licensure; and
- cite the average salaries for counselors and compensation by specialization.

CHAPTER OUTLINE

Introduction

Counseling as a Profession

Counseling Specializations
School Counseling
Clinical Mental Health Counseling
College Counseling
Career Counseling
Addictions Counseling

Rehabilitation Counseling
Marriage, Couples, and Family Counseling

Populations With Which Counselors Work
Children and Adolescents
Adults
Older Adults

Counseling Practice Settings

INTRODUCTION

New professionals joining the counseling profession often have questions: Why do people choose to enter the field of counseling? What will they do as counselors? Who will they work with? When will they be ready to practice counseling? Where might they work? and the question people are often afraid to ask, How much will they earn? These are all excellent questions that should be asked and answered. The profession of counseling is a dynamic field that offers opportunities to work with diverse individuals, families, groups, and communities in a variety of settings. This chapter provides you with answers to questions about the counseling profession using information from ours and other fields, recent data, and the voices of students and practicing counselors.

COUNSELING AS A PROFESSION

The questions, Why counseling and not psychiatry, psychology, or social work? or How is counseling different from psychiatry, psychology, or social work? are often asked of counseling professionals by family members, friends, clients, and community members. While all of these professions have an overall focus on enhancing human well-being, different training requirements and philosophical perspectives result in key distinctions for each discipline.

Perhaps the most notable distinction between psychiatrists and counselors is that psychiatrists are medical doctors (Bureau of Labor Statistics [BLS], 2009a). After finishing medical school, psychiatrists spend an additional four years completing residency training focused on preventing, assessing, diagnosing, and treating mental health concerns. Many of the approximately 40,647 clinically active psychiatrists (Center for Mental Health Services [CMHS], 2004) receive additional training in specialty practice areas, including child psychiatry, geriatric psychiatry, or addictions (BLS, 2009a). Psychiatrists can prescribe medication to treat mental health problems while counselors cannot (BLS, 2009a).

The primary distinction between psychologists and counselors is training. A doctoral degree is commonly required to become a licensed psychologist, although some states credential school psychologists with educational specialist degrees and industrial-organizational psychologists can be credentialed at the master's degree level (BLS, 2009b). Estimates suggest that by 2002, there were approximately 88,500 licensed psychologists in the United States (CMHS, 2004). Clinical and counseling psychologists often focus their practice in working with individuals who have severe mental health concerns (American Counseling Association [ACA], 2007a). Both psychiatrists and psychologists are trained to use psychotherapy to address mental health concerns among clients

(BLS, 2009a; BLS, 2009b), which is another distinction between these two professions and counseling. According to ACA (2007b), psychotherapy differs from counseling as a result of its emphasis on past events, personal insight, and the role of the therapist as the authority. There are two features that distinguish counseling from psychotherapy, according to ACA (2007b): length of service and setting. Counseling services are more likely than psychotherapy to be offered in outpatient settings (e.g., not residential treatment facilities or hospitals) and on a short-term basis (e.g., 8 to 12 sessions over no more than six months).

Data provided by state licensure boards indicates that as of 2007, there were 156,982 licensed social workers in the United States (ACA, 2007c). While social workers can practice with a bachelor's degree, a master's degree is required for licensure and clinical practice (BLS, 2009c). The educational requirements for clinical practice and licensure for social workers and counselors are similar, but their philosophical emphases have traditionally been more distinct. Social workers historically have emphasized the social and environmental contexts that contribute to problems in the lives of individuals and families (CMHS, 2004), while counselors appear to put emphasis on developmental, preventative, and educational approaches for promoting mental health (CMHS, 2004). Additionally, social workers frequently work with individuals facing significant issues (e.g., life-threatening disease, homelessness, unemployment) (BLS, 2009c), while counseling "believes that a person does not have to be sick to get better" (Smith & Robinson, 1995, p. 158).

Counseling is defined by ACA (2007b, p. 2) as a "relatively short-term, interpersonal, theory-based practice of helping persons who are basically psychologically healthy resolve developmental and situational problems." Mental health profession statistics indicate that as of 2007, there were 103,865 professional counselors licensed to practice in the United States (ACA, 2007c) and many more working toward licensure, reflecting the large presence of professionals committed to this profession. In 2000, there were approximately 20,000 students enrolled in graduate-level training programs in counseling, and anecdotal evidence suggests that this number has been increasing annually (CMHS, 2004). One student's perspective about why he chose to study counseling may also be helpful for understanding distinctions between counseling and related disciplines:

> Counseling uniquely brings together and balances the therapeutic component of traditional psychology with the case management and advocacy services typical within social work. Being involved in all aspects of a client's treatment has, in my experience, resulted in positive outcomes for both the client and the counselor. (Ryan Bruce, Graduate Student, Rehabilitation Counseling; personal communication, July, 16, 2007)

This personal account powerfully reflects the pride and professional identification of a student joining the counseling profession. *Professional identity* is a term that is often used by counselors that conveys their sense of commitment to and advancement of the philosophical foundations and principals of the counseling field. It is important to note, however, that in addition to developing an identity as a professional counselor, students are encouraged to learn more about related disciplines. Understanding what various helping disciplines offer in the way of team-based approaches to care, collaboration, and interdisciplinary communication is critical to effective service in our current healthcare system (Hoge, Jacobs, Belitsky, & Migdole, 2002). Recognition and utilization of the expertise of professionals from other disciplines is an important skill for both current and new professional counselors.

Active Learning Exercise 2.1

Describe your motivations for pursuing a career in professional counseling. Why did you choose to become a member of the counseling profession versus social work, psychology, or psychiatry? What types of professionals from related helping disciplines do you anticipate working with as a counselor? Review the Web sites of their professional associations. What can you learn about the expertise they have and services they offer? What skills might you need to collaborate and communicate with other professionals? In addition to your required coursework and clinical experiences, how else might you learn about interdisciplinary work (e.g., job shadowing, observation of interagency community meetings, volunteer work)?

COUNSELING SPECIALIZATIONS

The professional practice areas and roles of counselors are as diverse and dynamic as the persons they work with. Counselors work in a number of specialty practice areas (e.g., school, mental health, rehabilitation counseling) in different roles (e.g., direct service provider, administrator, advocate). The wide variety in practice areas and roles provides counselors with a number of choices in their training programs and careers. Following is a brief review of some specialty practice areas and key professional associations, along with narratives from the practicing counselors in these specialty practice areas. As you read, take a few minutes to reflect on what specializations and roles appeal to you.

School Counseling

According to the American School Counselor Association (ASCA, 2009a), school counselors provide a wide variety of services in educational settings such as elementary, junior high/middle, and high schools as well as postsecondary institutions. School counselors are certified (requirements vary by state) educators who provide responsive counseling, consultation, resource referral, and peer helping, as well as informational and systems support services, through delivery of a comprehensive school counseling program. Such comprehensive programs, guided by the ASCA National Model, are designed to improve academic, personal/social, and career outcomes for students. Specific issues often addressed by school counselors include conflict resolution, coping skills, peer relationships, career exploration and planning, substance abuse prevention, and academic skills support. A key mission for school counselors is the creation of equitable learning experiences for all students through leadership, advocacy, and collaboration. School counseling is an area of specialization for many counselors. Currently, 466 colleges or universities offer graduate training in school counseling. It appears that many more school counselors are needed, however, to meet ASCA's recommended ratio of 250 students to 1 school counselor; recent data indicates that this ratio is currently 479 to 1. Professionals interested in learning more about these and other current issues in school counseling may want to review recent editions of *Professional School Counseling*, the official journal of ASCA (ASCA, 2009b). The following narrative also provides some additional insights for new counselors considering this specialty area of practice.

> As students arrive at school, I try to be at the entrance to greet students and get a feel for the day ahead. Sometimes a student will come into school upset and my day will begin with taking that child aside to talk. Other days, I might have a guidance lesson scheduled first. As the day progresses, there might be a disagreement or an issue that requires me to diffuse the crisis. Although these events may seem chaotic, this is my job, and what I love about being a school counselor. Despite extensive planning, frequently my job requires my schedule to change due to a call from a concerned parent, a child walking into my office crying, or a call from the nurses' office that requires my attention. If you asked my students, all 620 of them, what my job is, you would probably get 620 different answers. I care for my students individually, know their names, and try to engage them at a personal level that makes a difference for them as well as provide them with a sense of community and family. (Megan Young, School Counselor, Carrolltowne Elementary School, Maryland, personal communication, July 16, 2007)

Clinical Mental Health Counseling

Many children, adolescents, adults, older adults, and families struggle with mental health concerns and are in need of specialized counseling services. According to the American Mental Health Counselors Association (AMHCA, 2009a), clinical mental health counseling is a unique specialty practice area with national standards for coursework, training, and clinical experience. Clinical mental health counselors provide services such as diagnosis and assessment, counseling, crisis management, and substance abuse treatment in settings such as hospitals, community agencies, and private practices. The *Journal of Mental Health Counseling* is a quarterly publication of AMHCA that provides counselors practicing in this specialty area with information and research related to the wide variety of services they offer (AMHCA, 2009b). Currently, 48 states license or certify clinical mental health counselors for independent practice, and a majority of managed care providers reimburse services delivered by clinical mental health counselors. In addition, counselors can also be credentialed as a Certified Clinical Mental Health Counselor (CCMHC) by the National Board of Certified Counselors (NBCC). Clinical mental health counselors work from a wide variety of different roles, including direct counselor, supervisor, and program administrator. The following narrative provides a brief overview of a typical day of practice in this specialty area from the perspective of a children's mental health counselor:

> While it often does not feel like it, when involved in the daily trenches, counselors do make a difference. I have learned that being a counselor is one way to make a

difference in the lives of troubled youth with mental health problems. I think back to a client that reminded me that what I do matters. I was completing a diagnostic assessment of a new potential client. This 17-year-old male was starting to have brushes with the court system, had been suspended from school, and was now attending an alternative school. The client was having every problem one could think of from social relationships, depression, suicidal ideations, family conflicts, and feelings that he didn't quite know what to do with. He was experiencing visual and auditory hallucinations, excessive paranoia, violent rages, and overwhelming feelings of anxiety. This client stands out to me because he presented with a tough exterior, not very open initially, and very skeptical that there would be anything that I, or anyone, for that matter would be able to do to help him. Well he was wrong, I did not give up on him, and showed him how not to give up on himself either. (Monica Parker, Coordinator of Child and Adolescent Services, Cobb County Community Services Board, Marietta, Georgia, personal communication, July 17, 2007)

College Counseling

According to the American College Counseling Association (ACCA, 2001) many students are confronted with feelings of stress, mental health concerns, and academic challenges related to the multiple life stressors and developmental demands that occur during the college years. College counselors provide brief, solution-focused, psycho-educational, and confidential counseling services to college students struggling with issues such as depression, substance abuse, homesickness, isolation, stress, and eating disorders. The *Journal of College Counseling* is published biannually by ACCA and provides counselors with key strategies and research related to addressing these and other issues with college students (ACA, 2009a). Counselors working in college settings often work in such roles as counselor, crisis responder, psychological test administrator, and consultant. ACCA (2007) reports a membership of approximately 1,412 college counselors, most of whom work at a college or university setting. A smaller number of college counselors work in junior/community colleges or private practice. Many members of ACCA are working in direct counseling roles, although a smaller number report working in a supervisory or administrative role within their work setting. College counselors often have professional credentials such as Licensed Professional Counselor, Licensed Professional Clinical Counselor, or National Certified Counselor. The following narrative from a counselor specializing in college counseling provides some additional insight into this unique profession:

A decade ago I completed an internship as a college counselor at a private university in Louisiana. My days were met with the challenges of giving students career assessments so that they might find a major and/or a career. I also had clients who were having relationship troubles, experiencing homesickness, or just generally needed help with exploring their values as they related (or in some cases did not relate) to those of their family. Ten years later, I am an assistant professor at a private university in New York, where I also work a few days a week as a college counselor in our campus-counseling center. Though the venue remains the same, my cases are quite different. My days are now met with crises, a full schedule of clients who always show up for their appointments, and many of my clients have diagnosable disorders. Some of my clients came to college having already been diagnosed, on psychotropic medications, and with a counselor at home. Today is not ten years ago. Issues seem more serious and students seem more affected by life's trials and tribulations. But for all the challenges I face as a counselor for this population, the benefits are incalculable. I am energized and enthused by these students who have sought counseling and gotten themselves the help they needed. I am impressed with their tenacity and their stick-to-itiveness. I am blown away by their resiliency. A typical day in the life of a college counselor is not what it used to be, but it is more rewarding than I ever could have imagined. (Morgan Conway, Assistant Professor, Niagara University, personal communication, July 25, 2007)

Career Counseling

The National Career Development Association (NCDA, 1997, p. 1) defines career counseling as "the process of assisting individuals in the development of a life-career with focus on the definition of the worker role and how that roles interacts with other life roles." NCDA (2007) indicates that career counselors use a variety of approaches, including counseling, test administration and interpretation, individualized career plans, exploratory activities, and psycho-education to help individuals identify and facilitate career and life strategies. Career counselors often have professional credentials such as Licensed Professional Counselor (LPC) or Licensed Professional Clinical Counselor (LPCC) that are issued by the state they practice in (requirements for licensure vary by state). In addition, some career counselors are also National Certified Counselors (NCCs), a national certification granted by the NBCC. Master Career Counselor (MCC) and Master Career Development Professional (MCDP) are two distinct membership categories offered by NCDA to recognize specific professional preparation and experience in career counseling. MCCs are professionals who, in addition to being members of NCDA for two or more years, have earned a master's degree in counseling or a related field, have three years of post–master's degree career counseling experience, and maintain such credentials as the LPC, LPCC, or NCC in additional to documentation of professional preparation in career counseling competencies. MCDPs have similar requirements as the MCC except they may not maintain credentials such as the LPC, LPCC, or NCC and their post–master's degree experience may not have been focused specifically on career counseling but instead on training, education, program design, or creation of materials related to career development. Counselors who are interested in learning more about current issues and research in career counseling may find review of recent editions of *The Career Development Quarterly* useful. This journal is the official journal of NCDA and provides its readership with up-to-date information about issues such as career coaching, work and recreation, and career education (ACA, 2009). In addition, the following narrative from a practicing career counselor provides more immediate insights about the benefits and challenges of practice in this specialty area.

As a career counselor, I have the opportunity to engage students in multiple ways throughout the year. I counsel students during hour-long individual appointments, present workshops on a variety of career topics, and meet with them at large career events held throughout the year. The common thread of all of these interactions is the chance to have a positive impact in assisting students with career planning. The majority of my time is spent counseling, where I help students through the journey of self-discovery, to gain knowledge of the world of work, determine how those two factors interact, and develop a plan to implement their career goals. One of the challenges of the work is to get students to realize that career planning is not a moment in time, but rather a process that requires them to be active, reflective, and to utilize good decision-making. The most interesting part of my work is the variety of the career activities I participate in; along with the range of individual students I see who are at various stages in the career planning process. (Holly Temple, Career Counselor, The Pennsylvania State University, personal communication, July 19, 2007)

Addictions Counseling

Counselors who work across a variety of settings are likely to encounter clients with addictive disorders. Many people struggle with addictions to alcohol, drugs, food, gambling, nicotine, the Internet, sex, shopping, and/or video games. As a result of the number of people who struggle with addiction, a specialization in addictions counseling was added to the most recent (2009) Council for Accreditation of Counseling and Related Educational Programs (CACREP) Accreditation Standards; CACREP develops standards for graduate training and accredits professional preparation programs in counseling that meet those standards (CACREP, 2009). Students graduating with this specialization can expect to deliver, in both addiction and mental health counseling contexts, treatment and prevention programming to clients, families, and others who are affected by addiction. Addiction counselors are responsible for screening and assessing for addictive disorders, addressing co-occurring (addiction and mental health) problems through individual and group counseling services, and advocating for equitable policies and practices related to preventing and treating addiction (CACREP, 2009). In addition to becoming an LPC, LPCC, or NCC, addiction counselors can also be certified as Master Addiction Counselors. Students who are interested in learning more about addictions counseling are encouraged to review the *Journal of Addictions and Offender Counseling*, published by the International Association of Addictions and Offender Counselors (IAAOC). This journal provides information about key strategies and research related to addictions and offender counseling (IAAOC, 2009). In addition, IAAOC also publishes a quarterly newsletter that includes information about emerging trends, professional development opportunities, and book reviews related to addiction counseling.

Rehabilitation Counseling

The American Rehabilitation Counseling Association (ARCA, 2007a, p. 1) defines rehabilitation counseling as "a systematic process which assists persons with physical, mental, developmental, cognitive, and emotional disabilities to achieve their personal, career, and independent living goals in the most integrated settings possible through the application of the counseling process." Rehabilitation counselors utilize approaches such as assessment, diagnosis, career counseling, counseling, case management, program evaluation, consultation, job development, rehabilitation technology, and removal of attitudinal, environmental, and employment barriers to help persons with disabilities realize their goals. The underlying values of rehabilitation counseling include independence, integration, inclusion, social justice, holistic care, respect for the worth and value of all individuals, and interdisciplinary care. The Council on Rehabilitation Education (CORE) accredits graduate training programs in Rehabilitation Counselor Education (CORE, 2009). Rehabilitation counselors, in addition to credentials such as the LPC, LPCC, or NCC, can also be credentialed as a Certified Rehabilitation Counselor by the Commission on Rehabilitation Counselor Certification (CRCC). To date, the CRCC has credentialed more than 35,000 rehabilitation counselors (CRCC, 2009). For counselors who are interested in this specialty practice area, review of the *Rehabilitation Counseling Bulletin*, a quarterly publication of ARCA (ARCA, 2009b) or *Rehabilitation Education*, a quarterly publication of the National Council on Rehabilitation Education (2009) may provide additional information about best practices in this field.

Marriage, Couples, and Family Counseling

The International Association of Marriage and Family Counselors (IAMFC, 2009a) indicates that counselors working in this specialty area can expect to deliver diverse services such as diagnosis and assessment; individual, couples, and family counseling; prevention programs; parent education; multifamily or couples group counseling; and crisis intervention. It appears that the issues addressed by marriage, couples, and family counselors are as varied as the services they offer. Individuals, couples, and families may request this type of counselor when they are experiencing relationship issues such as childhood trauma, substance abuse, infidelity, family violence, or communication problems. Marriage, couples, and family counselors are also trained to provide preventative services focused on communication, assertiveness, and time management to improve interpersonal relationships. Both intervention and prevention services are offered by marriage, couples, and family counselors in a variety of settings, including mental health agencies, hospitals, private practice, religious or spiritual institutions, or employee assistance programs. In addition to having professional credentials such as LPC, LPCC, or NCC, marriage, couple, and family counselors can also be certified in family therapy by the National Credentialing Academy or receive licensure as a Marriage and Family Therapist at the state level. IAMFC offers two publications, *The Family Journal* and *The Family Digest*, that provide information about current issues, research, and counseling approaches for professionals practicing in this specialty area (IAMFC, 2009b). In addition, counselors can find information about this specialty area of practice in publications of the American Association for Marriage and Family Therapy, which include the *Journal of Marital and Family Therapy* and the *Family Therapy Magazine*.

In addition to the specialty practice areas just described, counselors also specialize in such fields as gerontological, multicultural, and genetic counseling (BLS, 2007d). Gerontological counselors specialize in addressing the unique developmental concerns of aging persons and their family members. Employers can work with multicultural counselors to address issues specific

TABLE **2.1**

Areas of Specialization Within the Counseling Profession

Area	Description
School	Provides a wide variety of services in educational settings to support the healthy academic, social/emotional, and vocational development of youth. Approaches used include counseling, consultation, resource referral, and peer helping.
Clinical Mental Health	Focuses on work with individuals who have diagnosed mental disorders or who are at risk for developing such disorders. Uses approaches such as assessment and diagnosis, counseling, crisis management, and substance abuse interventions.
College	Provides brief, solution-focused, psycho-educational, and confidential counseling services to college students struggling with issues such as depression, substance abuse, homesickness, isolation, stress, and eating disorders.
Career	Focuses on helping individuals identify and facilitate career and life strategies through counseling, test administration and interpretation, individualized career plans, exploratory activities, and psycho-education.
Addiction	Provides intervention and prevention programming to clients, families, and others affected by addiction within addiction and mental health counseling contexts.
Rehabilitation	Focuses on helping individuals with disabilities realize their goals through utilization of approaches such as assessment, diagnosis, career counseling, case management, consultation, job development, and rehabilitation.
Marriage, Couples, & Family	Provides services such as couples and family counseling, parent education, and multifamily or couples group counseling to address relational issues such as infidelity, family violence, or communication problems.

to the increasingly diverse population in the United States. Finally, genetic counselors work specifically with families who are at risk for or are currently encountering birth defects or genetic disorders. It is also important to remember that there are opportunities to specialize within specialty practice areas (and you thought all of those acronyms were confusing). For example, a clinical mental health counselor may specialize in working with children with mental illness and their families, or a rehabilitation counselor may specialize in work with returning veterans. Whatever specialty area of practice you choose, there are many opportunities for a diverse and exciting career.

POPULATIONS WITH WHICH COUNSELORS WORK

A counselor's clientele is widely varied and is often influenced by such factors as area of the country (e.g., southern region, northeast), community (e.g., rural, urban, suburban), and master's degree program or specialty practice area (e.g., school, clinical mental health, career counseling). Because you may not yet be sure about the specific population you want to work with, learning more about the demographics and emerging counseling needs of children and adolescents, adults, and older adults in the United States may be useful to thinking more about the wide variety of people you are likely to encounter in your everyday practice.

Children and Adolescents

According to the Federal Interagency Forum on Child and Family Statistics (2006), the numbers and diversity of children in the United States are substantial. In 2006, children ages 0–17 represented 25% of the population, and among the 73.7 million children, 59% were European American, 19% Latino, 16% African American, and 4% Asian American. Of the estimated 73.7 million children in the United States, many (37.6 million, or 51%) live in low-income or poor families (National Center for Children in Poverty, 2006).

The impact of poverty on personal growth and opportunities of children and adolescents is a key challenge for many counselors working with this age group. Many school counselors have encountered the educational disparities that often impact children and adolescents from low-income backgrounds; only 67% of children in families with the lowest 25% of incomes will graduate high school, compared to 94% among families from the top 25% of incomes (American Youth Policy Forum, 2007). Estimates also suggest that many children and adolescents struggle with mental health concerns; 1 in 5 have a diagnosable mental illness or addictive disorder, and 1 in 10 have a serious emotional disturbance that impacts their ability to succeed at school, at home, and in the community (Knoph, Park, & Mulye, 2008). Perhaps more troubling than the large number of youth who are likely experiencing mental health issues is the realization that only 25% receive any mental health care (Huang et al., 2005). Counselors working in specialty practice areas such as clinical mental health; marriage, couples, and family; and school counseling can expect to encounter the challenges of helping children deal with very adult issues within the context of changing developmental stages.

Adults

According to the U.S. Census Bureau, in 2004 there were approximately 217.8 million people between the ages of 19 and 65 (U.S. Census Bureau, 2004). As with children and adolescents, the diversity of adults in the United States is also increasing; as of 2007, one in three residents of the United States was a minority (U.S. Census Bureau, 2007). More specifically, with a population of 42.7 million (as of 2006), persons of Latino origin are estimated to be the largest ethnic or racial minority in the United States (U.S. Census Bureau, 2006a).

It appears that the odds of struggling with a diagnosable mental illness increases with age. Estimates suggest that one in four adults (26%) over the age of 18 have a diagnosable mental illness (Kessler, Chiu, Demler, & Walters, 2005). A recent report by ACA (2009c), which cites a wide variety of research studies that document the need for counseling services, suggests that as of 2007, an estimated 23.2 million persons residing in the United States needed treatment of a substance use disorder, but less than 1% actually received help at a specialized treatment center. Addressing the unique and complex issues associated with addiction is likely to be a key issue for many counselors working with adults. Another timely concern for some counselors is recognition of the need for mental health services in rural areas. Citing recent research, ACA (2009c) reports that persons living in metropolitan areas are approximately

1.5 times more likely to receive mental health services than those who reside in rural areas with a population of less than 2,500 residents. Based on these estimates, there may be significant counseling needs in rural communities.

Older Adults

The U.S. Census Bureau (2006b) reports that the first cohort of baby boomers celebrated their 60th birthdays in 2006, signaling the beginning a population increase that is likely to double the number of Americans over the age of 65. More specifically, by 2030, one in five adults (72 million) in the United States will be over the age of 65. Counselors working in Florida, Pennsylvania, and West Virginia might specifically anticipate work with this population as these three states have the highest number of persons over the age of 65. Trends in the mental well-being of older adults also indicate some specific counseling needs for professionals specializing in this practice area.

Depressive illnesses (e.g., major depressive, dysthymic, or bipolar disorder) and symptoms are not uncommon among older adults, and older adults accounted for 18% of all suicide deaths in 2000 (National Institute of Mental Health, 2003). Citing a recent report by the Substance Abuse and Mental Health Services Administration, ACA (2009c) indicates that the number of persons age 65 and older with a diagnosable mental illness is also expected to double to over 15 million during the next 30 years. Counselors working with older adults should anticipate addressing a wide variety of role transitions that commonly occur during this stage of life. Retirement, death of partners and friends, isolation, and terminal illnesses are real issues that often impact the well-being of older adults.

COUNSELING PRACTICE SETTINGS

In addition to considering who you might work with, it is important to consider where you might practice as a counselor. Questions about practice often include both geographical location and workplace environment. Popular media often presents counseling as taking place in dimly lit, quiet offices furnished with comfortable couches and chairs in private settings, but the reality for many counselors can be quite different and exciting. Counselors address a variety of different issues (e.g., academic/employment, substance abuse, disabilities) across diverse settings (e.g., schools, homes, community agencies). In addition, it is important to reflect on where you might look for jobs once you graduate, considering both cultural and geographic characteristics of the location. For example, are you interested in working in an urban setting where many of your clients might have limited English proficiency? Or might you want to work in a rural setting where you may have to travel long distances to meet with clients who do not have access to public transportation? The key idea here is that you have many choices. As you read the following descriptions about the geographic locations and workplace environments for current practicing counselors, think about what appeals to you.

According to CMHS (2004), in 2002 over 50% of counselors practiced in the middle-Atlantic (e.g., New Jersey, New York, Pennsylvania) and east-north-central (e.g., Illinois, Indiana, Michigan, Ohio, Wisconsin) regions of the United States. With a rate of only 21.6 counselors for every 100,000 people, the east-south-central (e.g., Alabama, Kentucky, Mississippi, Tennessee) region may be in need of counselors. The area of the country with the highest rate of counselors per resident appears to be the mountain (e.g., Arizona, Colorado, Idaho, Montana, Nevada, New Mexico, Utah, Wyoming) region, with a reported 84.7 counselors per 100,000 residents. As you consider the state(s) where you are interested in practicing, you might also consider the type of community you would want to work in. Do you prefer an urban or rural setting? Liberal or conservative? Large or small?

The workplace environment of practicing counselors, according to CMHS (2004), appears to be almost as diverse as the geographic location. During 2002, approximately one third of counselors reported practicing in academic environments, with the majority of those individuals working in elementary and secondary school settings. Additionally, among counselors who practice in clinical settings (23%), 19% work specifically in mental health clinics. Other workplace environments for counselors include mental health hospitals (3%), other health settings (4%), social service agencies (3%), universities and colleges (14%), and independent practice (15%). What workplace setting appeals to you? Do you prefer to work in a setting where your clients spend most of their time (e.g., schools, prisons)? Are you called to work in the public sector within various social service agencies such as child welfare? Might you have a specific interest in working with individuals who are experiencing a mental health crisis and may be hospitalized in a psychiatric setting? Whatever your preference, it is clear that counselors practice in a wide variety of work environments, some of which you may already have experience working in.

Active Learning Exercise **2.2**

Create a professional objective statement. Describe in as much detail as possible the specialty area you are interested in practicing in, the role you would like to have, the setting, and/or the area of particular expertise.

Research your area of specialization and related training and professional development issues. Include library research from at least five recently published sources (the professional journals described previously may be useful) that provide information necessary to identify training needs and job functions. Summarize your findings. Then, list at least three professional training goals related to your specialty area of practice that you will achieve during your graduate training. Describe your specific action plans for meeting these goals, including utilization of both traditional (e.g., coursework, practicum) and nontraditional (e.g., local workshops, conferences) sources of learning in your plan.

COUNSELOR CERTIFICATION AND LICENSURE

In addition to your formal education and clinical training experiences, there are several issues that will influence when you will be able to counsel your first real client without formal supervision. Accreditation of your counseling training program, certification, licensure, and continuing education are all key issues that will impact your independent practice (e.g., practice without required clinical supervision) as a counselor. CACREP develops standards for graduate training and accredits professional preparation programs in counseling that meet those standards (CACREP, 2009). Attending a CACREP-accredited program can have a real impact on national certification and licensure, two key credentials for professional practice.

NBCC offers the NCC credential (NBCC, 2007a). Currently, over 40,000 counselors hold the voluntary NCC credential even though it is not required for independent practice. The NCC credential does, however, indicate to potential employers and clients that a counselor has met national standards developed by professional counselors, encourages professional identity, and provides access to reduced liability insurance rates. There are several different requirements that vary based on the accreditation statuses of universities or colleges where students receive graduate training in counseling. If counselors are graduates of CACREP-accredited programs, the two or more years of post–master's degree counseling experience and clinical supervision requirement is waived; this is just one of the benefits of attending a CACREP-accredited program. In addition to meeting specific educational and counseling experience requirements, to be credentialed as an NCC, counselors must past the National Counselor Examination for Licensure and Certification (NCE).

There is one more key benefit for many counselors credentialed as NCCs seeking state licensure. Satisfactory performance on the NCE is often one requirement for licensure as an independent professional counselor. Commonly referred to as Licensed Professional Counselors, Licensed Professional Clinical Counselors, or Licensed Mental Health Counselors, with more than 110,000 in 50 states and the District of Columbia, licensed counselors represent a large number of persons employed in community mental health centers, agencies, and military service settings (ACA, 2009b). Licensure is often required by employers and for reimbursement by third-party payer sources such as managed care. ACA's 2007 publication *Licensure Requirements for Professional Counselors* indicates that requirements for licensure vary from state to state but, in addition to examination requirements such as the NCE, typically include specific educational and supervised practice experiences. For example, Kentucky requires a minimum of 60 semester hours at a regionally accredited institution, across nine content areas; 400 hours of completed practicum and internship; and 4,000 hours of post–master's degree experience with 100 hours of individual supervision—in addition to satisfactory performance on the NCE—for independent licensure as a counselor. Maryland, on the other hand, requires a minimum of 60 semester hours at a regionally accredited institution; one course in alcohol and drug counseling; supervised field experience; and 2,000 hours of post–master's degree experience with 100 hours of individual supervision provided by a board approved supervisor—in addition to satisfactory performance on the NCE and the Maryland Professional Counselors and Therapists Act Exam—to become independently licensed.

To maintain national certification and state licensure credentials, professional counselors must participate in continuing education (NBCC, 2007b). According to NBCC (2007b), counselors must participate in 100 contact hours from nine approved areas every five years, and they must provide documentation of this participation if audited by the NBCC (10% of recertification applicants are audited). Similar to the variation in requirements for state licensure, continuing education requirements also vary by state. In addition to the necessity of continuing education for maintaining professional credentials, according to the 2005 ACA Code of Ethics standard C.2.f., Continuing Education,

> Counselors recognize the need for continuing education to acquire and maintain a reasonable level of awareness of current scientific and professional information in their fields of activity. They take steps to maintain competence in the skills they use, are open to new procedures, and keep current with the diverse populations and specific populations with whom they work.

Whether it is their need to engage in ongoing learning to maintain professional credentials or the ethical obligation to maintain and expand their boundaries of practice, counselors are not done with their training when they graduate from their professional preparation programs. Instead, members of this profession are committed to lifelong learning that will help them provide the most effective services and supports to a wide variety of individuals and families.

Active Learning Exercise **2.3**

Research how you can become an NCC. Ask the faculty members in your program if students are provided an opportunity to take the NCE at the end of their program. If so, work with other students in your cohort to develop a timeline, including group study opportunities, for taking the exam. If the exam is not offered at your current institution, find out when and where you could take it. How much will it cost? Does your current coursework meet the educational eligibility requirements for NCCs? If not, how can you meet those requirements? After considering these questions, develop specific actions along with timelines for applying for your NCC.

Then, research the licensure requirements for the state you plan to practice in and for your specialty area of practice. Is licensure typically required by your subfield? If not, are you still interested in taking the steps necessary to become licensed? What would be the benefits? Remember to think about whether clinical supervision is typically available in the organizations and sites that employ counselors in your specialty area of practice. If not, how might you obtain clinical supervision and what might it cost?

TABLE **2.2**

Median Annual Salary for Counselors by Area of Specialization (BLS, 2009d)

Area of Specialization	Salary
Rehabilitation counseling	$34,600
Substance abuse counseling	$39,670
Clinical mental health counseling	$40,270
Marriage and family counseling	$46,930
College counseling (colleges, universities, professional schools)	$50,690
School counseling	$53,540

COUNSELOR COMPENSATION

The BLS (2009d) recently published the mean annual earnings of counselors in 2008 for specialty areas of practice (see Table 2.2). Educational, vocational, and school counselors reported earning the highest salaries ($53,540) per year, while rehabilitation counselors reported earning the lowest ($34,600). If you are considering work as a marriage or family counselor, you might anticipate earning an annual salary of $46,930, while those interested in mental health counseling could expect to earn around $40,270 per year. Finally, counselors who specialize in substance use and behavioral disorders report mean annual earnings of $39,670.

It is important to note, however, that these are average salaries that often fluctuate greatly based on area of the country, licensure, years of practice, practice setting, and specialty certifications. Additionally, bilingual counselors are in high demand across many areas of the country where there have been sharp increases in the number of Spanish-speaking individuals. The ability to work with individuals and families who have limited English proficiency may result in higher annual earnings. The BLS (2009d) also notes that for counselors specializing in mental health, rehabilitation, or substance abuse, government employers typically offer higher salaries, while residential facilities tend to offer the lowest. Additionally, counselors who are self-employed in a solo or group private practice also tend to report higher salaries.

CONCLUSION

This chapter has highlighted reasons for joining the counseling profession. As a student joining the profession, you should understand how counseling is distinguished from related helping disciplines such as psychology and social work and develop skills for collaborative work with professionals from other disciplinary backgrounds. Counseling is a dynamic profession that provides a variety of options for specialization such as career, clinical mental health, rehabilitation, and school counseling. In addition to the different areas of specialization, the populations and practice settings counselors work in vary greatly. All of these factors, in addition to certification and licensure, can have a substantial impact on the annual salaries of counselors.

CHAPTER REVIEW

1. Professional counseling can be distinguished from psychiatry, psychology, and social work by its emphasis on developmental, preventative, and educational approaches for mental health and well-being.
2. Specializations within the counseling profession include career counseling; college counseling; clinical mental health counseling; marriage, couples, and family counseling; rehabilitation counseling; and school counseling. Each specialty area of practice has its own association and peer-refereed journal.
3. Counselors work with children and adolescents, adults, and older adults across a variety of settings, including schools, mental health agencies, hospitals, health settings, social services agencies, universities and colleges, and private practice offices.
4. Counselors can receive certification as an NCC. Certification, however, is not required for independent practice. Licensure is often required by employers and by third-party payer sources (e.g., managed care) for reimbursement of services.
5. The median salary for counselors across specialty areas of practice as of May 2006 was approximately $50,000. Salaries for counselors, however, vary greatly by state and specialization and can also be influenced by other factors such as licensure and specific skills such as Spanish language fluency.

REVIEW QUESTIONS

1. Describe the similarities and differences among psychiatry, psychology, social work, and counseling. How is counseling distinct from the other helping professions?
2. Identify and describe the areas of specialization within the counseling profession.
3. Describe the varying populations and issues related to their unique developmental level that counselors often encounter.
4. Identify and discuss the differences between certification and licensure for counselors.
5. Describe the range of salaries for counselors and associated influences on levels of compensation.

ADDITIONAL RESOURCES

- American Counseling Association (http://www.counseling.org/)
- American Counseling Association Divisions (http://www.counseling.org/AboutUs/DivisionsBranchesAndRegions/TP/Divisions/CT2.aspx)
- National Board for Certified Counselors (http://www.nbcc.org/)
- State Counselor Licensure Boards (http://www.counseling.org/Counselors/LicensureAndCert/TP/StateRequirements/CT2.aspx)

REFERENCES

American College Counseling Association. (2001). *College counseling advocacy booklet.* Retrieved July 16, 2007, from http://www.collegecounseling. org/pdf/Advocacy.pdf.

American College Counseling Association. (2007). *About us: Who we are.* Retrieved July 16, 2007, from http://www.collegecounseling.org/ wwa.html.

American Counseling Association. (2005). *Code of ethics.* Retrieved July 14, 2007, from http://www. counseling.org/Resources/CodeOfEthics/TP/Home/ CT2.aspx.

American Counseling Association. (2007a). An overview of counseling. *Crisis Fact Sheets.* Retrieved July 11, 2007, from http://www.counseling.org/ Resources/ConsumersMedia.aspx?AGuid= 8fa66290–45d6–4239–97aa-4a30b2f0ec62.

American Counseling Association. (2007b). Definition of counseling. *Crisis Fact Sheets.* Retrieved July 11, 2007, from http://www.counseling.org/Resources/ ConsumersMedia.aspx?AGuid=97592202–75c2– 4079-b854–2cd22c47be3f.

American Counseling Association. (2007c). *2007 Mental health professions statistics.* Retrieved July 11, 2007, from http://www.counseling.org/Files/ FD.ashx?guid=699735be-46d4-4156-954b- d7173ece8d31.

American Counseling Association. (2009a). *Journals.* Retrieved May 17, 2009, from http://www. counseling.org/Publications/Journals.aspx.

American Counseling Association. (2009b). *Important victory—California becomes 50th state to license professional counselors.* Retrieved October 26, 2009 from http://www.counseling.org/PressRoom/ NewsReleases.aspx?AGuid=32546ec2-a9aa-4734- 8d24-bda2d8fad70c.

American Counseling Association. (2009c). *The effectiveness of and need for professional counseling services.* Retrieved October 26, 2009, from http:// www.counseling.org/Files/FD.ashx?guid=dd88400 b-9fda-4e9f-8959-c6a770937fd1.

American Mental Health Counselors Association. (2009a). *Why use a mental health counselor?* Retrieved May 17, 2009, from http://www.amhca. org/public_resources/why_use_a_mental_health_ counselor.aspx.

American Mental Health Counselors Association. (2009b). *Member benefits.* Retrieved May 17, 2009, from http://www.amhca.org/become/ benefits.aspx.

American Rehabilitation Counseling Association. (2007a). *Scope of practice for rehabilitation counseling.* Retrieved July 17, 2007, from http:// www.arcaweb.org/Members/ScopeofPractice/tabid/ 65/Default.aspx.

American School Counselor Association. (2009a). *Careers/roles.* Retrieved May 17, 2009, from http://www.schoolcounselor.org/content.asp? pl=325&sl=133&contentid=133.

American School Counselor Association. (2009b). *Professional School Counseling journal.* Retrieved May 17, 2009, from http://www.schoolcounselor. org/content.asp?pl=325&sl=132&contentid=235.

American Youth Policy Forum, Inc. (2007). *The forgotten half revisited: American youth and young families, 1998–2008.* Retrieved July 12, 2007, from http://www.aypf.org/pressreleases/ pr18.htm.

Bureau of Labor Statistics. (2009a). Physicians and surgeons. In *Occupational outlook handbook, 2008–09 edition.* Retrieved May 17, 2009, from http://www.bls.gov/oco/ocos074.htm.

Bureau of Labor Statistics. (2009b). Psychologists. In *Occupational outlook handbook, 2008–09 edition.* Retrieved May 17, 2009, from http://www.bls.gov/ oco/ocos056.htm.

Bureau of Labor Statistics. (2009c). Social workers. In *Occupational outlook handbook, 2008–09 edition.* Retrieved May 17, 2009, from http://www.bls.gov/ oco/ocos060.htm.

Bureau of Labor Statistics. (2009d). Counselor. In *Occupational outlook handbook, 2008–09 edition.* Retrieved May 17, 2009, from http://www.bls.gov/ oco/ocos067.htm.

Center for Mental Health Services. (2004). *Mental health practioners and trainees.* In R. W. Manderscheid & M. J. Henderson (Eds.), *Mental Health, United States* (DHHS Publication No. [SMA] 3938) (pp. 327–368). Rockville, MD: Substance Abuse and Mental Health Services Administration.

Commission on Rehabilitation Counselor Certification. (2009). *About CRCC.* Retrieved May 17, 2009, from http://www.crccertification.com/pages/ about_crcc/112.php.

Council for Accreditation for Counseling and Related Educational Programs. (2009). *Home.* Retrieved May 17, 2009, from http://www.cacrep.org/.

Council on Rehabilitation Education. (2009). *Profile of CORE-accredited programs.* Retrieved May 17,

2009, from http://www.core-rehab.org/CORE%20Profile%202003-2004.doc.

Federal Interagency Forum on Child and Family Statistics. (2006). Population and family characteristics. In *America's children in brief: Key national indicators of wellbeing*. Retrieved November 9, 2006, from http://childstats.gov/pdf/ac2006/ac_06.pdf.

Hoge, M. A., Jacobs, S., Belitsky, R., & Migdole, S. (2002). Graduate education and training for contemporary behavioral health practice. *Administration and Policy in Mental Health, 29*, 335–357.

Huang, L., Stroul, B., Friedman, R., Mrazek, P., Friesen, B., Pires, S., et al. (2005). Transforming mental health care for children and their families. *American Psychologist, 60*, 615–627.

International Association of Addictions and Offender Counselors. (2009). *About IAAOC*. Retrieved June 17, 2009, from http://www.iaaoc.org/about.asp.

International Association of Marriage and Family Counselors. (2009a). *Is marriage and family counseling right for me?* Retrieved May 17, 2009, from http://www.iamfc.com/consumers.html.

International Association of Marriage and Family Counselors. (2009b). *Publications*. Retrieved May 17, 2009, from http://www.iamfc.com/publications.html.

Kessler, R. C., Chiu, W. T., Demler, O., & Walters, E. E. (2005). Prevalence, severity, and comorbidity of twelve-month *DSM-IV* disorders in the National Comorbidity Survey Replication (NCS-R). *Archives of General Psychiatry, 6*, 617–627.

Knoph, D., Park, M. J., & Mulye, T. P. (2008). *The mental health of adolescents: A national profile, 2008* [Research brief]. San Francisco, CA: National Adolescent Health Information Center.

National Board for Certified Counselors. (2007a). *About us*. Retrieved July 10, 2007, from http://www.nbcc.org/whoWeAre/About.aspx.

National Board for Certified Counselors. (2007b). *Guidelines for maintaining your credential*.

Retrieved July 10, 2007, from http://sbv.nbcc.org/guidelines.

National Career Development Association. (2007). *Need a career counselor?* Retrieved July 17, 2007, from http://associationdatabase.com/aws/NCDA/pt/sd/news_article/4927/_self/layout_details/false.

National Center for Children in Poverty. (2006). *Basic facts about low income-children: Birth to age 18*. Retrieved November 9, 2006, from http://www.nccp.org/publications/pub_678.html.

National Council on Rehabilitation Education. (2009). *NCRE publications*. Retrieved May 17, 2009, from http://www.rehabeducators.org/publications.htm.

National Institute of Mental Health. (2003). *Testimony*. Retrieved July 10, 2007, from http://www.hhs.gov/asl/testify/t030728.html.

Smith, H. B., & Robinson, G. P. (1995). Mental health counseling: Past, present, and future. *Journal of Counseling & Development, 74*, 158–162.

U.S. Census Bureau. (2004). Census Bureau estimates number of adults, older people, and school-age children in the states. *U.S. Census Bureau News*. Retrieved July 12, 2007, from http://www.census.gov/Press-Release/www/releases/archives/population/001703.html.

U.S. Census Bureau. (2006a). Hispanic heritage month. *Facts for Features*. Retrieved July 12, 2007, from http://www.census.gov/Press-Release/www/releases/archives/facts_for_features_special_editions/007173.html.

U.S. Census Bureau. (2006b). Dramatic changes in U.S. aging highlighted in new Census, NIH Report. *U.S. Census Bureau News*. Retrieved July 12, 2007, from http://www.census.gov/Press-Release/www/releases/archives/aging_population/006544.html.

U.S. Census Bureau. (2007). Minority population tops 100 million. *U.S. Census Bureau News*. Retrieved July 12, 2007, from http://www.census.gov/Press-Release/www/releases/archives/population/010048.html.

CHAPTER **3**

The Counselor's Roles and Functions

LEARNING OBJECTIVES

After reading this chapter you should be able to

- list the professional functions and roles involved in counseling;

- describe the processes and skills used in individual and group counseling;

- explain the importance of cultural sensitivity in counseling;

- explain the role of theory and research in the practice of counseling;

- explain the role of advocacy in the counseling profession; and

- differentiate between consulting and collaborating with other mental health professionals.

Group Counseling
Types of Groups
Stages of Group Development
Therapeutic Factors
Essential Skills for Group Counseling

Theory and Research in Practice
Theory
Research

Advocating for the Client and the Profession
Advocating for the Client
Advocating for the Profession

Consulting and Collaborating With Other Mental Health Professionals
Consultation
Collaboration

Conclusion

CHAPTER REVIEW
REVIEW QUESTIONS
ADDITIONAL RESOURCES
REFERENCES

INTRODUCTION

As a beginning counselor, one of the early challenges that you will encounter is explaining what counseling is. You might start with the explanation that counselors have advanced training to deal with mental, emotional, and behavioral issues and use the term *professional counselor* to distinguish themselves from the myriad of people who use the term *counselor*, as in financial counselor, retirement counselor, immigration counselor, and nutrition counselor. A more comprehensive explanation of counseling will take shape as you journey toward becoming a professional counselor. This chapter deals with the various activities that professional counselors deal with in their work. It begins with an overview of the professional functions and roles that counselors normally fulfill and the skills they utilize in individual and group counseling. Seeing that the counselor's use of those skills is influenced by the stages that comprise the counseling process, some attention is given to those stages. Attention is also given to the importance of theory and research in practice and the commitment to advocating for the client and the profession. Finally, the necessity of collaborating and consulting with other professionals is discussed.

PROFESSIONAL FUNCTIONS AND ROLES OF THE COUNSELOR

The direct services that counselors provide to clients may be categorized broadly as prevention, early intervention, and crisis intervention. The delivery of those services depends on the client's state of psychological well-being when counseling is initiated. In providing those services, counselors keep in mind that some degree of change and empowerment should be the natural outcome for their clients. Those services and intended outcomes underlie the functions inherent in professional counseling.

Prevention
Guided by wellness and developmental principles, the counselor is primarily a preventive practitioner. Transitions in childhood, adolescence, and adulthood

present a variety of developmental changes. Many people adjust to these changes successfully but some do not. When people are not successful in adjusting to changes, they could experience mental, emotional, and behavioral problems that interfere with their ability to function satisfactorily in their daily life. Using preventive action, counselors forewarn their clients of imminent developmental changes that could present problems in the future and prepare them to meet these changes successfully. Postpartum and parenting programs, premarital and preretirement counseling, and career preparation workshops are examples of preventive action. These counseling services are referred to as psycho-education. School settings are particularly beneficial locations for school counselors to provide children and adolescents with preventive actions relating to such issues as understanding and preparing for changes in the maturation process, managing the stress of school work and home chores, and the use of drugs. In the school setting, the term *group guidance* is commonly used instead of *psycho-education*.

Early Intervention

Although some leaders of the counseling profession have advocated that preventive counseling should become public policy in the way that preventive medicine has been for a long time (Levant, 2006), there seems to be little chance it will happen in the near future. Partially because the public does not view preventive counseling in the way they accept preventive medicine, clients often seek counseling after they have begun experiencing distress from mismanaging or failing to address the transitional challenges they face. In such cases, counselors intervene to help clients successfully deal with the psychological distress they are experiencing. The longer individuals remain in psychological distress without receiving help, the greater the chances of their distress becoming severe psychological problems. Thus, counselors are advocates of earlier rather than later intervention.

Crisis Intervention

In some cases, clients may be in such a critical state when they seek or are sent for help that they require crisis counseling. A student expressing suicidal thoughts or an adult suffering from the trauma of a recent natural disaster, for example, will need immediate attention to deal with circumstances that may quickly become more serious. The counselor must be more directive and move quickly in assessing the client's psychological state and immediate needs, developing a plan to respond to the circumstances, locating the necessary community resources, and referring to another level of care if necessary.

Client Change

In a comparative analysis of 16 major counseling approaches, Prochaska and Norcross (2007) found that change was an essential component in all of them. Inasmuch as counselors use these counseling approaches, they are involved in influencing change in their clients. As agents of change, counselors work with their clients to find new ways of thinking (cognitive), expressing and reacting to emotions (affective), acting (behavioral), or interacting with their environment (systemic). An example of the counselor as change agent might involve helping an unemployed client change his or her thinking from one of hopelessness to one of expectation. Another example might involve helping a student to discard inappropriate behaviors for better ones in the classroom. In the case of crisis counseling, the counselor might help the client to see the benefits of disregarding self-destructive plans and considering other actions that could produce profitable results.

Client Empowerment

Whether counselors have engaged in prevention, intervention, or crisis counseling with their clients, they leave them empowered to meet future life challenges with increased independence and confidence. Empowerment for clients should be a natural outcome of counseling; it is not something that counselors give to clients. However, the empowerment of clients can be facilitated when counselors pursue helping activities with a conscious and deliberate effort within the framework of wellness and human development. They do this by (a) conceptualizing their clients' problems as transitional challenges rather than pathologies, (b) understanding that their clients only need temporary help in managing or adapting to transitional challenges, and (c) recognizing that their clients are capable of learning from the counseling process the cognitive, affective, behavioral, and other skills they might require for their present needs and for the future.

Roles With Specific Responsibilities

In addition to the functions that are inherent to the practice of counseling, counselors might be called on to assume a variety of roles with specific responsibilities. The extent to which they get the opportunity to perform these roles depends on their experience and the setting where they work.

Outreach Worker

Counselors working in agency or school settings might be called on to give presentations in neighboring communities to such groups as adolescents, seniors, and the homeless.

Consultant

A school administrator might ask an agency to give assistance in dealing with bullying among students. Counselors with expertise in that area might be asked by their supervisors to work as consultants on behalf of their agency in helping the school set up an anti-bullying program.

Advocate

In their work activities or in volunteer positions, counselors may speak and act on behalf of marginalized clients, the need for support programs in schools and communities, and the promotion of the counseling profession.

Researcher

Because of the increasing requests from funding agencies, health insurance institutions, and school districts for proof of the success of counseling services, counselors might be involved in measuring counseling effectiveness and providing data to meet counselor accountability requirements.

Grant Writer

Depending on their experience and administrative position, counselors might be responsible for writing grant proposals for funds from various government and other institutions. Although school counselors write proposals for funds to supplement programs in their schools, many nonprofit agencies depend on obtaining funds as a crucial component in maintaining their existence.

Administrator

Counselors might be administrators, ensuring the effective functioning of the counseling programs where they work. Administrative responsibilities include overseeing the work of employees, conducting staff meetings, drawing up budgets, and making long-range decisions. It is common for the principal or assistant principal of a school, who is not a counselor, to be the administrative supervisor of a school counselor.

Clinical Supervisor

With sufficient experience and the necessary credentials, counselors might be called on to provide counseling supervision, which is different from administrative supervision. As a clinical supervisor, the counselor is responsible for overseeing the training and promoting the professional development of interns and beginning counselors in an agency or school setting. This involves such activities as reviewing the counseling sessions that the interns or beginning counselors have with clients and addressing current issues and trends in the profession of counseling.

Counselor Supervision

Although counselors should not be called on to be clinical supervisors until they have the required credentials and experience, which vary from one jurisdiction to the next, they will certainly be involved in the supervision process as supervisees during their professional preparation. Moreover, even fully licensed professionals may seek periodic supervision when faced with ethical or clinical dilemmas. Therefore, it is beneficial for you to have a greater understanding of supervision than what was provided in the preceding section.

Basically, supervision is used to further develop counseling skills and knowledge. It can be defined as an ongoing process in which one person gives assistance to one or more individuals to enhance the latter's professional competence (Bernard & Goodyear, 2004; Corey, Corey, & Callanan, 2007; Remley & Herlihy, 2007). Counselors-in-training and counselors with a preliminary or limited counseling license are required to complete a specified number of hours of supervision in their advancement toward obtaining full licensure. The number of hours and length of time required under supervision vary among counselor programs and licensure jurisdictions.

The first time counselors-in-training are exposed to supervision is in their practicum program, where they are assigned to their supervisors, who may be full-time or adjunct faculty members or other qualified mental health professionals contracted to provide supervision. The next supervision period typically occurs during internship, when the supervision is done by a qualified professional at the agency or school where the counselor-in-training is completing the internship. While counselors-in-training are accustomed to being assigned rather than choosing their supervisor, in the preliminary period before becoming fully licensed, novice counselors have the opportunity to select a supervisor who is not only qualified and competent, as all supervisors should be, but also meets the personal and professional goals and needs of the counselors who will become their supervisees.

Regardless of when supervision is provided, the supervisor's role includes two important responsibilities: (1) assisting in the development of the supervisee's counseling skills and knowledge and (2) ensuring that the welfare of the supervisee's clients is not put in jeopardy. Fulfilling those responsibilities involves being familiar with the supervisee's caseload and overseeing the supervisee's progress. This means that the supervisor may fulfill the role of teacher, model, coach, and advisor at various times. Also, the supervisor may need to address supervisee issues that are impeding the effectiveness of the supervisee's work with a client and, as a result, may at times have to fulfill the role of counselor to the supervisee. A caution that goes with the occasional counselor role: A therapeutic relationship between supervisor and supervisee should not become a substitute for supervision.

In many cases in practicum, and especially in internship, the supervisor is the individual who evaluates the supervisee's work, assessing his or her assignments, skills, knowledge, and professionalism in order to provide a final grade, or the major portion of the final grade, for the supervisee. This is an aspect of supervision that relates to a less obvious but still important reason for supervision: It is a gate-keeping mechanism for the profession. By attesting to the fact that the supervisee has successfully completed practicum, internship, or the preliminary period before full licensure, the supervisor is stating that at each stage the supervisee has attained an acceptable level of competence in the progress toward becoming a fully licensed professional counselor.

One of the central components in evaluating the supervisees' progress is analyzing their counseling sessions with clients. Various methods are used to do that. The most common ones include self-reports, process notes, audiotapes, videotapes, and live supervision. These methods vary in usefulness. In using self-reports, for example, the discussion in the supervisory session is based on the subjective information that emerges from the report that the supervisee gives of the counseling session(s). On the other hand, a videotape allows the supervisor to observe the nuances in the interaction between the supervisee and the client. The method of supervision to be used is one of the issues that counselors-in-training need to discuss with a prospective supervisor.

Other important issues for discussion include theoretical orientation, the type of supervision (individual or group), the frequency of supervision, and the supervisor's availability in crisis situations. The supervisor's personal style is a much more awkward topic but must be considered as well. A personal style to supervision may be influenced by such factors as the supervisor's personal values and the extent to which his or her approach would be directive (taking an active role in directing the content and pace of the session) or permissive (letting the supervisee take control of the session).

These dynamics contribute to the type of interpersonal relationship that develops between supervisee and supervisor and can be a crucial factor in whether the supervision is successful or not. Counselors-in-training need to determine what type of approach is most suitable for them. Successful supervision is a collaborative endeavor that should allow the supervisee to develop the competence to guide his or her clients through the activities that comprise the counseling process. A major component of counselor competence that underlies all aspect of practice is cultural sensitivity.

Cultural Sensitivity

Due to the increasing diversity of the client populations and client problems that counselors will continue to encounter, the importance of cultural sensitivity needs to be addressed. In doing their work, which we said could range from prevention to supervision, counselors need to keep in mind the impact that culture and history have on how people function. The culture in which individuals have been raised socializes them to look at and react to the world in a particular way. Historical events, such as wars, famines, storms, discrimination, and other man-made and natural occurrences, also influence how people experience events in the world around them. Consequently, counselors need to use their skills with an awareness of the unintended consequences they might have. Many of the traditional characteristics of counseling, such as clients' emotional expressiveness and openness to discussing intimate aspects of their lives, may not be consistent with the values of people from different cultures. Therefore, such skills as probing for hard-to-get information, challenging inconsistencies in a client's perceptions, or forming hypotheses about presenting problems must be done within a framework of cultural awareness. The importance of nonverbal communication in a cultural context must not be overlooked either, seeing that nonverbals may be interpreted differently by different cultural groups. Such behavior includes the distance clients prefer to have between them and the counselor and changes in voice level and intonation. Also, pauses and the rate and fluency of speech may not be indications of resistance, for example, but that English is not the client's first language.

Cultural sensitivity may be a particularly complex factor when working with groups, depending on the composition of the group. In group work, the counselor has to be attentive to the personal characteristics and issues of the group members and the dynamics they create. When the aspect of culture is added, the counselor's work is amplified by having to be aware also of the cultural characteristics and beliefs that members bring to the group. For example, a skill such as blocking may be used to promote turn-taking in speaking; however, a group member from a culture where conversations are conducted differently might see blocking as too intrusive and as an attempt to exclude or suppress.

Because the demographics of the school population are changing particularly rapidly, perhaps school counselors, among all counselors, face and will continue to face the greatest challenge with regard to practicing cultural sensitivity in their work. In addition to their customary guidance, counseling, and consulting responsibilities, many school counselors play a prominent role in assessing immigrant children for appropriate grade placement, bridging the cultural gap that might exist in various ways between the parents and the school, and developing multicultural awareness in the school. Such crucial responsibilities place many school counselors in the position of having much influence on minority families. As a result, school counselors need to be aware of the natural tendency to view and respond to such families through a monoculture lens. Arredondo et al. (1996) provide a model that describes the competencies counselors need to develop in order to provide culturally appropriate services to their clients. Counselors need to (a) become aware of their own cultural values and biases toward various forms of diversity; (b) increase their knowledge about the worldviews of people who are culturally and otherwise different from them; and (c) develop intervention skills that are culturally appropriate for a diversity of clients.

To be a culturally sensitive counselor, you need to be aware that the meaning of the term *culture* has widened beyond reference to race and ethnicity and includes sexual orientation, religion and spirituality, socioeconomic status, gender, and other factors. Seeing that some cultural markers are not visible, the presence of various kinds of cultural diversity may not be readily noticed among the clientele the counselor is serving. Thus, as you read the rest of this chapter, it is important to remember that the counseling skills, strategies, and other activities that you will learn about are not to be practiced in a cultural vacuum but with an awareness of the diversity among people.

INDIVIDUAL COUNSELING

Historically, one-on-one interaction has been the method employed in counseling. In carrying out this activity, practitioners usually follow a protocol that is referred to as the counseling process. The activities that comprise this process may be grouped into three broad stages or phases: building the counseling relationship, terminating the counseling relationship, and a middle stage in which the counselor accomplishes all the other interrelated activities that promote client insight and action toward reaching outcome goals (Gladding, 2007). Given that client and counselor engage in many different activities in the middle stage, there are some models that consist of more than three stages (Cormier, Nurius, & Osborn, 2009; Hackney & Cormier, 2004; see also the therapeutic procedures for the Adlerian and Reality Therapies in Corey, 2009). In all of the models, specific skills are more appropriate for some stages than others, but most skills can be valuable across all the stages if applied judiciously. Since the same skills may be used in different stages, the three-stage model provides a better framework for avoiding redundancy when describing the purposes of counseling skills. However, it is instructive to discuss, first of all, one of the models that outlines the counseling process in more than three stages. A more detailed map provides a better layout of the territory, so to speak, for the first-time traveler.

Stages in Individual Counseling

A comprehensive model with five stages may be conceptualized as follows (see Hackney & Cormier, 2004):

1. Establishing a therapeutic relationship
2. Assessing the client's problem, needs, and resources
3. Setting goals
4. Selecting and implementing strategies
5. Terminating counseling

These stages are generally conceptualized as predictable and sequential, with the completion of one stage preparing the counselor and client for the next. In actuality, however, the stages overlap. For example, maintaining an effective therapeutic relationship may continue into the later stages of the counseling process, and further assessment of client needs and resources may be necessary when goals and intervention strategies are being considered. Nonetheless, the developmental model of predictable and ordered stages provides a blueprint for new counselors as they and their clients work their way through the counseling process. An overview of the stages will help in understanding the purpose of the skills that will be discussed after.

Establishing a Therapeutic Relationship

This relationship facilitates progress through the various activities that counselor and client engage in during the counseling process. Depending on the theory of counseling that the counselor is using, the closeness of the therapeutic relationship between counselor and client will be at some point along a continuum, ranging from neutrality to friendly involvement.

Active Learning Exercise **3.1**

Reflect on occasions when you have met someone for the first time to discuss some issue or other. How did you go about establishing a relationship to begin the discussion? Was your approach different depending on the person's professional or other status?

Assessing Problems, Needs, and Resources

Assessment covers several integrated phases. It involves gathering and prioritizing information that includes health, family, and other data about the client's needs and resources. Counselors use this information to assist clients in gaining insight into their problems and developing goals to solve or alleviate them.

Setting Goals

Counselors help their clients turn the problems presented at the beginning of counseling into specific, positive, and measurable goals that reflect the clients' needs and capability. Well-defined goals facilitate the selection and implementation of appropriate intervention strategies.

Selecting and Implementing Strategies

Once a goal is set, a strategy is selected that would help the client reach the goal and, consequently, resolve the problem presented in counseling. The strategy is usually a technique or combination of techniques from one of the counseling approaches.

Terminating the Counseling Process

Ending the counseling relationship is as important as it was developing it in the beginning. Counselors need to ensure that bringing regular counseling sessions to an end does not undercut gains made by the client. For various reasons, early termination of the counseling process might be necessary, requiring referral to another practitioner in some cases.

Essential Skills for Individual Counseling

To move through the stages successively, counselors depend on specific skills to complete certain tasks associated with each stage. These skills may be categorized into three groups. *Nonverbal behavior* involves all communicative actions beyond the spoken and written word; *listening responses* include utterances that are not designed to influence the thoughts of the client but to encourage clients to tell their stories; and *influencing responses* are used to help clients move toward viewing their lives differently and acting accordingly. As much as these skills have been traditionally associated with counseling, they are based on ordinary interpersonal communication skills that have been enhanced and integrated into the counseling process (Egan, 2007). For example, two individuals in a conversation in North America would normally face each, have eye contact, and if they are not angry, would assume a relaxed and open posture. This instance of nonverbal communication was formalized into a framework for the counseling process under the acronym SOLER (Egan, 2007). Within this framework, counselors are encouraged to be intentional in their nonverbal communication of facing their clients *squarely* with an *open* posture, *leaning* forward slightly, keeping *eye* contact, and maintaining a *relaxed* manner. Since cultures differ in the ways they communicate nonverbal attentiveness, counselors need to be cautious in using this method too liberally. For example, because of their cultural background or customs, some clients might be offended by a counselor keeping constant eye contact.

Another contribution to adapting communication skills for the counseling profession came from Carl Rogers (1942, 1951, 1965), who initially saw the role of the counselor as not merely listening to clients but letting them know that he or she was listening. Therefore, such skills as paraphrasing client statements and giving nondirective prompts told clients that the counselor was listening and had heard, and that they could continue with their stories. Such skills became essential hallmarks of the Rogerian approach in counseling. Rogers later went on to emphasize the need for the counselor to reflect an accurate understanding of the underlying feelings that clients were not expressing but were implicit in their behavior, words, or attitudes. This counselor attitude, called empathy, is one of the core conditions in the person-centered approach that facilitates client growth in counseling. Also, it is the basis for the *empathic statement*, which is an influencing skill used to assist clients in moving toward deeper exploration of their issues. Traces of the empathic statement can be heard in such commonplace acknowledgements as "I can see that you are mad at me." Although it may be true that counseling skills are based on the nonverbal and verbal communication skills that the ordinary person possesses, it takes training for them to become highly developed, reflexive, and used judiciously in the counseling process.

As the terms *nonverbal*, *listening*, and *influencing* may indicate, some skills are better suited for certain stages of the counseling process than others. For example, challenging is an influencing response that is useful in helping clients undertake self-examination and identify the underlying causes of their problems. However, it could be counterproductive during the initial stage of counseling if a relationship of trust and understanding has not been established. On the other hand, a nonverbal behavior such as silence may be used effectively in different stages of the counseling process for different reasons. Therefore, counselors need to become competent in using the various skills so they can apply them where they are most productive and when circumstances require. Some of the skills necessary to facilitate progress through the counseling process are described in the following sections.

Initiating the Counseling Process

To provide effective and efficient help, counselors often need clients to disclose some of their most personal information. Many new clients are hesitant to take that step, so counselors need to develop the kind of relationship that will allow them to obtain much of this information as early as possible in counseling. Thus, building a relationship and eliciting information need to be done concurrently, with the skills used for both tasks effectively interwoven. Counselors use *nonverbal behavior* and *listening responses* particularly in the initiating stage of the counseling process to demonstrate that they are paying attention and to encourage clients to continue providing information. Counselors also use their knowledge of nonverbal behavior to monitor the attitudes and feelings of their clients, especially during this early period of the counseling process. Listening responses may range from very short verbal expressions to full sentences, while nonverbal behavior includes a wide range of voluntary and involuntary actions that do not involve the use of words:

- *Kinetics* (such as gestures, facial expressions, posture, and other bodily behavior)
  Example:
  A nod of the head confirms that the counselor heard and understood what the client said.
- *Observable automatic physiological responses* (such as blushing and paleness, quickness of breath, and dilation and constriction of pupils)
  Example:
  The counselor can be alerted to a client's inner conflict, for example, from observing the client's blush or a faltering in voice level while responding to a question.

Paralinguistics (voice level and intonation, rate and fluency of speech, emphases, pauses, and silence) and proxemics (physical distance between the counselor and client) are also types of nonverbal behavior. Sitting too close to clients from some cultures, for example, could cause the clients to raise defensive barriers that impede effective interaction. Counselors need to be aware also when clients are exhibiting nonverbal behaviors, given that these behaviors can confirm or contradict what the client said. For example, a client may deny that she or he is upset, but blushing, tightened jaws, or the intonation of the voice could indicate otherwise. The last example indicates that all nonverbal behaviors need to be "read" in the context of the spoken word.

- *Verbal prompt*—Verbal prompt (or *verbal encouragers*) is the very short expression or sound that counselors may make to let their clients know that they are listening.

  Examples:
  "I see."
  "Uh-huh."
  "Okay."

- *Paraphrase*—In paraphrasing (also referred to as *reflection of content*), counselors use their own words to rephrase the essential ideas or thoughts in a client's statement without changing the original meaning.

  Examples:
  "You are telling me that ..."
  "As I hear it ..."
  "What you are saying is ..."

- *Reflection of feelings*—This skill is similar to paraphrasing except that the focus is on the emotion instead of the client's ideas and thoughts. Discussing emotions too early in counseling could be threatening to some clients; in such cases, counselors should stick with the paraphrase.

  Examples:
  "It seems like you are really angry."
  "It sounds like you are really happy."

- *Summarization*—Whereas paraphrasing reflects one idea, summarizing reflects a collection of ideas. With summarization, counselors can set the tone and pace of the session by bring an end to rambling, listing the topics expressed, and giving focus to the dialogue.

- *Clarification*—Clarification is a request for elaboration or explanation when clients make statements that are vague, ambiguous, or confusing. It demonstrates that the counselor is interested in understanding, not merely listening to, what the client is saying. Clarification can be framed as a question or a statement.

  Examples:
  "Could you explain what you mean by masquerading?"
  "I am not sure I understand what you mean by masquerading."

Maintaining the Counseling Process

Once a facilitative relationship has been established and the client has begun to feel comfortable in providing information pertinent to the problem presented, counselors can begin assisting their clients in viewing their lives differently and acting accordingly. The skills commonly used for this period are referred to as *influencing responses* and include the use of questions, interpretation, information giving, immediacy, self-disclosure, and confrontation. The counselor also needs to become skilled in helping his or her clients set effective goals and in selecting interventions that are appropriate for the clients' needs. Taking on this role does not mean the counselor stops using the skills described in the last section.

- *Question*—Although clarification is usually framed as a question, it is different from open-ended and closed questions. Whereas clarification is used to ensure accurate understanding of a statement expressed, open-ended and closed questions are used to get new information. Closed questions are used to collect specific facts.

  Example:

  "Have you ever been hospitalized?"

  Open-ended questions, on the other hand, are used to encourage the client to give extended information.

  Example:

  "What were some of the responsibilities you had to take on when both of your parents were hospitalized at the same time?"

- *Probe*—Probes are more unsettling than closed and open-ended questions and are useful when encouraging clients to engage in examining how their problems might be influenced by their attitudes, beliefs, emotions, and behavior. Probes may be framed as closed questions, open-ended questions, or statements.

  Examples:

  After a client has stated how she is going to make her mother suffer, the counselor might ask, "Is making your mother suffer going to solve your problem?"

  "You say you are worthless; what experiences have you had that led to that opinion about yourself?"

  "You say you have done all you can; tell me about some of the things you have done to resolve the antagonism between both of you."

- *Empathic statement*—Empathic statements are advanced forms of reflection of feelings; they go beyond acknowledging the emotions expressed to embedding them in the context when or where the client felt them. One of the well-used formula for constructing the empathic statement is "You feel + emotion + because + experience."

  Example:

  "You feel angry because your father never acknowledged the financial help you gave the family when he was unemployed."

- *Challenge*—Also known as confrontation, a challenge is a response in which the counselor describes contradictions, discrepancies, or inconsistencies in the client's words, feelings, or actions. It promotes self-examination and is most successful when a high level of rapport, credibility, and trust has been developed between the counselor and client.

Example:

"On one hand, I heard you say that you would do anything to help your son, then on the other hand, I heard you say that you would never lift a hand to help him out. Help me understand how those two ideas fit together for you."

- *Self-disclosure*—Counselors share personal examples from their lives to help clients gain a better understanding of, or a different perspective on, their problems. If not used judiciously, self-disclosure could lead to attention being paid to the counselor's rather than the client's issues.

Example:

"I also struggled during my teenage years with shyness. But I realized that some people might be thinking that I didn't want to make friends, so I made an effort to approach the other kids in the school and slowly got over my fear of talking with people."

- *Immediacy*—Immediacy is a disclosure about something as it occurs in the session. It brings into the counseling process unexpressed issues and feelings that could impede progress.

Examples:

"Every time I mention your family, like just now, you back off from the topic."

"That statement makes me feel we are beginning to make some progress."

- *Interpretation*—Interpretation is a statement that counselors use to suggest possible meanings in the implicit messages and patterns that clients communicate through their ideas, attitudes, feelings, and behaviors. The suggestion promotes insight by helping clients consider deeper issues that might underlie their problems.

Example:

"I am wondering if your reluctance to speak to your spouse about it is not so much your fear of an argument as a fear of hearing the truth from her."

- *Information giving*—This skill is usually confused with advice giving, which is a recommendation or prescription of a specific solution to be taken. With information giving, counselors provide factual information to dispel myths and provide options for making choices.

Example:

"I understand your unhappiness at seeing your son having to find new employment for the second time in just four years, but research shows that the shifting emphasis in our modern society calls for the average person to change jobs roughly five times before he or she retires."

- *Identification of outcome goals*—Counselors use this skill to help clients determine what they want from counseling. Identification of outcome goals can be more effective after counselors have information that allows them to put into context the clients' issues to be dealt with.

Examples:

"At the beginning of counseling you said you wanted to _____. Tell me more specifically, what do you expect to accomplish from counseling?

"At the end of counseling what would be different from the way things are now?"

- *Development of outcome goals*—Developing effective goals involves specifying the behavior to be changed, the conditions or circumstances in which the changed behavior will occur, and the amount or level of change to be made.

Examples:

"In what situations do you want to be doing this?"

"You say you would like to _____; compared to now, how much more would you like to be doing it?"

- *Selection and implementation of strategies*—This involves having knowledge of and skill in using techniques drawn from various counseling orientations, such as the psychodynamic, cognitive-behavioral, feminist, and other approaches. Techniques vary in their complexity and should be chosen to fit the needs and capability of the client.

Terminating the Counseling Process

The termination stage includes addressing counselor-client feelings resulting from the counseling process, evaluating the progress made by the client, reinforcing changes made, and planning for the maintenance of change after counseling ends.

- *Evaluation*—It is important for counselor and client to evaluate the outcome goals that were mutually agreed upon. Other factors, such as client satisfaction with the counseling process in general, can be evaluated as well.
- *Summarization*—Recapping highlights from the counseling experience gives counselors the opportunity to support clients' future autonomous efforts by validating progress made and pointing out behaviors that clients might need to monitor.
- *Generalization*—The counselor helps the client understand how the new behaviors acquired during counseling can be used to deal with future situations similar to those that precipitated the problem presented in counseling.

GROUP COUNSELING

In many ways, group counseling is not unlike individual counseling. In both contexts, the counselor establishes an appropriate therapeutic relationship, uses client information to conceptualize presenting problems, assists clients in working to attain outcome goals, employs specific skills to facilitate the counseling process, and prepares clients for termination. However, interacting with about 10 individuals in the same place and at the same time compounds these tasks. For example, while a statement or nonverbal behavior might elicit one interpretation from the lone client in individual counseling, that same piece of communication has the potential to produce as many interpretations and reactions as there are members in the groups. In spite of the complexity and effort associated with group counseling, it is used in a wide variety of situations and settings. Group counseling is not the only type of group work with which the counselor may be involved, however. The next sections deal with some of the benefits of group work in general and three types of groups with which the counselor might be involved.

Types of Groups

Group work is used instead of individual counseling for a variety of reasons. It can be used in such settings as schools and residential homes where there is a large clientele with a common problem, thus saving time and money; in the aftermath of catastrophic events that require quick dissemination of information or counseling; and for the psychological assistance that group members can get from each other. Group counselees can find some relief in realizing that they are not abnormal, unique, or alone in their problems and that they can make positive use of other members' behavior and experiences.

There are several types of counseling groups (Corey & Corey, 2006), but the three with which you should be familiar are *psycho-education*, *counseling*, and *psychotherapy*. Commonly called *group guidance* in schools, psycho-education involves imparting information that can help group members with a wide range of issues, including stress, study skills, timidity, parent-adolescent relationships, employment, and caring for the severely disabled. This assortment of issues indicates that some approaches to this type of group work can provide information for enhancing personal growth as well as preventing and coping with emotional and behavioral problems.

In *group counseling*, group members deal with similar issues that are adversely affecting their lives and need intervention rather than preventive service. The counselor encourages and facilitates group interaction as an essential strategy in helping members learn, try, and receive feedback on new behaviors. *Group psychotherapy* (or therapy) is concerned with more severe psychological problems such as disorders relating to obsession and compulsion, posttraumatic stress, and narcissism.

The line between psycho-education and counseling and between counseling and psychotherapy is as unclear in group work as in working with individuals, resulting in the terms often being used interchangeably for different types of groups. Regardless of the labels used, however, research indicates that from the first meeting of the group, the dynamics of group work begin generating certain forces that the counselor can harness to enhance group progress. The stages that groups go through in their development and the group interaction that leads to curative experiences for the members are examples of these forces in group work. These forces are not equally strong or noticeable in all types of group work; however, with knowledge of the *stages of group development* and the *therapeutic factors* that result from group interaction, counselors can use their skills accordingly to help members get the most out of these aspects of group work.

Stages of Group Development

Theorists propose that groups progress through stages or phases that can be identified by the activities that group members engage in. It is important to note that there are numerous competing models of group development, but

TABLE **3.1**

Stages		Characteristics of Formative Stages in Group Development
Stage 1	Forming	Dependency, anxiety, concerns about acceptance
Stage 2	Storming	Power, authority, counter-dependency, status, competition
Stage 3	Norming	Trust, group cohesion, group procedures
Stage 4	Performing	Work, task oriented, feedback
Stage 5	Adjourning	Separation issues

you are most likely familiar with the one that has been popularized as *forming, storming, norming, performing,* and *adjourning* (Tuckman & Jensen, 1977; see Table 3.1).

In this model, the first stage is characterized by group members' anxiety, concerns about acceptance, and dependency. In the second stage, issues shift to power, authority, status, counter-dependency, and competition. In the next stage, trust and group cohesion develop, and negotiations about group procedures take place. In the fourth stage, the group is more task oriented, with feedback given and received more freely and sincerely. Adjournment, the final stage, introduces separation issues and emotions that might give rise to positive as well as negative feelings. As with the stages in individual counseling, the formative stages for groups are not linear but recursive, with the group often regressing to an earlier stage before moving forward to the next stage.

Therapeutic Factors

While the stages of development may occur in most group work, the therapeutic factors may not be present in psycho-educational group work where interactions for remedial or restorative purposes are usually not needed or encouraged. With regard to counseling and therapy, Yalom (2005) has identified 11 therapeutic factors:

1. Installation of hope (the belief that professional group work will help)
2. Universality (the realization among group members that they are not abnormal because of their problem)
3. Imparting information (therapeutic information received during group counseling)
4. Altruism (sharing experiences to help others in the group)
5. The corrective recapitulation of the primary family group (reliving and coming to terms with past family conflicts)
6. Development of socializing techniques (learning about oneself for interaction with others in society)
7. Imitative behavior (emulating the positive behaviors of other group members)
8. Interpersonal learning (working through problems by interacting with others in the group)

9. Groups cohesiveness (developing close relationships with other group members)
10. Catharsis (expressing emotions freely)
11. Existential factors (addressing issues such as one's purpose in life, one's mortality, and responsibility for one's life)

The therapeutic factors and the stages of group development are inherent aspects of group work that counselors can use as sign posts in moving group members toward change or their intended goals. However, counselors must still acquire a set of essential skills for intentional use in group work. The group skills described in the next section represent a basic inventory on which additional training in group work can be built.

Essential Skills for Group Counseling

As in individual counseling, listening and influencing responses facilitate progress through the counseling process. Although it is ultimately the responsibility of the group counselor to ensure that counseling is productive, participation by group members is important in creating interactions that move the process forward. The counselor encourages group interaction by modeling listening and influencing skills. Even if the counselor is not actively trying to demonstrate certain skills, some members will pick up on them and try to use them, especially if they see these skills having positive effects. Paraphrasing and asking for clarification are good examples of listening responses that the counselor might want group members to emulate early in group counseling to encourage group interaction. Skillful modeling and guidance are needed to have group members try influencing skills such as challenging.

Facilitating

It is the counselor's responsibility to ensure not only that communication takes places among group members, but also that a safe and accepting environment is created for unguarded and honest communication to lead to group goals. All of the following skills contribute to facilitating group counseling in one way or another.

Initiating

It is the counselor's responsibility to intervene when group communication breaks down, there is a need to move onto new material, or group members are not focused on meaningful interactions.

Modeling

Emulation is a natural by-product of interaction in such contexts as group counseling. Therefore, counselors need to ensure that they model adeptly the particular values and skills that they want group members to copy.

Paraphrasing

Successful modeling of this skill will result in quick duplication of its use by group members. When group members let each other know that they are listening and understanding, communication becomes more fluent and meaningful.

Clarifying

This is another skill that can be easily picked up by group members. Clarifying ensures that they understand what each other's statements mean, especially since an act of communication, verbal or nonverbal, can mean one thing to one member and something else to another.

Reflecting Feeling

Because the exact emotion and its intensity are not always easy to determine, reflecting people's feelings is more difficult than reflecting what they say. Furthermore, it may be discomforting for some group members to hear their emotions identified too early in counseling, especially among a group of strangers. Therefore, the counselor needs to be alert as to how and when feelings are being reflected by group members. When done appropriately, however, reflection of feelings by group members can be a powerful device for enhancing group cohesion.

Questioning

Questions that draw out information from members are as essential in group counseling as they are in individual counseling. However, those that result in yes or no answers are not productive and may sound like an interrogation. Therefore, the group counselor needs to guide members away from using this skill too much.

Disclosing

Counselors may reveal personal information from their own lives to encourage group members to share personal material and make themselves known to the others. For counselors, knowing what and when to self-disclose is the essential component of this skill. Revealing too much personal information too soon could have a negative reaction since some members might not be ready for such openness.

Linking

Group counselors can increase group communication and cohesion by making connections between what one group member says and the concerns of another member. Identifying common concerns can be initiated by the counselor's inquiry as to whether anyone else shares the anxieties, feelings, or beliefs expressed.

Information Giving

There may be situations when information, suggestions, and even directives will be helpful for a group member or the entire group. Information giving should be done sparingly, however, since group members will very likely want to copy you and start telling people what to do.

Giving Feedback

Feedback is useful since it gives an honest and realistic assessment of how group members are perceived by each other. As with other skills, it is preferable to get other members to give feedback rather than the counselor. The success of feedback lies in the counselor's skill in helping the group member receive the feedback.

Interpreting

Interpretation is a suggestion offered as an alternative explanation for a group member's behaviors. The intent is to promote deeper understanding and insight, but the counselor has to gauge the readiness of the group member for such suggestions.

Challenging

This is used to encourage members to reflect on the discrepancies in their statements, emotions, and behavior. Coming from other members, rather than the "leader," it can be more effective. However, inasmuch as challenging can result in varying degrees of embarrassment, it must be modeled skillfully and used judiciously.

Blocking

Although the counseling process is enhanced when group members emulate the counselor in such skills as challenging, the counselor needs to remember that the psychological and physical safety of the members is paramount. Therefore, blocking is necessary to stop such harmful behaviors as scapegoating, inappropriate personal questioning, and gossiping.

Supporting

Experiencing painful emotions and taking risks with new behaviors are beneficial for group members. During these times, the counselor provides support, in the form of encouragement and reinforcement, to help group members through their struggles and let them know that they are not on their own. However, counselors should be on the alert for group members who, in the guise of giving support, might want to "protect" others from painful emotions, thus inadvertently depriving them of beneficial therapeutic experiences.

Summarizing

During any session, the counselor may want to help members pull together the elements of a discussion to provide focus, take stock of where they are so they can decide where to go next with the discussion, or provide provisional closure to an issue before moving on to the next predetermined topic. Summarizing is also effective at the beginning of sessions, when the highlights of the previous session may be reviewed, as well as at the end, when members reflect on what they have gained from the session.

Setting Goals

Although the purpose of the group will have been established before it begins, group members should identify their own personal goals within the general goal that brought the group together. The counselor needs to help each member work on personal goals.

Assessing

Keeping track of each member's progress makes the task of assessment difficult in group counseling. The behaviors of all group members must be observed to provide interventions such as supportive and corrective feedback when necessary.

Evaluating

Evaluating the sessions and their effect on group members is also important. It is important for counselor and group members to evaluate each session or a series of sessions to ensure that group interactions are therapeutic and that the goals of the group are being addressed.

Terminating

Bringing group counseling to an end involves several considerations. The counselor helps group members understand how the new behaviors they have acquired can be used to deal with future situations similar to those for which the group was organized. In addition to validating the progress made by group members, counselors must take the time to review behaviors that individual members need to continue to monitor. In its general purpose of summarizing and evaluating the strategies used and the outcome achieved over the life of the group, termination also provides an opportunity for counselors to begin participating in research at a fundamental and practical level.

THEORY AND RESEARCH IN PRACTICE

Conducting research creates anxiety for counselors even before they graduate (Heppner, Kivlighan, & Wampold, 2005), and unless they proceed to a doctoral program, they are likely to leave research and theory behind once they receive their master's degree and begin their professional career. Research, as well as theory, seems to lack relevance to the everyday activities of the counselor. Yet, theory and research are fundamental aspects of the procedure that counselors follow in their work. The relevance of theory to counseling practice will be discussed first.

Theory

In scientific circles, a theory is defined as an organized set of principles that helps us to understand, predict, and control events in a consistent manner in a given area of life. Therefore, in the field of counseling, theories help in understanding, predicting, and managing the developmental and associated psychological problems that clients experience. For example, one of the first decisions counselors make in the counseling process relates to the nature of the therapeutic relationship they should develop with their clients. The effectiveness of some counseling approaches is based on the theory that a strong relationship with clients is crucial to facilitating behavior change. In other approaches, the counselor-client relationship is not deemed to be as important as other factors, such as the techniques that comprise the intervention strategy. When counselors choose to emphasize or deemphasize the therapeutic relationship, they are relying on theory to make a decision on an important aspect of the counseling process. Counselors who understand that they are relying on theory to make such significant decisions in their practice can be more intentional and effective.

Counselors' use of theory is also evident in the assessment stage of the counseling process. Counselors are instinctively hypothesizing about the causes that underlie the problems their clients have presented. Although in helping clients deal with behavior health problems such as drug and alcohol addiction, many counselors may not give much attention to underlying causes, even those counselors may find it helpful to uncover motivating factors in the case of other problems. For example, in helping a client who has initiated counseling because of several failed marriages, the counselor may conceptualize the state of affairs in terms of object relations, cognitive distortions, the existentialist concepts of isolation and loving, and so forth. Hypothesizing about clients' problems in this manner is an example of theory in action because, in doing so, counselors call into play theories that offer explanations of human behavior. Such explanations are central to the counseling process. They not only help counselors understand behavior but also influence the choice of which strategies are used in dealing with the behavior.

To provide effective counseling, it is important for counselors to not only have a clear understanding of various counseling theories, but also keep abreast of new insights into their applicability. As beneficiaries of the interactive relationship between theory and research, counselors need to be avid consumers of research and take advantage of published and presented reports on how theories, as well as the strategies resulting from them, are being applied to problems that may be new or old and persistent. The academic underachievement of students from underserved groups and the growing problems of obesity among all children continue to be persistent challenges. On the other hand, the increasing use of the Internet; the availability of self-help books, text-messaging, and CDs; and the numbers of first-generation, foreign-born, and native minority students in universities and the public school system are some of the issues creating new challenges to how current theories are utilized in counseling.

Research efforts are constantly being used to test theories and assess their applicability to different problems and clients. To make use of current modifications and adaptations that will make their services more accessible, relevant, and effective to a diverse group of clients, counselors need to keep abreast of these research efforts as they are reported in professional journals and at national, regional, and state conferences.

Research

As in the case of theory, discussing the importance of research in practice can begin with its fundamental role and early application in the counseling process. When a client presents a problem in counseling, one of the early activities in which counselors engage is assessment. Counselors collect as much data or information as they can about the client, including childhood experiences, medical history, family dynamics, social relationships, educational and career background, and what the client has done before in an effort to solve the problem. After completing a thorough exploration of the client's background and current status, counselors research the literature that is relevant to the client's problem. Depending on their knowledge and experience, counselors also research the client's cultural background so they can consider experiences and worldviews that might be germane to understanding the problem and, therefore, be important in developing appropriate goals and intervention strategies.

From that research, counselors put the problem in context and define it in such a way that allows them to develop a hypothesis, or explanation, about its origin. In collaboration with the client, counselors then set goals and develop a strategy that would solve or alleviate the problem. As shown in Table 3.2, when compared from this perspective, the procedure counselors follow in counseling is similar to the research process counselors-in-training learn in their research courses. These are generalized procedures in the counseling and research processes. All approaches to counseling and research are not developed in exactly the same way, but most approaches in both disciplines include some of the components described earlier. The comparison not only demonstrates that the research process is inherent in the practice of counseling, but it also suggests that if this inherent function is recognized, intentionality in carrying out the activities in the counseling process can be enhanced and, overall, counseling made more effective.

At another level, research can be viewed as a separate activity that evolves from the counseling process. Even if counselors do not intend to become researchers primarily, they may want to approach research from the perspective of the scientist-practitioner. This approach provides the framework for counselors to engage in research (as the scientist) while providing counseling services to their clients (as the practitioner).

In the course of their work, counselors develop outcome goals, keep track of their clients' progress, and analyze the data they collect to evaluate the extent to which the strategy they are using is effective. These activities can help counselors determine such questions as which strategy works with which problem or client. For the beginning counselor, early research activity can be as practical as using such data to compare behavior before and after treatment (the A-B design). Also, observing and recording the progress of a client throughout counseling can result in case study research. You can review

TABLE **3.2**

Comparing the Counseling Process and the Research Process

Steps in Counseling Process	Steps in Research Process
Presentation of problem	Subject or problem to be studied
Background research (assessment)	Background research (literature research)
Definition of the problem	Definition of the problem
Explanation of the problem	Hypothesis
Setting of goals	Research objectives
Implementation of strategy	Implementation of experiment
Evaluation of counseling	Interpretation and conclusion

research designs of varying sophistication for the counseling discipline in such texts as Heppner et al. (2005).

The sophistication with which the scientist-practitioner research is done depends on the complexity of the problem and the answers required by the counselor. However, even such relatively straightforward research designs as the case study can reveal new insights worth disseminating for the benefit of others in the profession. Indeed, with the persistence of old challenges and the introduction of new ones, as mentioned previously, the potential exists for the adaptation of traditional strategies to produce new perspectives that can be shared with other counselors.

It is also important to realize that research impacts counseling on an economic level as well. With school districts, government agencies, and third-party reimbursement organizations requiring proof that counseling services are producing expected outcomes, the scientist-practitioner model can produce research to make the case for the effectiveness of a specific counseling plan for particular clients and the effectiveness of counseling in general. Research used for these purposes also fulfills one aspect of the counselor's role as advocate, which is discussed in the next section.

ADVOCATING FOR THE CLIENT AND THE PROFESSION

Being an advocate is another important role that is gaining recognition as an essential aspect of counseling. Advocacy has a long history in the helping disciplines that goes back to the social activism of the late 1880s, when America's first *settlement house* was founded in New York City. The term for these houses came from the philosophy that people interested in social justice should settle (live) in economically depressed and underserved neighborhoods to offer services and assess the conditions for social reform. At the turn of the 20th century, Clifford Beers (1908, 1981) wrote *A Mind That Found Itself* about his experiences as a patient in a mental institution and used it to advocate for a better social perception of, and treatment for, the mentally ill. In the 1990s, practitioners of counseling and therapy, such as Derald Wing Sue and Patricia Arredondo, advocated for multicultural competencies and standards to improve counseling services for clients from diverse backgrounds (Sue, Arredondo, & McDavis, 1992). These examples not only give an idea of the lengthy history of formal advocacy in the helping fields, but also demonstrate that it can be used in a wide range of situations, such as working to strengthen community services, improve treatment for special groups, and bring about improvement within the counseling profession itself.

On account of the various purposes for which it can be used, advocacy has been defined in different ways. You can develop a comprehensive understanding of the term from the following statement: Advocacy involves increasing a client's sense of personal power and influencing those with power toward greater responsiveness to the needs of individuals, groups, and communities (Kiselica & Robinson, 2001; Teasdale, 1998). Under this broad definition, counselors can advocate for their clients and their own profession from positions in educational, corporate, and community settings and at the local, state, and federal levels.

Advocating for the Client

From the foregoing definition, advocacy may be viewed as occurring at different levels of deliberate and direct involvement by counselors. In this context, advocacy includes empowering clients, which, as stated earlier in the chapter, is an underlying principle in counseling. This empowering may be seen in the case of a client gaining insight from counseling and, as a result, developing the confidence to approach colleagues, teachers, supervisors, and others when a conflict arises and needs to be resolved. At another level, advocacy is a more premeditated and direct activity that involves, for example, teaching a client specific skills for an interpersonal problem that involves a power differential. Providing assertiveness training for a client to deal with sexual harassment or other types of victimization falls into this category.

A more direct form of advocacy occurs when counselors take action on behalf of their clients by speaking to a person who is in a decision-making position with regard to the client. This type of advocacy involves reframing the client's problem so that the decision maker obtains a better understanding of and responds favorably to the needs of the client. The necessity for advocacy at this level might come from a situation in a home where a 13-year-old child takes care of three younger siblings after school while the parents are at work; in a high school where a coach is not including on a school team those students whom he perceives as having an alternative sexual orientation; or in a company where minorities are being passed over for promotion. The last two examples indicate that advocacy involves working on behalf of groups as well, not only individuals.

In cases in which social perception and public policy are the barriers to underserved groups being provided with health care services, effective advocates ensure that the situation is seen not as a result of the shortcomings of the group, but of a limitation in the social and cultural structures of the community. In such cases, community participation may be necessary to strengthen advocacy efforts. Counselors can take leadership positions in nonprofit organizations, participate in community outreach efforts, and initiate letter-writing campaigns to promote valid causes on behalf of underserved populations.

Active Learning Exercise **3.2**

Advocacy requires conviction and courage. To what extent do you see yourself being involved in advocacy relating to such issues as homelessness, unemployment, and teenage pregnancy?

Advocating for the Profession

In addition to advocating for individuals and groups, counselors advocate on behalf of the profession itself. The community activities already presented as being constructive in advocating for groups and their needs can also be beneficial in advocating for the profession. However, advocating for the profession presents opportunities for different activities. For example, counselors can participate in their professional associations at the local, state, or national levels to promote public understanding of the purpose of counseling and the role of counselors. They can do so as community relations or outreach committee members, as speakers at public hearings on counseling issues, and as delegates providing clarity and information to legislative representatives on the effect of upcoming legislation on the counseling profession. Such work on behalf of the profession has resulted in the enactment of licensure legislation that recognizes professional counselors as mental health providers in most states.

While meeting with a legislator or even speaking on counseling issues at a public forum can seem too remote an activity for beginning counselors, it must be noted that advocacy begins with becoming a member of the American Counseling Association and its divisions and their state associations. Furthermore, as a counselor-in-training, you can become a member of student-oriented organizations such as the Graduate Counseling Students Association or a chapter of Chi Sigma Iota (the international honor society for the counseling profession); if neither organization exists on your campus, your first efforts in advocacy for the profession can begin with organizing one or the other. By inviting speakers to discuss such topics as the roles of counselors, the value of mental health services, and the current status of counseling licensure legislation, counseling students' organizations can help to not only provide professional development for trainees in the department, but also change the perception about the counseling profession that is held by many students attending the university and individuals in surrounding communities.

Inasmuch as counselors can advocate for change in society's perception of the profession, they can also advocate for change within their own associations to keep them dynamic and responsive to the social and cultural changes occurring in their local or regional jurisdictions. The effect of advocacy within professional organizations is reflected in the work that Sue, Arredondo, and others did at the national level for multiculturalism in counseling and therapy. The contrary feedback, and at times unfriendly debate, that resulted on account of their efforts demonstrate the persistence and resilience that is often required for success in advocacy.

Being an advocate is a challenging role. Persistence and resilience are only two of the factors that contribute to success in advocacy. Advocacy also requires skills in effective communication, problem assessment, problem solving, and partnership building. Two other types of professional interactions that the counselor will experience and that require similar skills are collaboration and consultation.

CONSULTING AND COLLABORATING WITH OTHER MENTAL HEALTH PROFESSIONALS

Although mental health professionals share some skills and may do the same work in some settings, there are important differences in the primary activities for which they have been trained. Because of the existence of these similarities and differences, tensions have traditionally existed (and still do) among the professions over who can or should have the exclusive right to perform certain helping activities. In some jurisdictions, for example, counselors are not allowed to administer and interpret certain psychological tests. Such sources of tension are fuelled to an extent by economic considerations, because many health insurance companies will only reimburse clients for services received from mental health practitioners who can prove that they are qualified to provide those services.

In spite of these differences, all mental health practitioners are mindful of their obligation to respect the various approaches to helping in which each has been trained and to ensure that their clients receive the best mental health services possible. Since the problems of many clients are multidimensional and a single practitioner may not be qualified to offer the array of services required, helping clients effectively necessitates a working relationship among mental health practitioners that utilizes the specific knowledge and skills they received from their professional training. This relationship is necessary for the success of work being done, whether in one setting or across settings.

Consultation

Consultation and *collaboration* are two types of interactions that evolve from the relationships in which practitioners often participate to provide services for their clients. Consultation involves an expert in a particular discipline or field providing insight to help an individual or group prevent or solve a problem. In general terms, the word *consultation* refers to commonplace interactions, for example, calling upon an interior designer for assistance in remodeling a home. The interior designer (the consultant) gives advice about structural changes, for instance, walls that can be removed to make rooms larger and where cabinets can be installed. However, the designer/consultant does not implement these changes. He or she may assist the homeowner in arranging for the necessary building codes if any are needed, identifying suitable fixtures, and selecting companies where they can be purchased, but leaves it up to the homeowner to proceed with getting the changes made.

In a counseling context, this situation would involve a third person, the client. Examples of consultation in a counseling situation include the following scenarios:

- A supervisor helps a counselor-in-training to identify the difficulty in treating the problem that a client has presented and developing strategies or skills that could help the client.
- A counselor assists a teacher with strategies to deal with a student with ADHD in the classroom.
- A social worker advises a counselor about resources for a client with a rare or unusual need.
- A psychiatrist outlines to a counselor the effect of a drug on a client so that the counselor can provide effective counseling.

As in the case of the interior designer, the consulting practitioner would not implement the strategy. For example, in the second scenario just listed, the counselor would provide the strategy and coach the teacher in its use, but leave the teacher to implement the strategy in the classroom.

Much of the consultation that a counselor may do involves a single occasion or a few brief discussions. However, some consultations undertaken by counselors are long term. The more involved and formal the consultative relationship is, such as being hired as a consultant by a business company, an agency, or a school, the greater the need for counselors to be acquainted with the consultative process and determine if they have the required competence. In these circumstances, counselors would have a written contract that spells out the terms of the consultation to be given. Recommendations for what should be in such a contract include the following points (Remley, 1993):

- The service that is to be completed by the consultant
- Any materials that the consultant needs to provide
- A time frame for the completion of the consultation
- The person to whom the consultant is responsible
- Payment and method of payment for the consultation

Active Learning Exercise **3.3**

Consultations are very common. Think of an experience that you, a family member, or a friend has had involving any kind of consultation (such as with a mechanic, event planner, or landscape designer). What was the process like?

Collaboration

Collaboration is not as formalized a process as consultation. Also, collaboration is a more inclusive term that suggests a variety of activities, ranging from sharing information to developing a program. Specifically, the process of collaboration assumes that no one practitioner in the relationship has all the knowledge necessary to bring about a solution or realize the intended goal. Rather, it assumes that the practitioners participating are functioning as an interdependent team. This teamwork occurs when they are all in one agency providing services for a client, as well as when they are involved in different settings providing complementary services for the same client. The school is a typical setting where the need for collaboration might bring together a counselor, psychiatrist, psychologist, and social worker to develop a plan and provide services to assist a student.

For example, in dealing with a student who is exhibiting severe behavioral problems, a psychologist might be involved in administering and interpreting tests, a psychiatrist in prescribing medication, and a social worker in investigating reported conditions in the student's home. Meanwhile, the school counselor might be involved in counseling the student on an ongoing basis. Or, depending on the severity of the problem, the student might be receiving treatment from a psychologist, while the school counselor is concentrating on the student's academic needs.

Collaboration also includes the development and implementation of programs. A school counselor might team up with a drug and alcohol counselor to create and deliver a preventive program for students graduating from middle school to high school. Or a marriage and family counselor might collaborate with a psychologist to present a series of psycho-educational workshops for parents of children with conduct disorder. Collaborating to bring about these projects is just as essential an aspect of providing mental health services as collaborating on services for the individual client.

Success in all types of collaboration and consultation requires counselors to develop an attitude of mutual respect and cooperation in their relationship with other professionals. Furthermore, for counselors to take optimal advantage of working with other mental health professionals, it is important for them to be knowledgeable about what various practitioners are trained to do and what their state's licensing statues allow them to do. Having this information enables counselors to know who to contact for specific assistance in helping their clients.

Active Learning Exercise **3.4**

Make arrangement to speak with a professional counselor in a school setting, community agency, and a rehabilitation center. Ask the counselor about the various professionals with whom he or she consults and collaborates in providing services to clients. Who is involved? To what extent are they involved? Are you familiar with the functions and roles of those professionals? Develop a list of resources for learning about them.

CONCLUSION

This chapter has outlined the various functions, roles, and activities that you are likely to experience on your journey from a counselor-in-training to a licensed and experienced professional. Your workplace and the roles for which you become responsible in that setting will determine to a large degree the roles and activities you will concentrate on. Group counseling, crisis intervention, administrative work, and clinical supervision are a few examples. Furthermore, regardless of the setting or organizational responsibilities, with the demographic changes in the population resulting in an increasingly diverse clientele and workplace, enhancing your multicultural counseling competency should remain a commitment throughout your career.

Even as a counselor-in-training, you will find opportunities to evaluate traditional theories and treatment in terms of their efficacy in addressing the challenges of your nontraditional clients and clients in general. Moreover, in dealing with some of those challenges, you will realize the importance of collaborating and consulting with other professionals who contribute different services to the overall health care of your clients. Advocacy on behalf of your clients and profession sometimes becomes necessary in these circumstances. A further step in advocacy entails publicly addressing social practices and policies that negatively affect clients and the counselor's ability to provide them with appropriate service. Most likely you may not get the opportunity to experience all of the roles and activities that comprise the practice of counseling. Nonetheless, their presentation in this chapter is intended to make them familiar to you as you encounter or hear about them on your journey in the counseling profession.

CHAPTER REVIEW

1. Although the term *counseling* is widely used to describe many types of help giving, the term *professional counseling* signifies the activities that you will be involved in when dealing with the mental, emotional, behavioral, and other developmental issues that clients present in counseling.
2. In fulfilling their professional roles and functions, counselors utilize a repertoire of intervention skills to assist clients in addressing their problems. Counselors also utilize the processes and dynamics inherent in the interaction between the counselor and client or group members.
3. The increasing diversity among clients requiring various types of counseling services makes cultural awareness a necessity for counselors. Along with race and ethnicity, it is important to consider sexual orientation, religion and spirituality, socioeconomic status, gender, and age as differences that require cultural sensitivity.
4. A fundamental aspect of being a professional counselor involves participating in research and keeping abreast of changes in theoretical approaches to the problems that clients have. Research and theory are integral aspects of counseling that can enhance practice when they are undertaken intentionally and with forethought.
5. Seeing that no single practitioner may be qualified to offer the array of services that a client might require, counselors collaborate and consult with other professionals to ensure that clients receive the best possible mental health care.

REVIEW QUESTIONS

1. Discuss the functions involved in professional counseling and the roles counselors might have to fulfill in their work.
2. Discuss some of the developmental challenges individuals might encounter at different stages in their lives.
3. What are some of the differences among preventive, intervention, and crisis counseling?
4. Explain why cultural sensitivity should be an important aspect of providing counseling service.
5. Identify situations in which group counseling might be more effective than individual counseling.
6. Explain the relationship between theory and research in the profession of counseling.

ADDITIONAL RESOURCES

- Lowen, A. (1958). *The language of the body.* New York: Macmillan.
- Parsons, F. (1909). *Choosing a vocation.* Boston: Houghton Mifflin.

- Rogers, C. R., Perls, F., & Ellis, A. (1965). *Three approaches to psychotherapy* 1 [Film]. Orange, CA: Psychological Films, Inc.

- Rogers, C. R., Shostrom, E., & Lazarus, A. (1977). *Three approaches to psychotherapy* 2 [Film]. Orange, CA: Psychological Films, Inc.

REFERENCES

Arredondo, P., Toporek, R., Brown, S. P., Jones, J., Locke, D. C., Sanchez, J., & Stadler, H. (1996). Operationalization of the multicultural counseling competencies. *Journal of Multicultural Counseling and Development, 24,* 42–78.

Bernard, J. M., & Goodyear, R. K. (2004). *Fundamentals of clinical supervision* (3rd ed.). Boston: Pearson Education.

Beers, C. P. (1908). *A mind that found itself.* New York: Longman Green.

Beers, C. P. (1981). *A mind that found itself.* Pittsburg: University of Pittsburg Press.

Corey, G. (2009). *Theory and practice of counseling and psychotherapy* (8th ed.). Pacific Grove, CA: Brooks/Cole.

Corey, M. S., & Corey, G. (2006). *Groups: Progress and practice* (7th ed.). Belmont, CA: Brooks/Cole.

Corey, G., Corey, M. S., & Callanan, P. (2007). *Issues and ethics in the helping professions* (7th ed.). Belmont, CA: Brooks/Cole, Cengage Learning.

Cormier, S., Nurius, P. S., & Osborn, C. J. (2009). *Interviewing and change strategies for helpers: Fundamental skills and cognitive behavioral interventions* (6th ed.). Belmont, CA: Brooks/Cole.

Egan, G. (2007). *The skilled helper* (8th ed.). Belmont, CA: Brooks/Cole.

Gladding, S. T. (2007). *Counseling: A comprehensive profession* (5th ed.). Upper Saddle River, NJ: Merrill Prentice Hall.

Hackney, H. L., & Cormier, S. (2004). *The professional counselor: A process guide to counseling* (5th ed.). Boston: Allyn & Bacon.

Heppner, P. P., Kivlighan, D. M., & Wampold, B. E. (2005). *Research design in counseling* (3rd ed.). Belmont, CA: Wadsworth.

Kiselica, M. S., & Robinson, M. (2001). Bringing advocacy counseling to life: The history, issues, and human drams of social justice work in counseling. *Journal of Counseling and Development, 79,* 387–397.

Levant, R. F. (2006). Making psychology a household word. *American Psychologist, 61,* 383–395.

Prochaska, J. O., & Norcross, J. C. (2007). *Systems of psychotherapy: A transtheoretical analysis* (6th ed.). Belmont, CA: Brooks/Cole.

Remley, T. P., Jr. (1993). Consultation contracts. *Journal of Counseling and Development, 72,* 157–158.

Remley, T. P., Jr., & Herlihy, B. (2007). *Ethical, legal, and professional issues in counseling* (updated 2nd ed.). Upper Saddle River, NJ: Merrill Prentice Hall.

Rogers, C. R. (1942). *Counseling and psychotherapy.* Boston: Houghton Mifflin.

Rogers, C. R. (1951). *Client-centered therapy.* Boston: Houghton Mifflin.

Rogers, C. R. (1965). *Client-centered therapy: Its current practice, implications and theory.* Boston: Houghton Mifflin.

Sue, D. W., Arredondo, P., & McDavis, R. J. (1992). Multicultural counseling competencies and standards: A call to the profession. *Journal of Counseling and Development, 70,* 477–486.

Teasdale, K. (1998). *Advocacy in health care.* London: Blackwell Science.

Tuckman, B. W., & Jensen, M. A. C. (1977). Stages in small group development revisited. *Group & Organizational Studies, 2,* 419–427.

Yalom, I. D. (2005). *The theory and practice of group psychotherapy* (5th ed.). New York: Basic Books.

CHAPTER 4

Ethical and Legal Standards in Counseling

LEARNING OBJECTIVES

After reading this chapter, you should be able to

- recount the development and background of ethics and ethical standards;

- discuss the role of ethics for professionals in the counseling field;

- understand ethical decision-making and the differences between ethics and law;

- describe the impact of counselor ethics on diverse groups of individuals, families, and communities;

- discuss the ethical issues involved in group work; and

- understand the ethical boundaries in counseling and counselor supervision.

CHAPTER OUTLINE

Introduction

Context, Perspective, and History
Universality of Ethics
Ethics Becomes a Key Force in Counseling
Ethics Defined

Ethical Decision-Making
From Knowledge to Wisdom
Responsibility for Decisions
Adhering to Ethical Standards
Ethics and Law
A Model for Ethical Decision-Making
Ethics as a Means of Empowerment
Avoiding Harm and Doing Good

INTRODUCTION

This chapter moves from general attention to the history, pertinence, and universality of ethics and ethical behavior, through general and specific attention to ethical issues, ethical standards and ethical practice for counselors and other mental health practitioners, to limited attention to legal issues related to counseling. The goal of the chapter is to afford entry-level counseling students fundamental knowledge and perspectives of ethics as a means to inform and empower all facets of student learning and practice. Following an introduction and contextual overview, the narrative focuses on ethics, ethical decision-making, ethical standards, and ethical behavior of individual counselors, counselor educators, and counseling organizations. This chapter also includes selective attention to legal issues as these relate to ethics and ethical practice. After attending to the preamble of the American Counseling Association (ACA) ethical standards (ACA, 2005), the focus moves to discussions of selected aspects of the ACA ethical standards, concluding with a focus on ethical decision-making and implications for ethical knowledge and practice, with an eye to lifelong learning.

CONTEXT, PERSPECTIVE, AND HISTORY

This chapter is predicated on the assumptions that lifelong learning is essential for all professionals and that numerous quality resources exist for continuing education and sustained inquiry aimed at enhancing comprehension and application of ethical standards for ethical practice. This approach aims at affording stimuli here that lay a groundwork for students and new professionals to chart their own course in subsequent study, supervised practice, and continuing education for life. With these perspectives in mind, this section now moves to the history and context of ethical issues, principles, and applications.

Ethics originated as a branch of philosophy with emphasis on virtue and positive human behavior manifest in respect and good works toward self and others. A central question of ethics asks, "What is the good life?" Aristotle, Plato, and their colleagues focused a body of oral tradition, and subsequent publications discerned general ethical principles articulated as a means to enhance the dialogue and extend this ethical facet of philosophy's pursuit of truth (Beauchamp & Childress 2001; Hutchins & Adler, 1952a, 1952b, 1952c; Kitchener 1986; Stewart-Sicking, 2008). One dominant manifestation of this aspect of ethics is discernable in the wish of someone to be remembered in death as "a good and decent person," to wit, an ethical person.

Universality of Ethics

Over the centuries, ethics has taken on increasing importance in individual and social direction and the governance of human behavior for individuals and societies at all levels, local, national, and international. Recent unprecedented ethical breaches in business scandals associated with corrupt investment managers such as Bernard Madoff and corporate leaders at Enron, Tyco, and Worldcom, to name only four, revealed ruthless abandon in excessive executive misbehavior, bringing financial ruin for corporations and millions of shareholders. Such dereliction gave rise to renewed attention to ethics in all public and private sectors of society (Zuckerman, 2004).

Today, ethics is an overt distinguishing characteristic of learned and other societies and professions, including professional organizations and their members. While counseling students might focus primarily on ethical codes for counselors, it is important to appreciate the universality of many ethical principles and standards for all professions. For example, counseling students and counselor educators generally study ethical standards and codes from a variety of mental health professions and organizations, such as ACA (2005), the American Association for Marriage and Family Therapy (2001), the American Psychiatric Association (2001), the American Psychological Association (2002), and the National Association of Social Workers (1999), as well as standards emanating from smaller entities comprising ACA and other mental health associations. What may be less obvious to mental health practitioners is the universality of ethical principles and standards and points of focus in ethical standards of organizations ranging from computer societies and national and multinational businesses to ethics courses in the military, such as the ethics course at the United States National Defense University, also known as the National War College (Johns, 1988).

Across these ethical standards, codes, and courses in these varied environments, one sees considerable attention to such ethical principles as confidentiality, fidelity, respect, integrity, responsibility, and accountability. Suffice it to say, businesses, professions, governments, and societies require ethics and ethical standards, and many ethical principles appear universal in their meaning and importance in Western society and many other areas of the world. Hopefully, this contextual view encourages both confidence and curiosity in the study of ethics as a prelude to ethical personal and professional behavior. The authors hope this overall theme of ethics as encouraging and empowering becomes engaging and contagious with all readers and their clients. In setting the stage by considering your own personal perspective, please review and reflect on Active Learning Exercises Considering Your Personal Ethical Code.

Active Learning Exercise **4.1**

Consider your personal ethics code. How do you behave positively toward others? How would you promote good works toward yourself and others? How would you refrain from harming someone else? What information or personal experiences do you use to help you make good and virtuous decisions?

Ethics Becomes a Key Force in Counseling

In the late 1970s, the first author (Engels) served on the American Personnel and Guidance Association (APGA; now ACA) Ethics Committee for three years, circa 1978–1981. Ethics committees of professional mental health associations and learned societies are typically responsible for member and public education and adjudication of allegations of member unethical behavior, and APGA/ACA's committee responsibilities were and remain no exception (Kocet, 2006). Thus, the committee provided an annual educational ethics program, but oral tradition on the committee indicated that no one had come to the programs for many years, and this tradition proved the rule for 1978 and 1979. In the first author's experience at that time, counselors paid attention to programs focused on legal issues, but largely ignored ethics programs.

In 1980, however, this tradition was shattered when approximately 35 APGA members attended and stayed for the duration of the ethics committee's content program, which focused primarily on ethical issues with limited attention to legal issues in school counseling. Moreover, a number of those at that program, including Wayne Huey, then American School Counselor Association (ASCA) Ethics Committee chair, decided to initiate what became a longstanding and richly applauded tradition of sponsored ethics and ethical/ legal programs for ASCA at every APGA/ACA conference for at least 15 years. Similar increases in interest and participation in ethics programs and discussions throughout ACA and ACA-affiliate conferences may be attributable to state licensure laws requiring continuing education in ethics, Council for Accreditation of Counseling and Related Educational Programs (CACREP, 2001) accreditation requirements, major publications, and other factors, including increasing counselor dedication to ethics.

The key point is that ethics has become an increasingly major force and stimulus in counseling and other mental health disciplines and professions, and this expanding tradition of attention to ethics is manifest in all facets of counselor preparation and counseling practice. In brief, one can see major increases in the volume of literature and conference programs related to ethics, and this added attention to ethics and jurisprudence seems a most healthy approach to good practice by good practitioners. Of course, at the heart of literature lie definitions.

Ethics Defined

Dictionary definitions of ethics contain elements relating to

- the branch of philosophy or knowledge that deals with moral principles—right and wrong;
- the study of standards of conduct and moral judgment;
- moral precepts;
- values;
- rules of conduct;
- a system or set of moral principles of a particular person, religion, group, or organization;
- moral principles that govern a person's or group's behavior; and
- moral correctness of specified conduct. (*Random House Dictionary*, 2001, p. 243; *Webster's New World Dictionary*, 2002, p. 217; *Concise Oxford American Dictionary*, 2006)

In light of these definitions, one can see both personal and organizational aspects of ethics. A common definition might hold that professional ethical standards constitute a consensus value statement of a profession, providing guidelines or standards governing the conduct of members of a profession. Seen in this light, constituent input is mandatory for maximal validity in the form of consensus. Aspirational ethics is on a plane above and beyond ethical standards, something of an individual matter focused on the most and best a counselor can ethically do with and for a client while also complying with the ethical standards of the profession. This perspective of going beyond standards and minimal requirements is reminiscent of altruism and noble acts of human kindness, of human character in action.

ETHICAL DECISION-MAKING

John Rothney, an eminent counseling pioneer with more than 200 major publications on counseling (Engels, 1975), defined counseling as a process aimed at helping clients increase their self-awareness and self-knowledge, notice opportunities for choice, and learn to make decisions so that, when facing important decisions in life, clients were better able to decide wisely than they would have been without the counseling. Rothney's extensive, numerous, and rigorous follow-up studies documented the lasting effectiveness of counseling for a duration of at least five years through his focus on client self-report and rigorous longitudinal studies of decision processes and outcomes related to counseling (Engels, 1975). Rothney's keen attention to decision-making is pivotal to this discussion of ethics in that decision-making is central to most counseling. Moreover, Rothney's emphasis on important decisions is a point worth noting here.

Like Rothney, Janis and Mann (1977) observed that ethics is a central component of all important decision-making in counseling, noting attention to ethics as a distinct and defining aspect of any important decision. Janis and Mann's perspective on decision-making holds that important decisions have an ethical component, while lesser decisions might not. T. S. Eliot's discussion in "Choruses from *The Rock*" (Eliot, 1934, p. 7), affords a similar perspective. Eliot asks, "Where is the Life we have lost in living? Where is the wisdom we have lost in knowledge? Where is the knowledge we have lost in information?" In raising these graduated questions, Eliot is noting levels of decision-making. Eliot's questioning and insights afford a perspective for counselors and clients, noting that some decisions are more important than others and that the most important choices in life require the most rigorous sifting, winnowing, and decision-making. A hierarchy ranging from data to wisdom serves to illustrate this point.

From Knowledge to Wisdom

Sometimes we only need data to make a relatively trivial decision, for example, What is the cost? At times we need information, for example, How much does it cost and will it hurt anyone? At times, knowledge suffices for good choices, but for vital decisions, people need wisdom; we need to make the best possible, wisest choices. If knowledge tells one how to build a runway, wisdom helps one weigh pros and cons in deciding whether one needs a runway or an airport at a particular place. A friend with prostate cancer noted the importance of finding the single best qualified, wisest surgeon, rather than merely finding someone who was able to perform the surgery. One sees parallel elements in counseling involving matters of grave human importance and consequence such as marriage, life partner, and progeny decisions. This perspective holds that this final level, wisdom, is the level where ethics is a prominent element and requirement of wise decision-making.

Responsibility for Decisions

One additional aspect of decision-making focuses on jurisdiction and responsibility for decisions and their consequences. Much of counseling focuses on responsibility, emphasizing the crucial dimension of taking responsibility for one's decisions and their consequences. Before deciding, one needs to review who owns responsibility for the choice. Once one acknowledges responsibility for a decision, he or she should also accept responsibility for the outcome(s) and consequences of that decision. Certainly, clients need to take responsibility for client choices. At times, however, counselors may determine that someone else is more appropriate for and has jurisdiction over and responsibility for a decision, for example, a school counselor may note that a school principal has fiduciary and other responsibility regarding determination of parental custodial rights regarding school records. Counselors may also need to take responsibility for a client deemed at risk to self or others, to include the possibility of involuntary commitment for needed care. Guidance for such weighty matters can be found in ethical standards.

Active Learning Exercise **4.2**

Consider and list the characteristics of an ethical counselor. If you were this counselor, how would you manage counseling relationships with your clients? What values, morals, and good behaviors would guide you to be the best ethical counselor? What would you do if you were unsure of a decision? How would you explain the importance of counselor ethical behavior to someone who is not a counselor?

Adhering to Ethical Standards

Formal professional ethical guidelines or standards have been part of ACA's history for more than 50 years, with considerable constancy in terms of principles and major additive emphases related to crucial issues. For example, the 1988 ACA ethical standards added a major emphasis on technology in terms of electronic records and privacy protection, as well as client access to vital tools of technology. In 1988, it seems many counselors had little or no idea there was a national insurance data bank that shared information to guard against fraud and protect insurance companies, and the committee found it imperative to expand coverage of the standards to include such matters. The year 1995 yielded two sets of standards, one called "practice standards" and the other inaccurately referred to as "aspirational standards." The 1995 standards added specific topical emphasis on sexual matters and prohibitions against counselor sexual intimacy with clients. Most recently, the 2005 standards emphasize and amplify many facets of multicultural and diversity issues as means to enhance counselor ethics and counseling practice (Kocet, 2006). In the current authors' view, the 2005 standards constitute a dramatic improvement over the false dichotomy between principles and practice depicted in the 1995 dual *Code of Ethics and Standards of Practice* (ACA, 1995). Having one single set of standards from the flagship organization seems prudent. As noted later, however, some other entities within ACA publish their own ethical standards, echoing the ACA standards and adding points of emphasis pertinent to members of these other ACA organizations. Additionally, legal matters can complicate ethical decision-making.

Ethics and Law

In brief, ethics and law seem to have more in common with one another than either has in exclusion from the other, perhaps most notably a focus on morality, fairness, and justice. However, differences between ethics and law are important in substance and in practice. Generally, law is more explicitly and intentionally definitive, with acute attention to specific statutes, nuances emanating from statutes, interpretations, precedents, and decisions arising from the study and adjudication of legal principles and proceedings. The language of ethics is typically less specifically definitive and focused on principles and guidelines for good practice, with minimal attempt at exhaustive coverage regarding the propriety of the complex range of human behavior connected with an ethical issue or principle. As noted earlier, ethical standards constitute consensus value sets that stipulate the least one must do. Practitioners are expected to comply with ethical standards and appropriate local, state, national, and international law in all their professional work.

In their collective 70 years of professional practice, the authors have noted and experienced consistently positive ethical and legal behavior of counselors and other mental health practitioners, with allegations of illegal and unethical behavior and adjudication by licensure boards and ethics committees restricted to a select minimal number of cases per year. In Texas, for example, periodic reports from the Board of Examiners of Professional Counselors routinely report single-digit numbers of disciplinary and related adjudication matters from more than 12,000 Licensed Professional Counselors (Texas Board of Examiners of Licensed Professional Counselors, 2006). Statistics from ACA and the American Psychological Association seem quite similarly indicative of ethical and legal practitioner behavior. While appreciating that some victims do not come forth and while one infraction or transgression via omission or commission is too many, one could infer ethical behavior and ethical decision-making in the overwhelming majority of practitioners who are not and have never been accused of unethical and/or illegal activity. At the same time, however, healthy skepticism must also acknowledge estimates that only a low percentage of victims of mental health practitioner malpractice bring charges against their assailants, and yet lower percentages of practitioners acknowledge such malpractice in formal survey research (Welfel, 2010, p. 190).

When ethical standards and law are parallel, practitioners can proceed in relative comfort regarding both areas. However, areas and points of difference between ethics and law can be vital yet problematic in determining a counselor's course(s) of action in a particular counseling decision or set of decisions. For example, scenarios may pose *neither* legal nor ethical concerns or *both* legal and ethical concerns. Such situations may afford clarity and pose no apparent contradictions for practitioners. Again, it is worth noting that, in the authors' combined 70 years of practice, these two quadrants account for and describe the vast majority of counselor behavior. On the other hand, scenarios in which *either* ethical or legal but *not both* sets of concerns are represented, pose concerns, quandaries, and potential problems of varying magnitude as practitioners grapple with competing factors of ethics and law (Engels, Wilborn, & Schneider, 1990). In Texas, for example, the state supreme court's multiple rulings, most recently in the case of *Thapar v. Zezulka* (1999), indicate that a client's right to privacy in counseling trumps a counselor's ethical duty to warn an intended victim, as stipulated in the ACA code and in the well-known Tarasoff cases (1974/1976). Thus, a Texas Licensed Professional Counselor (LPC) or other mental health professional faces a dilemma when considering appropriate action in these and similar cases. Avoiding or minimizing informed consent for clients, while likely legal, can be seen as a violation of ethical standards. While the ACA ethical code lists specific prohibitions against sex with clients, state laws restricting sexual intimacy between two consenting adults seem relatively rare. However, a state licensure board might publish rules regarding such matters that could prohibit sexual intimacy with a client. In these and similar cases, one sees complexities that require attention in counselor preparation programs and in practice. Moreover, these complexities necessitate that counselors have and maintain a sound understanding of ethical principles and standards as well as appropriate laws as a basis for professional judgment.

Licenses and other governmentally issued credentials for counselors constitute legal sanctions for counseling primarily as means to protect the public. Seen in this light, counselor licensure and other government-issued credentials, such as school counselor certification, place counselors in positions of trust and responsibility that require legal and ethical knowledge and practice. To this end of protecting the public and reminding counseling practitioners of their legal and ethical obligations, some states, such as Texas, are requiring jurisprudence examinations as well as continuing education, including required study of ethics, for license renewal.

Thus, legal and ethical issues, principles, codes, and statutes are vital for counseling practice, and counselors must comply or risk losing their credentials or organizational memberships. This negative reinforcer of losing a privilege is one factor in motivating ethical and legal compliance. On the side of positive reinforcers, adherence to the ethical standards and a solid grasp of ethical principles underlying the standards can empower counselors and clients. There are also considerations when ethics and law appear at odds, and counselors are tasked with deliberating contrasting obligations. However, one of the 2005 *ACA Code of Ethics*, H.1.B. (ACA, 2005), stipulates that when a counselor is faced with contradictions between law and ethical standards, ultimately, "counselors may adhere to the requirements of the law, regulations or other legal authority," presumably without being deemed to have violated the ethical standards. The authors find such a standard problematic in and of itself, in that, ultimately, this standard seems to risk undercutting any legal or ethical defense a counselor might put forth that stems from following the ethical standards as a guide to professional behavior and as a positive reinforcer. Counselors need to know pertinent aspects of law that sanction and govern counseling practice; however, counselors also must stay current with ethical standards. In brief, one can see major increases in the volume of literature and mental health conference programs related to ethics and law, and this added attention to ethics and jurisprudence seems a most healthy stimulus for ethical practice.

A Model for Ethical Decision-Making

The profession has a number of models to help counselors make ethical decisions. Welfel (2010) has posited an adaptation of Kitchener's ideas (1986), yielding a 10-step model of ethical decision-making, moving from heightened ethical awareness and sensitivity; through context, delineation of central issues, study of pertinent ethical and legal standards, and consultation with colleagues and supervisors; to the actual decision, its documentation and reflective processing regarding the decision made and future implications (Welfel, 2010, p. 30). The authors recommend this or a similar approach as a starting point and a deliberate mode of ethical decision-making that exceeds reliance on intuition or other less deliberate and less balanced approaches.

Ethics as a Means of Empowerment

Along with heightened attention to and respect for ethics, the authors infer an emerging view of ethics as empowering and encouraging. This theme of empowerment moves beyond avoidance of violations and a sense of duty and obligation to a counselor's continuing commitment to good and "the good life" based on ethical principles such as worth, dignity, uniqueness, potential, autonomy, temperance, and fidelity. Through this chapter and other outlets, the authors join those who work to advance ennobling and guiding dimensions of ethics and ethical standards. Readers are encouraged to keep this overriding focus on client worth and empowerment in mind throughout this chapter and in all their studies of ethics.

Human worth, dignity, uniqueness, and potential are focal principles in the preamble to the *ACA Code of Ethics* (2005). This preamble states that counselors are dedicated to promoting human worth, dignity, uniqueness, and potential. Can one imagine or create a more empowering or ennobling premise and basis for action? Each of these principles is a vital dimension of human existence, and this preamble can truly be seen as a beacon for the standards and principles that follow, and, in turn, for counselors who abide by the standards. The authors routinely prompt classes, interns, and practicing counselors to consider adherence to these principles as a litmus test for finding an ethical course of action. In effect, if one can say that one is taking a course of action with one's client to promote the client's worth, dignity, uniqueness, and potential, one can have a sense of confidence, albeit without a guarantee, that the course of action is ethical in intent. Keeping one's "eyes on the prize" of human worth, dignity, uniqueness, and potential seems a core pursuit and quest for mental health professionals and vital language and concepts for the preamble. Adding these principles to those promulgated by Plato (1977), Aristotle (Hutchins & Adler, 1952a, 1952b, 1952c), Kitchener (1986), Beauchamp and Chidress (2001), and so many others yields an impressive positive basis for ethical perspective, motivation, empowerment, and action.

Avoiding Harm and Doing Good

Two cornerstones of ethics for all professions are do no harm, and do good, non-maleficence, and beneficence. Avoiding harm is vital to the work of counselors. Sanctions for risk of harm vary with client disposition, but, generally speaking, counselors and other health practitioners must err on the side of avoiding harm. At the same time, beneficence seems the ultimate statement of constructive ethical principle and behavior, the rationale for empowerment. These two principles constitute the foundation for ethical practice. Related principles point to client autonomy, integrity, fidelity, and respect for self and others, potential elements of a good life (Beauchamp & Childress, 2001; Kitchener, 1986). These and related principles constitute the genesis and provenience of ethics and ethical standards for the counseling profession.

Moving to specifics, the remainder of this chapter focuses on the major area of confidentiality, as well as all sections of the 2005 *ACA Code of Ethics*, with expanded attention on selected sections. A summary, conclusions, and attention to implications round out this discussion.

ETHICAL STANDARDS FOR COUNSELORS

As one readily sees, many counselors and many counseling settings are multi-disciplinary in focus and practitioner credentials, resulting in sometimes confusing and perplexing variation in requirements and a need for due deliberation by the practitioner. For the purposes of this chapter, emphasis is primarily on the 2005 *ACA Code of Ethics*, while acknowledging the proliferation of ethical standards even within the ACA family of organizations, for example, the National Career Development Association (NCDA) *Ethical Standards* (2007). While counselors need to know of this proliferation and master elements pertinent to a counselor's practice specialty, such knowledge could also be highly distracting or confusing for students in counselor preparation programs. Hence, this chapter's earlier mentioned singular general focus is intended to help keep the readers' eyes on the prize of more global ethical principles, including client worth, dignity, uniqueness, and potential, while attending to what might otherwise seem compartmentalized topical points of focus in sections of the varying ethical standards and laws pertaining to counseling. The authors hope readers will appreciate the proliferation of standards, while concentrating on the ACA standards and the key ethical principles underlying all counseling ethical standards.

Major sections of the *ACA Code of Ethics* are

A. The Counseling Relationship;
B. Confidentiality, Privileged Communication, and Privacy;
C. Professional Responsibility;
D. Relationships with Other Professionals;
E. Evaluation, Assessment, and Interpretation;
F. Supervision, Training, and Teaching;
G. Research and Publication; and
H. Resolving Ethical Issues.

Confidentiality is a major factor in affording clients a sense of security and confidence in the privacy of the intimate encounter that is counseling. Empathy, warmth, genuineness, and informed consent are key elements in establishing a counseling relationship based on counselor-client rapport, borne of trust in the confidentiality of the counseling process. Confidentiality can be seen as arising from canon law dictating strict and irrevocable requirements on priests to safeguard any and all facets of a penitent's confession, including the very occurrence of that confession. Over time, laws have respected this seal of confession and similar areas of privileged communication between clergy and penitent, lawyer and client, physician and patient. While counselors do not enjoy privileged communication in this legal sense, counselors can ask legal authorities that counselors not be compelled to testify or otherwise compromise what a client shares in counseling. There is, however, no certainty that a court or other authority will comply with such a request.

As noted earlier, ethical standards constitute a consensus value set for a profession, borne of a professional organization's ethics committee working vigorously to construct and promulgate drafts of the standards for member review and input, culminating in a consensus for the organization. Because these standards constitute rules and guidelines that form a consensus for ethical behavior, multiple opportunities for member input are essential. As noted previously, typically, these standards are configured topically in sections, with the ethics committee's best effort to articulate major points relevant to each section. For example, ACA's 2005 ethical standards stipulate that counselors maintain confidentiality in all instances except those in which a client reveals information regarding harm to self or others. Although subpoenas and similar court orders could also require that counselors break confidentiality or face legal complications, the sense of the standard is counselor protection of all facets of client privacy, including privacy after a client's death. Each section of the standards covers vital aspects of the counseling process, with general and specific principles and guidelines for ethical practice. Discussions and examples of specific sections of the ACA and Association for Specialists in Group Work (ASGW, 1998) standards and guidelines are included here for purposes of elaborating some key points.

ETHICAL AND PROFESSIONAL ISSUES IN GROUP WORK

Ethical standards can be seen as the central anchor in any profession and any professional specialty. Ethically minded group workers adhere to moral and ethical codes, standards, and principles held by their professions and professional associations dedicated to the practice and promotion of group work. In this regard, group counselors actually find more than one anchor or ethical base, in that the ASGW uses the *Best Practice Guidelines* (ASGW, 1998), while maintaining its membership in ACA and adherence to the ACA ethical standards. In 1998, ASGW published the *ASGW Best Practice Guidelines* to replace previous versions which were written as self-regulating guidelines for group workers. Pederson (1998) has noted that "ethical guidelines are a necessary but not sufficient condition for promoting ethical behavior" (p. 23). Guidelines have the tendency to relate to the common, everyday situations of practice rather than unusual incidents that professionals encounter. The *ASGW Best Practice Guidelines* (ASGW, 1998) provide more specific guidance for group workers than may be possible in the general *ACA Code of Ethics*.

Selected aspects of the *Best Practice Guidelines* are offered here to highlight the depth and breadth of the standards, while affording some practitioners a refresher. Section A, "Best Practices in Planning Group Work," outlines responsibilities and expected behaviors of group workers in the planning of groups (ASGW, 1998). This section says group workers must actively know, understand, and apply standards, codes and guidelines, and competencies of regulatory organizations, such as the *ACA Code of Ethics* (2005), *ASGW Best Practice Guidelines*, and Association for Multicultural Counseling and Development Multicultural Counseling Competencies. Group workers must identify types of groups to be offered, screen prospective group members, give basic information about the group to prospective members prior to beginning groups, select members, and set group goals. Informed consent means group workers must inform prospective group members of the goals, purpose, techniques, theoretical orientation, rules, procedures, and limitations of counseling (ASGW, 1998).

Group workers must assess their skills and knowledge, and choose techniques and leadership styles specific to each type of group offered. Additionally group counselors must have a professional disclosure statement that addresses confidentiality and its limits, theoretical orientation, basic information about the group and professional qualifications of the leaders, goals and purpose of the group, and roles and responsibilities of group members and leaders. Group workers have the responsibility to educate members about confidentiality and its limits, and encourage members to respect and maintain confidentiality. Open and honest discussion in the group can help attain and maintain these values. Finally, group workers must seek appropriate assistance for their own personal problems, seek consultation and supervision, and actively pursue their professional development.

Section B, "Best Practices in Performing," details responsibilities and expected behaviors of group workers during the course of group counseling sessions (ASGW, 1998), including the group workers' primary commitment and responsibility to implement, adapt, and modify knowledge, skills, and techniques in the group plan to fit situational demands of the group (Trotzer, 2006). Group workers are aware of and monitor their strengths and weaknesses (ASGW, 1998). They explore their own cultural identities, develop cultural awareness of group members served, and use culturally relevant techniques in their group practice. Group workers have adequate understanding and knowledge of skills used for the group specialty area (psychotherapy, counseling, task, psycho-education), and are able to perform core group competencies as described in the *ASGW Professional Standards for the Training of Group Workers*. Group workers understand and implement models of group development, process observation, and therapeutic conditions. They facilitate and manage group communication and disclosures, and protect members from physical, emotional, or psychological trauma. Relationships with the group members, other than the counseling relationship, must be avoided to prevent compromise, loss of professional objectivity, or group member exploitation. Group workers assist members to make meaning of their group experience, develop individual goals, and evaluate the group experience between sessions and at the conclusion of the group. Group workers utilize an ethical decision-making model in responding to ethical challenges and issues concerning behavior of the leader or members.

Section C, "Best Practices in Group Processing," details responsibilities of group workers in processing, reflecting, and evaluating group process and outcomes (ASGW, 1998). To productively guide the group forward, group workers must engage members, supervisors, or colleagues in processing and assessing group and member goals, leader behaviors, and group dynamics and interventions (Trotzer, 2006). Processing with clients may take place within sessions, before and after sessions, between sessions, at the time of termination, and during later follow-up, as appropriate (ASGW, 1998). Group workers provide consultation to other organizations and seek out consultation from competent professionals when necessary.

In this section, the authors raise some ethical and professional issues in group work from the *ASGW Best Practice Guidelines* providing a fundamental ethical knowledge base for the beginning counseling student. Taken together, one's knowledge, technical skills, and personal qualities can help one develop and refine the ability to make sound ethical decisions. Becoming an ethical-minded group worker requires willingness to raise questions, think through the ethical considerations, determine a course of action to follow, and acknowledge responsibility for consequences of these determinations and actions. As noted earlier, ethical codes and standards are modified as society continues to change; therefore, counselors need to develop their own ethical stances about group issues that affect the welfare of the group and its members.

ETHICAL AND PROFESSIONAL ISSUES IN MULTICULTURAL AND DIVERSITY COUNSELING

Many diverse cultural and ethnic groups live in the United States. The effectiveness of counseling with clients from these sometimes distinct cultural and ethnic groups depends on many factors, but the most basic is for the counselor and the client to understand and relate to each other. Weinrach and Thomas (1996) noted that people find it easier to understand and relate to others when they share similarities with others, such as age, culture, religion, education level, gender, language, sexual orientation, physique, and socioeconomic background. It is rare that counselors will share all these similarities with their clients at any given time. Therefore it is important that counselors be sensitive to clients' different cultural backgrounds, special needs, values and beliefs, and other differences. It is equally important that counselors have knowledge of clients' backgrounds, be competent in skills and techniques, and have awareness of their own biases, values, beliefs, and prejudices.

Cultural competence begins with self-understanding and learning how one comes to view oneself in relation to others. Understanding and defining one's own value system and exploring personal prejudices and biases can improve one's ability to understand and appreciate client value systems. In recent years, multicultural competence has been emphasized as an important aspect of ethical counseling practice. "Multicultural counseling refers to preparation and practices that integrate multicultural and culture-specific awareness, knowledge, and skills into counseling interactions" (Arredondo et al., 1996, p. 42).

According to the 2005 *ACA Code of Ethics* counselors should not discriminate on the basis of age, disability, religion, ethnicity, race, social status, or sexual orientation. While counseling interactions may involve a white (Euro-American) counselor with clients of color or others from distinct backgrounds, counselors counseling with clients who are culturally different from themselves need competence to work successfully with these clients (Corey, Corey, & Callanan, 2003; Herlihy & Watson, 2003; Remley & Herlihy, 2005). A brief review of three multicultural competencies cited by Arredondo et al. (1996) is offered here, but students are encouraged to acquire additional knowledge from other resources.

The first of these three multicultural competencies is "Counselor awareness of own cultural values and biases." Culturally skilled counselors believe that cultural self-awareness and sensitivity to one's own cultural heritage is essential. They are also aware of how their own cultural background and experiences have influenced their attitudes, values, and biases about psychological processes, and how these affect their work with clients. It is important to realize the limits of one's own multicultural competence and expertise, and recognize sources of discomfort with differences between counselor and client in terms of race, ethnicity, culture, sexual orientation, religion, socioeconomic background, physique, and language. Culturally skilled counselors also seek educational, consultative, and training experiences to improve their competence, understanding, and knowledge in order to effectively work with culturally different clients and clients of diverse backgrounds (Arredondo et al., 1996).

"Counselor awareness of client's worldview" is the second multicultural competency. Counselors need awareness of how their negative and positive emotional reactions toward other racial and ethnic groups may be harmful to the counseling relationship. The authors encourage students to be aware of stereotypes and preconceived notions they may hold toward other racial and ethnic minority groups and to explore these stereotypes to gain more awareness and understanding. Counselors need to obtain specific knowledge about different cultural groups, especially the groups that clients represent. This knowledge may be about, but not limited to, client life experiences, values, beliefs, and assumptions. Culturally skilled counselors are also advised to become knowledgeable, through literature and relevant research, about mental and other disorders that may affect various ethnic and racial groups (Arredondo et al., 1996).

The third multicultural competency, "Culturally appropriate intervention strategies," details the importance of counselors valuing and appreciating bilingualism and having an awareness that the overall Western understanding of the characteristics of counseling may clash with the values of clients from various cultural groups. Culturally skilled counselors have knowledge of family structures, hierarchies, community values, and beliefs of the clients with whom they counsel. It can also be important to seek consultation with traditional healers or spiritual leaders in the treatment of culturally different clients when appropriate (Arredondo et al., 1996).

Emphasis throughout these competencies is on positive individual change. To become ethically minded, culturally skilled counselors, students should engage in a self-examination process, assess knowledge pertaining to other cultures and clients from diverse backgrounds, and become aware of and combat personal and social stereotypes and prejudices. Keeping client worth, dignity, uniqueness, and potential as primary foci can be especially helpful in respecting clients within the context of client cultures.

MAINTAINING ETHICAL BOUNDARIES IN COUNSELING

Ethics helps counselors remember that counseling is not focused on counselors, but on people seeking assistance with a range of human concerns. While some clients need help narrowing positive opportunities, others may need help in enhancing self-knowledge, making sense of life, and/or responsible self-governance. Vulnerable and trusting, clients may look to counselors for guidance and direction. It is the counselor's responsibility to guard that trust and never use it to the counselor's personal advantage. ACA's standards indicate that relationships outside the client-counselor relationship need to be avoided whenever possible.

Counselors may minimize or not recognize the power differential between themselves and clients, while clients may readily and routinely defer to their perceptions of counselor comments. The following example was experienced by one of this chapter's authors: A woman shared how she had encouraged her newly married 20-something son and his young wife to seek counseling for their troubled relationship. After two months, the son told his mother he and his wife were getting a divorce. Surprised, the mother asked how they came to that decision. Her son proceeded to tell his mother that the counselor said they should just get a divorce since it seemed they could not resolve their conflict. Among this author's thoughts were the following: What was the context for these alleged counselor comments? Might the son have interpreted the counselor in that way because of what he wanted to hear? If this client inference was accurate, where was this counselor educated and what had the counselor learned about client autonomy? Whatever the actual occurrences in this example, one sees here a manifestation of counselor power/influence over clients. Seen in light of this example, counselors must remind clients of the responsibility to make their own decisions and accept responsibility for their choices. Counselors who decide for clients or tell a client what to do cross a vital ethical counseling boundary.

Only in the rarest of cases, for example, when a client appears incapable of self-governance or poses a risk to self or others, would a counselor tell a client what to do. Rather, counselors communicate via empathy, warmth, genuineness, and other appropriate interventions that help clients notice opportunities for choice, learn means of deciding, and accept responsibility for decisions and their consequences. The counselor's role is not about making decisions for clients, but about helping clients see life and life problems from varying perspectives affording increased client self-awareness, a clearer picture of choices and consequences, and a sense of responsibility. Steps for ethical decision-making by counselors are mentioned very near the end of this chapter, with attention to Welfel's (2010) model.

Counselors also have a tremendous responsibility to take care of their own needs outside their work so they do not inadvertently meet counselor needs at client expense. Although client exploitation may take many forms, one of the most common transgressions cited by licensing boards is sexual contact with a client (Texas Board of Examiners of Licensed Professional Counselors, 2006). Counselors are taught that sexual intimacy is inappropriate, yet it occurs with some frequency in mental health professions (Texas Board, 2006). How do counselors miss signs that lead to this most grievous act of impropriety with clients? Laaser (1998) outlines "warning signs" of therapists who offend. Counselors need to be increasingly aware of potential acts that break the bounds of the client-counselor relationship.

Laaser (1998) notes 14 warning signs addressing the issue of crossing sexual boundaries between counselor and client. Some of these could also be warning signs a counselor needs to be introspective in addressing concerns in the counselor's own life as a means to avoid meeting personal needs at client expense:

1. Absence of supervision and accountability in the counselor's life,
2. marital or relationship concerns,
3. presence of sexual addiction including pornography,
4. presence of chronic low level depression in life,
5. trauma from early life that is unrecognized and unresolved,
6. agreeing to give certain clients special time and attention outside the regular bounds of the client-counselor relationship,
7. seeing certain clients at odd times,
8. looking forward to certain clients toward whom a counselor might have a sexual attraction,
9. posting in client record notes that a client is seductive,
10. having feelings of anger toward one gender,
11. sitting close to clients and hugging or otherwise touching inappropriately,
12. carrying feelings of entitlement for meeting personal needs through one's client,
13. using sexual humor frequently, and
14. having a disproportionate amount of stress and work (Laaser, 1998, p. 60).

All counselors might acknowledge some of these signs, stressing the importance of counselors' taking inventory in their own lives and deciding what they need to do to bring balance to themselves so they can be fully present for a client's needs. Counselors are encouraged to have healthy relationships outside the profession and be involved in community-related activities and groups that give them a well rounded life. Healthy friendships and hobbies can provide that balance counselors need to decrease the chances of developing inappropriate relationships with their clients. Certainly, personal counseling for a counselor can be a highly insightful means of and for processing issues related to any aspect of meeting a counselor's needs at the expense of one's clients. Constant practitioner self-monitoring and frequent recommitment and rededication to client worth, dignity, uniqueness, and potential could be helpful and systematic means to staying focused on client well-being, especially at those times when a counselor might notice that he or she is experiencing these warning signs. Suffice it to say, counselors occupy a vital position of trust requiring constant and strict adherence to requirements of this trust.

Ethical Boundaries in Counselor Supervision

Another area counselors need to be aware of is ethical boundaries associated with the supervisory relationship. Supervisors have a responsibility to supervisees to practice ethically and treat supervisees with respect and dignity. The following describes qualities that a supervisee should expect in a supervisor: (1) well-educated and experienced in supervision, (2) involved in continuing education, (3) appropriately licensed and approved, (4) adherence to an established theory of supervision and ability to articulate it to a supervisee, (5) appropriate malpractice insurance, and (6) informed consent with supervisees (Association for Counselor Education & Supervision [ACES], 1995).

Post-degree supervisees, such as LPC interns, have an ethical responsibility for the following: (1) completed academic requirements for an advanced degree, (2) provision of transcripts and letters of reference to one's supervisor, (3) appropriate malpractice insurance, (4) provision of a statement of counseling philosophy to the supervisor, and (5) adherence to an informed consent agreement with the supervisor (ACES, 1995).

Supervisor and supervisee should jointly decide mutual expectations for the supervision experience. For ethical administration of supervision, the following need to be in place at the start of the supervision experience: a formal contract should be signed by both supervisor and supervisee regarding the supervision experience (Bernard & Goodyear, 2004). Second, clients need to be informed that their counselor is being supervised and is not yet licensed to practice independently. Third, if applicable, the person responsible for paying the counseling fee should be notified that the counselor is under supervision. Fourth, written permission from clients for audio or video taping their sessions should be in place from the start of the supervision experience. The supervisor and supervisee also need to have contingency plans in case of emergencies for the supervisee's clients (ACES, 1995).

Avoiding Multiple Relationships

Potential problems with multiple roles with clients need early identification as a first step in resolution. Counselors in small communities commonly experience multiple relations difficulty, but it can also happen with counselors in churches and other communities within communities. Multiple roles between supervisee and supervisor in all phases of counselor preparation should be discussed before they become problematic. Peer status is the eventual goal for supervisors and supervisees, but during the supervision process, supervisors are responsible for keeping the boundaries. One of this chapter's authors had an experience with an intern in an entry-level counseling program that illustrates an effective boundary placed by the supervisor. The supervisee came to the faculty supervisor after an ethics lecture and asked if this orientation were required of all counselors. The faculty supervisor responded, "Yes," and the student supervisee went on to say, "So that's why our practicum supervisor would not go shopping and to the movies with us. We thought she just didn't like us." Another key area for supervisors is awareness of supervisees' personal issues that are interfering or have the potential of interfering in working with a particular client or clients. The supervisor may need to suggest outside counseling for the supervisee (Borders & Brown, 2005).

CONCLUSION

In closing, readers are encouraged to "keep their eyes on the prize," to read, discuss, and practice the *ACA Code of Ethics*, guided by the principles cited earlier. One fundamental, necessary skill highlighted in the U.S. Labor Secretary's

Commission on Achieving Necessary Skills report (1993) stipulates the need for learning to learn in an age when learning must be continuing and lifelong. Valuable tools abound for lifelong learning about ethics, including textbooks, workshops, professional conferences, and a number of poignant and timely papers and related stimuli on the ACA home page. On ACA's home page, for example, one finds the standards, topical interviews on aspects of the standards, and related papers and discussions on ethics.

Additionally, individuals are encouraged to consider and embrace aspirational ethics as a means of enhancing the profession and the counseling each practitioner provides each client. In turn and in so doing, counselors can move toward continuous rededication to self, clients, and the counseling profession. As counseling students and counselors increase their own self-understanding, they can also clarify their values and principles as part of a journey of actively implementing these values and principles in modeling counselor support for human worth, dignity, uniqueness, and potential.

CHAPTER REVIEW

1. Ethics is universal and has origins in ancient history with philosophers such as Aristotle, Plato, and Moses.
2. Ethics in counseling serves to guide the profession in providing direction for practice with the intent of protecting the client.
3. Ethical standards were developed by mental health professional associations to guide new professionals and practicing counselors in the field of counseling. ACA, ASCA, ACES, and NCDA are among counseling related professions with specific codes of ethics for counselors to follow. ACA's *Code of Ethics* applies to all counselors, ASCA's code of ethics is designed specifically for school counselors, ASGW's *Best Practices Guidelines* provides direction in working with groups, Multicultural Counseling Competencies denote necessary skills needed by all counselors, ACES' code of ethics focuses on counselor supervision practice, and NCDA's code emphasizes standards for career development practitioners and career counselors.
4. Specific issues in counseling include multiple relationships, confidentiality, and legal aspects in counseling.
5. Ethical decision-making models assist beginning and seasoned professionals in determining a path to deal with ethical matters from a linear perspective by providing direction for counselors who may find themselves in a situation where an ethical violation is encountered.

REVIEW QUESTIONS

1. How has ethical decision-making evolved over time?
2. What are some elements of ethics that pertain to business and other environments?
3. Define and explain ethical and legal behavior as it relates to counselors and other mental health professionals.
4. Why are ethical standards important for professions and professional organizations?
5. What are the focal principles in the preamble to the 2005 *ACA Code of Ethics*?
6. What are some ethical guidelines for group workers?

7. What are the three multicultural competencies for counselors?
8. What are the warning signs of counselors who offend the counseling relationship?
9. What are three elements of Welfel's ethical decision model?

ADDITIONAL RESOURCES

- American Association for Marriage and Family Therapy: *Code of Ethics* (http://www.aamft.org/resources/)
- American Counseling Association: *Code of Ethics* (http://www.counseling.org/Resources/CodeOfEthics/TP/Home/CT2.aspx)
- American Psychiatric Association: *Principles of Medical Ethics With Annotations Especially Applicable to Psychiatry* (www.psych.org/MainMenu/PsychiatricPractice/Ethics/ResourcesStandards/)
- American Psychological Association: *Ethical Principles of Psychologists and Code of Conduct* (http://www.apa.org/ethics/code.html)

- Association for Multicultural Counseling and Development: *Multicultural Competencies and Standards* (http://www.counseling.org/Resources/)
- Association for Specialists in Group Work: *Best Practice Guidelines* (http://www.asgw.org/PDF/Best_Practices.pdf)
- National Association of Social Workers: *Code of Ethics* (http://www.socialworkers.org/pubs/Code/code.asp)
- National Career Development Association: *Ethical Standards* (www.ncda.org/pdf/ethicalstandards.pdf)

REFERENCES

American Association for Marriage and Family Therapy. (2001). *Code of ethics*. Washington, DC: Author.

American Counseling Association. (1995). *ACA code of ethics and standards of practice*. Alexandria, VA: Author.

American Counseling Association. (2005). *Code of ethics*. Alexandria, VA: Author.

American Psychiatric Association. (2001). *Principles of medical ethics with annotations especially applicable to psychiatry*. Washington, DC: Author.

American Psychological Association. (2002). *Ethical principles of psychologists and code of conduct*. Washington, DC: Author.

Arredondo, P., Toporek, R., Brown, S. P., Jones, J., Sanchez, J., Locke, D. C., & Stadler, H. (1996). Operationalization of the multicultural counseling competencies. *Journal of Multicultural Counseling and Development, 24*, 42–78.

Association for Counselor Education & Supervision. (1995). Ethical guidelines for counseling supervisors. *Counselor Education & Supervision, 34*, 270–276.

Association for Specialists in Group Work. (1998). *Best Practice Guidelines*. Author.

Beauchamp, T. L., & Childress, J. F. (2001). *Principles of biomedical ethics* (5th ed.). New York: Oxford University Press.

Bernard, J. M. & Goodyear, R. K. (2004). *Fundamentals of clinical supervision*. Boston: Allyn & Bacon.

Borders, L. D. & Brown, L. L. (2005). *The new handbook of counseling supervision*. Mahwah, NJ: Lawrence Earlbaum Associates.

Corey, G., Corey, M. S., & Callanan, P. (2003). *Issues and ethics in the helping professions* (6th ed.). Pacific Grove, CA: Brooks/Cole.

Concise Oxford American dictionary. (2006). New York: Oxford University Press.

Council for the Accreditation of Counseling and Related Educational Programs. (2001). *CACREP accreditation standards and procedures manual*. Alexandria, VA: author.

Eliot, T. S. (1934). The rock: A pageant play, written for performance at Sadler's Wells Theatre, 28 May–9 June, 1934, on behalf of the Forty-five Churches Fund of the Diocese of London. *Book of Words*. New York: Harcourt, Brace.

Engels, D. W. (1975). *John Watson Murray Rothney: Development of his published thought*.

Unpublished dissertation, University of Wisconsin–Madison.

Engels, D. W., Wilborn, B. L., & Schnieder, L. J. (1990). Ethics curricula for counselor preparation programs. In *Ethical standards casebook* (pp. 111–126). Alexandria, VA: American Association for Counseling and Development.

Herlihy, B., & Watson, Z. E. (2003). Ethical issues and multicultural competence in counseling. In F. D. Harper & J. McFadden (Eds.), *Culture and counseling: New approaches* (pp. 363–378). Boston: Pearson.

Hutchins, R. M., & Adler, M. J. (1952a). Aristotle I. In *Great books of the western world*. Chicago: Encyclopedia Britannica.

Hutchins, R. M., & Adler, M. J. (1952b). Aristotle II. In *Great books of the western world*. Chicago: Encyclopedia Britannica.

Hutchins, R. M., & Adler, M. J. (1952c). Plato. In *Great books of the western world*. Chicago: Encyclopedia Britannica.

Janis, I. L., & Mann, L. (1977). *Decision-making: A psychological analysis of conflict, choice, and commitment*. New York: Free Press.

Johns, J. (1988). *Ethics course syllabus*. Unpublished manuscript, U.S. National Defense University, Washington, DC.

Kitchener, K. S. (1986). Teaching applied ethics in counselor education: An integration of psychological processes and philosophical analysis. *Journal of Counseling and Development, 64*, 306–310.

Kocet, M. M. (2006). Ethical challenges in a complex world: Highlights of the 2005 *ACA Code of Ethics. Journal of Counseling and Development, 84*, 228–234.

Laaser, M. (1998). Therapists who offend. *Christian Counseling Today, 6*, 17–62.

National Association of Social Workers. (1999). *Code of ethics*. Silver Springs, MD: Author.

National Career Development Association. (2007). *Ethical standards*. Tulsa, OK: Author.

Pederson, P. B. (1998). The cultural context of the American counseling association code of ethics. *Journal of Counseling and Development, 76*, 23–28.

Plato. (1977). *Plato complete works* (J. M. Cooper & D. S. Hutchinson, Eds.). Indianapolis, IN: Hackett Publishing Company.

Random house dictionary. (2001). New York: Ballantine Books.

Remley, T. P., & Herlihy, B. (2005). *Ethical, legal, and professional issues in counseling* (2nd ed.). Upper Saddle River, NJ: Merrill Prentice Hall.

Stewart-Sicking, J. A. (2008). Virtues, values, and the good life: Alasdair Macintyre's virtue ethics and its implications for counseling. *Counseling and Values, 52*, 156–171.

Tarasoff v. Regents of the University of California, 13 Cal. #d 177,529 p. 2d 553 (1974), vacated, 17 Cal. 3d 425, 552 p. 2d 334 (1976).

Texas Board of Examiners of Licensed Professional Counselors. (2006, April). *LPC board meeting with counselor educators at Texas universities*. Austin, TX.

Thapar v. Zezulka, 994.S.W. 2d at 635. Austin: Texas Supreme Court (1999).

Trotzer, J. P. (2006). *The counselor and the group* (4th ed.). New York: Routledge.

U.S. Department of Labor. (1993). *Secretary's commission on achieving necessary skills executive summary*. Washington, DC: U.S. Department of Labor.

Webster's new world dictionary and thesaurus. (2002). New York: Wiley Publishing.

Weinrach, S. G., & Thomas, K. R. (1996). The counseling profession's commitment to diversity-sensitive counseling: A critical reassessment. *Journal of Counseling and Development, 73*, 472–477.

Welfel, E. R. (2010). *Ethics in counseling and psychotherapy: Standards, research, and emerging issues* (4th ed.). Pacific Grove, CA: Brooks/Cole.

Zuckerman, M. B. (2004, January 19). Editorial: Policing the corporate suites. *U.S. News & World Report*, p. 72.

CHAPTER 5

Counseling With Diverse Clients

LEARNING OBJECTIVES

After reading this chapter, you should be able to

- recount the history of multicultural and pluralistic trends;

- understand multiple identities and their development, including the roles of specific acculturative experiences;

- describe characteristics and concerns among diverse groups of individuals, families, and communities;

- discuss strategies for developing cultural self-awareness, social justice, and advocacy; and

- understand a counselor's role in eliminating intentional and unintentional bias, prejudice, oppression, and discrimination.

CHAPTER OUTLINE

Introduction

History of Multiculturalism

Cultural Identity Development
Multiple Identity Development Theory

Multicultural Competence

Racial and Ethnic Diversity
Blacks or African Americans
Latinos or Hispanic Americans
Asian Americans
Whites or European Americans
Other Ethnic Groups
Acculturation and Ethnic Identity

Other Forms of Diversity
Gender and Sexual Orientation
Religion
Age
Disabilities
Socioeconomic Status

Advocacy and Empowerment
Barriers
Becoming an Effective Advocate

Conclusion

CHAPTER REVIEW
REVIEW QUESTIONS
ADDITIONAL RESOURCES
REFERENCES

INTRODUCTION

The terms *diversity* and *multiculturalism* are often used interchangeably. In this chapter, we define *diversity* as the *condition* of a population whereas *multiculturalism* is a *movement* that advocates recognizing and celebrating the diversity within a population. Each person's culture is multifaceted, in that it includes demographic variables such as age and gender; status variables such as social or economic status; formal and informal affiliations such as professional organizations or personal groups to which one belongs; and ethnographic variables such as nationality, ethnicity, language, and religion (Pedersen, 1991). When counselors and clients meet, they bring to the counseling relationship their differences and similarities (C. C. Lee, 1997). Being multiculturally aware requires that counselors recognize these factors and their influence on the counseling process. In this chapter, we will provide an overview and definitions of multiculturalism, diversity, and other relevant concepts; provide information and counseling considerations for specific client groups; introduce the larger context of individual identity development; and finally, discuss the need for social action and the critical role of counselors within that process. In setting the stage by considering your own personal perspective, please review and reflect on the following active learning exercise.

Active Learning Exercise **5.1**

Consider your first impressions of going into a public place, like your university, a library, or a sports auditorium. How about your counseling program or class? Imagine looking around you at the other people who are there. What are they like? In what ways are they similar to you? In what ways are they different? What information or personal experiences do you use to arrive at your conclusions? Given the dramatically changing demographic landscape of the United States, professional counselors need to be well aware of the population dynamics not only within their own communities, but in their states, regions, and the nation, as well.

One Step Further: Make a table, with yourself and five or six others (e.g., in your classroom, your workplace, your softball team) listed along the left-hand column; the Racial and Ethnic and Other Forms of Diversity categories (or selected descriptors from them) along the top row of the next column to the right. Fill in as much information as you know about each person. We'll ask you to revisit this table as the chapter goes along.

HISTORY OF MULTICULTURALISM

There is a reciprocal influence between people and culture. Although people shape culture, culture also influences individuals and shapes their belief systems and ways of living. The influence of culture on individuals has been recognized by social anthropologists and psychologists for decades (see Willey & Herskovits, 1927), but only recently has multiculturalism been recognized as a vital force in understanding human development (Pedersen, 1991).

In the earlier days of the multiculturalism movement, *race* and *ethnicity* represented primary areas of focus. The term *race* has historically been described as a biological and geographic concept. Different races, based on biological and genetic distinctions, were first identified in the 15th and 16th centuries among European and non-European peoples. Some believe that these differences, along with the perception among Europeans that their non-European counterparts were inferior, served as support for enterprises such as colonization, slavery, and even extermination. Contemporary scholars consider race as a social construct, and that genetic within-group variations outnumber those between groups, widely disputing scientific support for earlier notions of racial differences in characteristics such as temperament, personality, and disorders (Zuckerman, 1990). More researchers are turning their attention to specific racial or ethnic characteristics, such as skin color (e.g., Nassar-McMillan, McFall-Roberts, Flowers, & Garrett, 2006), and studying the meaning of those characteristics among individuals and groups. *Ethnicity*, on the other hand, is more often thought of as individuals and groups sharing a bond with a homeland or historical past, such as kinship patterns, geographical concentrations, religious affiliation, language, or physical differences. *Race* and *ethnicity* are often used interchangeably, although they represent overlapping, yet distinct constructs.

More recently, additional characteristics such as gender (e.g., Carter & Parks, 2001; Robinson, 1999; Ross-Gordon, 2003), sexual orientation (Hutchins, 2006; Logan 2006; Mostade, 2006), religion (e.g., Nassar-McMillan, in press; Richards, Keller, & Smith, 2004), socioeconomic status (e.g., Liu & Pope-Davis, 2004; Nassar-McMillan, Karvonen, & Young, 2006), disabilities (e.g., Elliott & Mullins, 2004; Nassar-McMillan & Algozzine, 1999; Nosek & Hughes, 2004), and age (e.g., Davison, 2004) have emerged as important topics in better understanding our clients and their human development. Moreover, some scholars have proposed that specific intersections of such demographic characteristics may explain human development and behavior better than others, for example, race, class, and gender (e.g., Pope-Davis & Coleman, 2001) or race, ethnicity, and gender (e.g., Robinson, 2005). Others still view the relationships between risks and resiliencies among specific clients or client groups as predictive of their healthy adaptation, or functioning (e.g., Jamil, Nassar-McMillan, & Lambert, 2006).

These demographic combinations may prove especially useful in the current era in which the United States is rich with various diversities, but in which the census data on race and ethnicity is extremely limited. For example, "Whites" are defined, by the U.S. Census Bureau, as individuals having origins from Europe, the Middle East, or North Africa, including people who are Irish, German, Italian, Lebanese, Near Easterner, Arab, or Polish (Census, 2001). It also includes all Latino or Hispanic individuals who do not fall into the "some other race—Mexican, Puerto Rican, or Cuban"—group. Such individuals may not consider themselves White but are legally designated as such. Therefore, classifying different ethnic groups has been confusing and difficult. To address this difficulty, the U.S. Census Bureau has begun to collect data on respondent ancestry. Figure 5.1 depicts the fifteen largest ancestry groups reported in the 2000 census.

Governmental or other efforts to define or categorize individuals are considered *etic* classifications made by entities outside of those groups for

Fifteen Largest Ancestries: 2000

(In millions. Percent of total population in parentheses.
Data based on sample. For information on confidentiality protection,
sampling error, nonsampling error, and definitions, see
www.census.gov/prod/cen2000/doc/sf3.pdf)

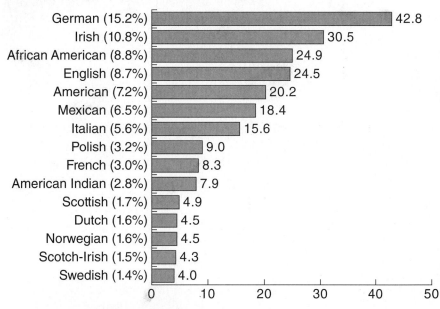

Source: U.S. Census Bureau, Census 2000 special tabulation.

FIGURE **5.1** Largest Ancestries in the United States

scientific or other purposes. At the same time, individuals from within those groups may not define themselves in the same way, therefore, such classification systems, particularly from a counseling perspective, may not do justice to individuals representing those groups. *Emic* distinctions, or those made from within specific demographic groups, may serve as more useful in understanding human development and behavior.

CULTURAL IDENTITY DEVELOPMENT

The counseling profession is largely based upon the notion that individuals go through developmental phases as they grow and change. Skilled professional counselors, therefore, must be able to identify the current stages of their clients in order to help them progress in their identity development. Developmental theories address the process of these changes, or development (Miller, 2001). These theories help to make meaning out of clients' lives in terms of their respective developmental levels, whether those are biological, cognitive, moral, or psychosocial. Moreover, definitions of development tend to be based on value judgments (Reeves, 1999). For example, Western (i.e., White or European) culture might define individualistic or self-reliant characteristics as more positive than collectivistic, or non-Western, ones.

Erik Erikson, in his foundational identity development theory, expanded Freud's psychoanalytic theory of psychosexual development (Erikson, 1968). Erikson's theory offered the world a model through which to help "normal" people find meaning in their daily lives and through everyday situations. Each stage in his eight-stage theory (Erikson, 1968) is comprised of a conflict with two oppositional outcomes, with the goal of each stage being that the conflict is worked out in a constructive and satisfactory manner. If so, the positive quality associated with the conflict becomes integrated into one's ego-identity. Conversely, if the conflict is not worked out satisfactorily, the associated negative quality becomes integrated. These developmental stages encompass the lifespan of individuals.

Although Erikson recognized the influence of culture on the psychosocial development of individuals, W. E. Cross (1971) developed the first psychosocial model of identity development focusing on individuals within a specific culture. He labeled his model the Nigrescence, or Black Racial Identity Model (1971). Cross' (1971, 1978, 1995) Nigrescence model introduced five distinct but overlapping stages that describe the process of development for individuals of African descent: Pre-Encounter, Encounter, Immersion/Emersion, Internalization, and Commitment. According to Myers et al. (1991), common stages among this model and many of those developed subsequently as appropriate for other specific multicultural groups include (1) a denial or lack of oppression awareness identity; (2) a questioning of their own oppressed identity; (3) a stage of immersion into the oppressed subculture; and (4) a self-realization of the limitations of that immersion and a concomitant integration of all known parts of self into a holistic being. Other models were subsequently developed to conceptualize the development of Asian Americans (Sue & Sue, 1973); women (Avery, 1977; Downing &

Roush, 1985); gay, lesbian, bisexual, and trangendered individuals (Cass, 1979; McCarn & Fassinger, 1996; Troiden, 1989), and minority groups in general (Atkinson, Morten, & Sue, 1989). There also is a White Racial Identity Model (Helms, 1990). Some researchers, in fact, have found relationships between White racial identity attitudes, corresponding to this model, and multicultural counseling competencies (Ottavi, Pope-Davis, & Dings, 1994) in that higher levels of development are related to higher levels of multicultural counseling competence.

Multiple Identity Development Theory

In recent years, as the multicultural counseling movement has made strides in understanding the development of individuals as cultural beings, theorists have recognized the limitations of unidimensional cultural assessments. For example, expanded models for understanding those with mixed-race backgrounds (Chideya, 1999) or with bicultural identities have been developed (Phinney, 1996). Still others have theorized identity development processes across the lifespan for multiethnic individuals and groups that allow for different identities to emerge and develop within different spheres, such as daily public social interactions versus the sphere of private life at home (Hermans, 2001). This relatively new line of thinking offers the potential for developing greater self-understanding and understanding of others, thereby also providing the potential for more effective counseling services.

Active Learning Exercise **5.2**

Using the table you developed earlier in this chapter, add President Barak Obama to the column on the left side. What do you know about his Racial and Ethnic and Other Forms of Diversity characteristics? Fill in the information that you know. Consider the sources from which you learned this information. Are the characteristics self-reported by President Obama or ascribed to him by another party or entity? What else can you research and learn about him to fill into the table?

MULTICULTURAL COMPETENCE

Multicultural competence is critical for professional counselors. To provide adequate services and overcome barriers in counseling, professional counselors must recognize and address the differences between themselves and their clients (Sue & Sue, 1990). Without awareness and the ability to address these similarities and differences, "counseling becomes an uncomfortable, unpredictable interaction for both parties, and the likelihood of a second session, let alone productive change, becomes low" (W. M. Lee, 1999, p. 2). Given the vast differences among people, it is likely that professional counselors *will* indeed be different from their clients. Moreover, a likely scenario will involve racial, cultural, and other types of diversity. For example, the average counselor might be older than the average client, more likely to be female than male (given the demographics of the counseling profession), and have higher levels of education, and thus higher levels of income, than her or his clients.

Developing multicultural competence typically involves focusing on three general areas: self-awareness, other awareness, and operationalizing the differences between the first two (Sue, Arredondo, & McDavis, 1992). Each of these three areas requires an in-depth self-analysis of attitudes and beliefs, knowledge, and skills. We believe that each of us is a multicultural being, and, like all of our personal characteristics, our multiculturalism is a part of ourselves that we bring into each and every counseling session. Thus, the more informed we are about our own culture, the more effective we will be in working with all of our clients. Multicultural competence will be revisited in the Advocacy and Empowerment section of this chapter.

RACIAL AND ETHNIC DIVERSITY

Each individual or family counseling client represents a rich cultural identity that needs to be explored without preconceived notions or judgments on the professional counselor's part. At the same time, it may be helpful to have some general information related to specific cultural groups, such as statistics about historical challenges faced by specific populations. Thus, this section focuses on ethnically based cultural groups and cultural groups based on other aspects of diversity. We hope to demonstrate how different groups may have similar or different needs and values. We also hope that the insights gained here can be transferred to better understand the dynamics and issues of other populations. Please keep in mind that self-identification is "a state of mind, not an inherited trait, and its acquisition often requires considerable effort" (W. E. Cross, 1991, p. 149). For example, a client could be born as a Jew, but may not practice the Jewish religion or identify with Jewish traditions (W. E. Cross, 1991). If a counselor were to greet a Jewish client when they first met with "Shalom," it might seem clever to the counselor, but it would demonstrate the opposite of multicultural competence. In other words, multiculturally competent counselors avoid labeling their clients and allow them to define their own cultural identities and affiliations. Moreover, the information provided here is extremely brief and only provides a snapshot of a much greater context. In short, we recommend further exploration into the unique and complex cultural backgrounds of your respective clients.

Earlier, we explored the complexity of immigration and census classifications. You may have seen or heard the term *people of color*. We believe that this term allows for more flexibility and autonomy on the part of individuals or groups for self-definition and self-determination in terms of their own race and ethnicity. With the vast number of diverse groups represented in the United States, we will present specific information to the four largest populations. Therefore, in the next section we present cultural information that may be relevant to individuals who define themselves as being either African American (or Black), Hispanic or Latino American, Asian American, or European American (or White); and quite possibly as a person of color.

Blacks or African Americans

African American and *Black* are terms used interchangeably to categorize Americans who are descendents of people born in Africa. Most African Americans are descendents of Black slaves brought over from Africa during the slave trades from the 15th and 19th century. "African Americans/Blacks" comprise approximately 12 percent of the U.S. population (U.S. Census Bureau, 2001).

The poverty rate of Blacks is 24.4 percent higher than that of other ethnic groups (U.S. Census Bureau, 2004). Those who live in impoverished environments may show adaptive behaviors that are not considered healthy in mainstream culture. Behaviors may be related to survival and, therefore, adaptation, rather than representing mental health issues: "Aggression, strong emotions, and cunning are aspects of adaptation developed through life in a particular environment" (A. Cross, 1974, p. 165). Therefore, the experiences and environment of specific clients, along with historical oppressions of African Americans in general, must be taken into account by professional counselors in order to best understand the behaviors, attitudes, and perceptions of their African American clients. The Black identity model (W. E. Cross, 1991) may be a useful tool to both clients and counselors to understand where clients are in their identity development.

Latinos or Hispanic Americans

The terms *Hispanic* and *Latino* are often used interchangeably, but there are differences in both the actual origins of each, as well as individual preferences for terms among the population, based on sociopolitical or other issues. Hispanics comprise the largest minority group in the United States, at 12.5 percent of the overall population (U.S. Census Bureau, 2001). Hispanics include Spanish-speaking individuals and families, such as those with origins from Mexico or South America, but include other languages and many subcultures.

Hispanic groups share similar values and issues such as familismo, personalismo, and machismo (Andres-Hyman, Ortiz, Anez, Paris, & Davidson, 2006). Familismo is the cultural value of including extended family members such as godparents or close friends in family life (Andres-Hyman et al., 2006; Cox & Monk, 1993; Sabogal, Marin, Otero-Sabogal, Marin, et al., 1987). It represents a collectivistic view in which elders are respected and the focus of daily life is on the needs of the family rather than the individual. Personalismo is addressing each other in an informal manner (Andres-Hyman et al., 2006), signifying closeness and respect. Lastly, machismo is an attitude that men should be masculine and behave in a certain manner. Machismo is found in many cultures (Fragoso & Kashubeck, 2000), and although it is often viewed as negative and associated with being controlling of women and children, others view it as a strength of Hispanic men in terms of their role in providing and caring for the family (Mayo, 1997).

Asian Americans

Asian Americans represent ethnic groups from Asian countries such as China, Japan, Korea, Thailand, Laos, Vietnam, and Cambodia, among others. Asian

Americans comprise 3.6 percent of the United States (U.S. Census Bureau, 2001). This cultural group also represents a wide array of languages and subcultures. Furthermore, some Asian groups have been established in the United States for generations, while others are new immigrants or refugees (e.g., Laotians, Hmong, Vietnamese, Cambodians); thus, counseling issues for some Asians may be linked to acculturation or immigration. For example, different reasons for immigration such as economic pursuit versus political asylum or refuge are likely to have a great impact on the daily life and functioning of an Asian American client or family. Thus, the term *model minority* sometimes used to describe later generation Asian Americans who are professionally, economically, and in other ways "successful" may not accurately describe the needs of Asian Americans who are struggling in educational, employment, and other arenas due to their recent immigration challenges.

Important in most Asian cultures are filial piety and the collectivistic view that one must respect elders and work to better the family and group rather than the individual. "Respect for self-control" and "shame avoidance" are also important values of Asian culture (Kim, 1995). Bear in mind that, although the majority of Asian Americans may hold these values, generational and acculturation experiences in the United States may have shaped the values and views of others. Similar to our belief that people have the right to self-identify, individuals also have the right to choose their values and views. Comedian Margaret Cho, who makes jokes around being an L.A. "valley girl" of Korean descent, might serve as a good example of personal self-identification in a generational and acculturational context.

Whites or European Americans

European Americans, also referred to as *Whites*, comprise about 75 percent of the population of the United States. Although European Americans are the majority and may hold certain privilege and power (McIntosh, 1998, 2003; Sullivan, 2006), it is important to understand the specific needs of the European American individuals and families in counseling. This view has recently been brought to light for a variety of reasons. Contemporary scholars and practitioners interested in multicultural competence believe that the omission of "White" from the discussion inadvertently omits the discussion of White privilege—that is, the social, economic, and political advantages of being White in the United States (Krieger, Williams, & Zierler, 1999; C. Lee, 1997; Sullivan, 2006). As a professional counselor it is important to understand cultural issues related to being White, or European American, regardless of one's own ethnicity or cultural background. Furthermore, counselors should also be aware of the needs and issues of economically and educationally disadvantaged Whites.

Other Ethnic Groups

In the 2000 U.S. census, a Some Other Race category was incorporated to capture data from groups not identified as African American/Black, Asian, Native American, or White. This group included Moroccan, South African, Belizean, or Hispanic origin such as Mexican, Puerto Rican, or Cuban.

Moreover, the government defined *White* as individuals with origins in Europe, the Middle East, or North Africa, including people who are Irish, German, Italian, Lebanese, Near Easterner, Arab, or Polish (U.S. Census Bureau, 2001). Individuals with such ancestries may or may not consider themselves White. Furthermore, U.S. census definitions may be fluid for many groups, meaning that the designations have changed many times over the course of U.S. history. For example, Arab Americans have been defined in the last century as being from Turkey in Asia, Syrian, Asiatic, Colored, Other, and, recently, White (Samhan, 1999). This phenomenon aptly illustrates the importance of self-identification for individuals and families with whom we work as professional counselors.

Native Americans comprise a special designation within the U.S. government classification system. Although not among the four largest population groups (in fact, representing slightly less than 1 percent of the U.S. population) according to census data, this population represents an alarming array of risk factors. For example, the annual income level among Native American Indians is approximately 62 percent of the national average. Economic poverty can lead to an array of counseling-related issues (e.g., lack of hope, substance abuse, low self-esteem, lack of educational opportunities). Among the strengths of this group are the spiritual focus of the cultural beliefs and values.

Learning about and assessing client issues from a cultural context involves knowing something about your clients' cultural origins. In order to better understand our clients and to help them arrive at an understanding of their own ethnicity, we introduce the important constructs of *acculturation* and *ethnic identity*.

Acculturation and Ethnic Identity

Acculturation is typically characterized as the level to which first generation immigrants and, in some contexts, their offspring shift from their country of origin to the new host country, in terms of a variety of variables such as values, beliefs, and attitudes (Berry, 1980, 1990). It typically denotes an affiliation with the new culture, while either foregoing the former one or integrating it into the new value structure.

In contrast to acculturation, ethnic identity is characterized as an affiliation with the country of origin, rather than the new or existing host culture (Phinney, 1996). It is more typically associated with later generations of immigrants of particular origins. The higher a person's identification with and pride in their country or culture of origin, the higher his or her ethnic identity with that culture.

Although the constructs of acculturation and ethnic identity are independent of one another and represent dichotomous viewpoints—such as identification with new culture versus culture of origin or beliefs about culture and other external concepts versus beliefs about self and self-concept—both constructs represent ways of reconciling values and other aspects of two, sometimes competing, cultural perspectives and experiences. Generational gaps are often found between recent and later immigrant and refugee ethnic groups.

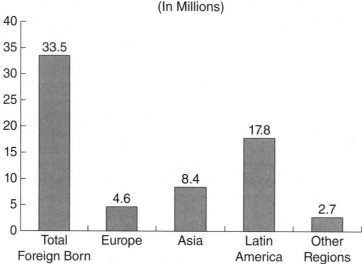

Foreign-Born Population by World Region of Birth: 2003
(In Millions)

Source: Current Population Survey, Annual Social and Economic Supplement, 2003

FIGURE **5.2** U.S. Foreign-Born Population by World Region

For example, U.S.-born individuals may be more likely to have encountered a broader range of bicultural experiences. In such a case, then, counseling parents may require different considerations than counseling children because of the different experiences and levels of acculturation. In any case, contemporary theorists believe that successful acculturation and resolution of personal ethnic identity development and identity within the host culture appear to be critically important aspects of overall wellness and adjustment, particularly among earlier generations of immigrants (e.g., Berry, 1986; Phinney, 1996; Oppedal, Røysamb, & Sam, 2004). Figure 5.2 depicts the distributions of the U.S. foreign-born population by world region.

OTHER FORMS OF DIVERSITY

The diversity among us reaches far beyond race or ethnicity. As a counselor, you may be different from your clients in terms of gender, sexual orientation, religion, and age but represent the same or similar ethnic backgrounds. Although the diversity issues between you and your clients are limitless, we will cover only selected major diversity issues in this section.

Gender and Sexual Orientation

According to federal statistics, males and females represent the total population almost equally (U.S. Census Bureau, 2007). Historically, biological sex was viewed as dichotomous, in that biological males were boys or men, and biological females as girls or women. Fairly recently, this biological predetermination has been refuted by social scientists, who tend now to approach gender as a social construct. As such, society has a heavy influence on how each gender should think and behave. Women in most cultures are expected to be nurturing. Men are expected to provide for the family financially. These roles are particularly associated with heterosexual relationships. Although some gender roles are slowly dissipating in the Western culture, some immigrants, refugees, and more traditional Americans may still uphold them. In addition, the disparities between men and women in arenas such as educational attainment, salaries earned, and career opportunities are still present with women continuing to experience more barriers to advancement than men. Thus, in counseling individuals, couples, or families, professional counselors need to be aware of gender issues within a larger context. For example, with the current trend of dual career households, helping family members or couples to discuss partner equity such as completing household tasks may improve marital satisfaction (Saginak & Saginak, 2005).

Active Learning Exercise **5.3**

Review the group table you developed earlier in this chapter. As you consider each group member's gender, speculate on how being male or female, or some other self-identified gender, has influenced his or her life at various developmental points. Perhaps you could interview specific individuals to learn more about this influence. How has your own gender influenced your development at various points throughout your life? How would your own life have been different, at various points in time, if you had been born a different gender?

Although individuals who are lesbian, gay, bisexual, or transgendered (LGBT) exist within different ethnic groups, they are still minorities in our society. There are 8.8 million gay, lesbian, and bisexual persons in the United States (Gates, 2006). Lesbians and gays prefer sexual partners of the same sex while bisexuals prefer both genders. Transgenders are individuals who were born as one gender but identify themselves as the opposite gender. In the United States, persons who are LGBT, and their needs, are often invisible. They often face isolation and discrimination due to their sexual orientation and self-identity as a male or female (Fassinger & Arseneau, 2007).

Despite these challenges, same-sex marriages are increasing (Gates, 2006). Additionally, one in nine unmarried partners are of the same sex (U.S. Census Bureau, 2003). This increase in same-sex partnerships may be due to individuals being more willing to choose and disclose their preferences (Gates, 2006) and the changing views of society. When counseling LGBT clients, culture of origin and its views toward sexual orientation must be considered along with the oppression faced within mainstream U.S. society (Savage & Harley, 2005).

Religion

Christianity remains the most predominant religion in the United States, reported by over 75 percent of U.S. Americans. In a telephone survey of 50,281 individuals in 48 states, the four top religions indicated were Christianity (76.5 percent), Judaism (1.3 percent), Islam (.5 percent), and Buddhism (.5 percent) (Kosmin, Mayer, & Keysar, 2001). In the world population, there are 19 religions with several hundred subdivisions (Barret, Kurian, & Johnson, 2001). Thus, religious diversity needs also to be considered in our work with clients. Religions are practices and beliefs of individuals, which may affect behaviors related to gender, sexual orientation, and many other aspects of diversity. Because many professional counselors may be a part of the Christian majority, it is especially important to be aware of how one's own faith or religious practices might interplay with preferred counseling theories, techniques, and interventions, as well as one's own values and lifestyle choices. It is equally important to consider clients' degree of religiosity or lack of identification with a specific religion. Not every client will identify with a religion at all or with a single religion. In fact, a recent survey conducted through Trinity College in Hartford, Connecticut, revealed a drop in religious affiliation over the past decade (Kosmin & Keysar, 2009). Thus, clients' religious self-identification as well as level of religiosity need to be explored in the context of their daily coping preferences and strategies.

Age

Different age groups may have different developmental and life-stage issues. Individuals' developmental issues and perceptions of life are based on the abilities with which they were born (nature) and the influences of their environment (nurture). When professional counselors understand the developmental and environmental influences on their clients, they may be able to distinguish between what is a developmental, environmental, or a problematic health condition. It is important to take into consideration the physical, cognitive, emotional, and social development of clients of any age (Berk, 1998). In addition to developmental factors, the environment is equally important in shaping individuals. Environmental issues include living conditions, available resources, and any relevant past or present experiences such as trauma or life changes, among others.

Clients in the *older* age group, often described as individuals aged 65 and above, may be facing the end of a long career or experiencing physical or cognitive deterioration. Many older adults who may not be well educated or may not have had professional careers may lack financial stability, putting them below the poverty level. Individuals in the United States today are expected to live as long as 85 or 90 years old (Berk, 1998). Specific issues to be aware of in the elder adult groups are their cognitive, physical, and sexual abilities, and their access to resources. Older clients may become disabled due to illnesses or deterioration in their development such as immobility or dementia. Furthermore, those who are immigrants or refugees may experience emotional stress relating to their acculturation experiences or financial situation (Haley, Robb, Jang, & Han, 2003).

Disabilities

Approximately 20 percent of individuals in the United States have a disability, with more than half of those representing severe disabilities (McNeil, 1997). Individuals with disabilities present diverse issues. Individuals with disabilities experience issues that are both similar to and different from individuals without disabilities. For example, individuals who are blind may see the world differently than those who are not blind because they see the world through different senses. Often, individuals with disabilities are capable of living a normal life if they have access to places and things that individuals without disabilities have. Our society, however, has a habit of developing cities and products for the majority. As a result, those in the minority—in this case individuals with disabilities—are at a disadvantage; for example, those who are wheelchair bound may not be able to access buildings with stairs, and those who are blind may not be able to see the computer screen or use the Internet without installing extra and costly programs.

Socioeconomic Status

Poverty, with impacts on issues such as homelessness, family structure, and educational achievement and attainment, among others, afflicts one in four children (Flaxman, Schwartz, Weiler, & Layey, 1998). In 2005, 13 million people in the United States lived below the poverty line (U.S. Census Bureau, 2006). Hispanic Americans and Blacks represent the highest percentage of individuals living in poverty, with Hispanic Americans at 21.8 percent and Blacks at 24.9 percent (U.S. Census Bureau, 2006a). Whites and Asian Americans were at 8.4 percent and 10.9 percent respectively (U.S. Census Bureau, 2006b). Low socioeconomic status has been associated with lower academic achievement (Flaxman et al., 1998).

Low socioeconomic status directly restricts accessibility to educational, health care, and other resources (Caldwell-Colbert, Henderson-Daniel, & Dudley-Grant, 2003). Low socioeconomic status relates to experiencing more stress and poor health (Gallo & Matthews, 2003), among a host of other critical risk factors. Lack of financial stability, in essence, causes a domino effect that may prevent individuals from obtaining an education, accessing better careers and occupations, and receiving adequate health care.

ADVOCACY AND EMPOWERMENT

Advocacy can be defined as "action taken on behalf of clients and/or the counseling profession to support appropriate policies and standards for the counseling profession and promote individual human worth, dignity, and potential and to oppose or work to change policies and procedures, systemic barriers, long-standing traditions, or preconceived notions that stifle human development" (Council for Accreditation of Counseling and Related Educational Programs [CACREP], 2009).

Each of the diversity issues presented earlier can, in and of itself, pose a potential *barrier* for certain individuals or groups. More than likely, multiple diversity issues are interrelated. For example, individuals representing a minority status in ethnicity, gender, sexual orientation, or socioeconomic status may face multiple forms of oppression or synergistic barriers. Social or cultural, political, educational, employment, or language/accessibility are among the potentially resulting barriers.

Barriers

Prejudice and *discrimination* refer to the judgments and attitudes that we hold toward others based on their known characteristics, such as race, ethnicity, sexual orientation, and the like. Such *stereotyping*, or *prejudice*, with the intent to classify the world around us often causes us to make untrue and unwarranted assumptions about others. Subsequent actions that we take toward other individuals with similar characteristics, based on these assumptions, are called *discrimination*. These discriminatory acts are the historical precursors to the barriers identified earlier, and the outcome is manifest in systemic *oppression*, primarily enforced or sustained by majority groups but sometimes even *internalized* by those individuals representing minority statuses or issues. This oppression underlies each barrier.

Hays (1996) proposed a view of diversity that includes age, disability, religion, ethnicity/face, sexual orientation, social status, indigenous cultural heritage, national origin, and gender. In his Addressing Model, he defines *oppression* as "biases with power" (Hays, 1996, p. 74), in the form of ageism, racism, classism, heterosexism, colonialism, and sexism. Somewhat later, Robinson (1999) identified *dominant discourses* in today's society and their discriminatory consequences (e.g., racism, sexism, homo prejudice, able-bodyism, and class elitism) in shaping individuals' *visible* and *invisible identities*. Beginning to unravel the identity development process will require that we look at the intersections of these various oppressions and discourses and their impacts on each individual client.

Becoming an Effective Advocate

In terms of advocating for and empowering clients, professional counselors must develop multicultural counseling competencies as we mentioned in the introduction to this chapter. We will briefly review those here, but first we encourage you to reflect upon the concepts of *privilege* and *power* as they relate to your own cultural context. *Privilege* is the manifestation of the belief that one group is superior to another. Individuals often are oblivious to their own beliefs about such relationships. For example, ableism, or prejudiced attitudes or discriminatory practices toward individuals with disabilities, are based on the idea that individuals without disabilities are stronger, healthier, and therefore, superior to individuals with disabilities. McIntosh (1998) discusses invisible privileges and poses statements that reflect a lack of awareness of such power. For example, "If I should need to move, I can be pretty sure of renting or purchasing housing in an area which I can afford and in which I would want to live," and "I can go shopping alone most of the time, fairly well assured that I will not be followed or harassed by store detectives," or "I can be fairly sure of having my voice heard in a group in which I am the only member of my race." The *power* that goes along with having such privileges, due simply to who we are or what characteristics we were born with, is that which leads to oppression of others. This power does not belong to just young, middle-class, and straight Whites. Each of us may have certain powers, such as physical beauty, that may allow us certain privileges. Thus, becoming aware of our personal privileges, or lack thereof, is the first step in becoming multiculturally competent.

Active Learning Exercise **5.4**

Brainstorm lists of both power and privileges (such as those identified by McIntosh, 1988) that you have experienced throughout your life. Come up with at least two examples of ways in which the specific privileges on your list have benefitted you in the last several years. Imagine and explore the ways in which your life might be different today if you had not had the same privileges that you identified. Review the table you have been making. Make an additional column on the right-hand side of the table, labeling it Possible Privileges on the top row. Speculate on the privileges that may have been enjoyed by various group members on your table. Be sure not to make assumptions, but rather, consider the possibilities.

Before moving on, please review the Active Learning Exercises accompanying this section of the chapter. Both personally and professionally, you may find it useful to consider the role of privilege in your daily life. For example, in developing *self-awareness* of cultural values and biases, professional counselors can move from levels of unawareness to levels of awareness by learning about their own cultural heritages, resulting biases and values, and limits to their own current levels of cultural competence, and by developing comfort with differences between themselves and "different" others. In terms of *knowledge development*, professional counselors can learn more about how their own culture both personally and professionally impacts their definitions of normality in learning and development; how oppression, racism, discrimination, and stereotyping impact their own work; and how their own communication style may be received by various individual clients. And in terms of *skills*, professional counselors can seek out education, training, and consultation to improve their effectiveness in working with culturally different populations.

In developing more comprehensive *awareness of others'* attitudes and beliefs, professional counselors can become more aware of differences between themselves and their clients or students they serve. In terms of *knowledge*, professional counselors can learn more about their clients' cultural and historical heritage, how those factors can play into their learning styles, their communication styles, and even their help-seeking behaviors; and how these issues can come into play within the counseling relationship. And in terms of *skills*, professional counselors can become more familiar with relevant research regarding learning and communication styles of their culturally diverse clients.

The ideal end result of developing these competencies is that you will become a more multiculturally proficient professional counselor who is able to use effective and culturally competent counseling strategies in the counseling you provide. More specifically, by becoming more aware of your *attitudes* and *beliefs*, you can gain increased respect for your clients' culturally different backgrounds, experiences, and values. In terms of *knowledge*, you can learn and understand more about how traditional counseling settings may be incongruent with the cultural values of various cultural groups, how the help-seeking behaviors required to function effectively within many counseling environments might also be incompatible with the help-seeking behaviors of various culturally diverse groups, and how testing and assessment tools may be culturally biased. And in terms of *skills*, you can become more conversant with a wider range of verbal and nonverbal communication styles and responses, develop comfort in seeking consultation with supporting personnel, and work to eliminate biases, prejudices, and discriminatory practices in counseling settings and communities. In terms of the latter, in advocating effectively for the counseling profession, we need to develop and support policies and procedures that promote social justice and oppose "systemic barriers, long-standing traditions, or preconceived notions that stifle human development" (CACREP, 2009).

CONCLUSION

Together we have explored the history of multiculturalism, leading up to contemporary society in which we view individuals and families as having multiple cultural identities. In this context we learned about the importance of multicultural competence, particularly for counselors and other helping professionals. We learned about various population groups comprising racial and ethnic diversity. In addition, we considered other types of diversity, such as gender, sexual orientation, religion, age, disabilities, and socioeconomic status.

Ethnic and other minorities are often in the lower socioeconomic strata, limiting their access to resources necessary for their advancement. In addition to experiencing limited access to resources, ethnic minorities also face discrimination and racism, which often affects their emotional well-being and often limits their opportunities for professional success. Moreover, some ethnic minorities do not have adequate written or verbal English language skills, which, in itself, can prevent them from obtaining access to higher education and to some occupations. Professional counselors are obligated to empower and advocate for those facing barriers and to influence policy makers to develop equitable legislation to address the needs of all people. Empowerment dictates the development of accessible services and resources within our own communities, states, regions, and the nation to meet the needs of all clients.

In this chapter, we learned about the importance of becoming an advocate, as well as strategies for doing so. Perhaps the most important aspect of this chapter was to begin to engage in the important process of cultural self-exploration, without which achieving true multicultural competence is not possible.

CHAPTER REVIEW

1. Early concepts of multiculturalism, such as race and gender, have expanded over the decades to include characteristics such as ethnicity, gender, sexual orientation, religion, socioeconomic status, disabilities, and age.
2. The multicultural counseling movement includes expanded models for understanding individuals as multidimensional cultural beings.
3. The four largest identifiable ethnic population groups in the United States include Black or African Americans, Hispanic or Latino Americans, Asian Americans, and European Americans, although individuals representing a wide array of ethnic and other demographically diverse categories, such as Native Americans, older clients, or people with disabilities, may present unique sociocultural counseling issues as well.
4. Developing multicultural counseling competence, along with taking the role of advocacy, are critical initiatives for counselors to take in helping their clients overcome barriers such as prejudice and discrimination.

REVIEW QUESTIONS

1. How has the concept of race evolved over time?
2. Define and explain some of the different classifications used to categorize individuals (e.g., etic, emic).
3. What are some of the obstacles to accurate classification of individuals by government and other groups?
4. Describe the process of multicultural identity development.
5. Describe the attitudes/beliefs, knowledge, and skills that are important in understanding self and others in a cultural context.
6. What would it mean for you to become multiculturally competent?

ADDITIONAL RESOURCES

- Association for Multicultural Counseling & Development: Multicultural Competencies and Standards (http://www.counseling.org/Resources/)
- Association for Multicultural Counseling & Development : Cross Cultural Competencies and Objectives (http://www.counseling.org/Resources/)
- Advocacy Competency Domains (Lewis, Arnold, House, & Toporek; endorsed by American Counseling Association Governing Council, 2003; http://www.counseling.org/Resources/)
- Guidelines on Multicultural Education, Training, Research, Practice, and Organizational Change for Psychologists (American Psychological Association, 2002; http://www.apa.org/pi/multiculturalguidelines/formats.html)

REFERENCES

American Psychological Association. (2002). *Guidelines on Multicultural Education, Training, Research, Practice, and Organizational Change for Psychologists*. Retrieved November 30, 2009 from http://www.apa.org/pi/multiculturalguidelines/homepage.html.

Andres-Hyman, R., Ortiz, J., Añez, L., Paris, M., & Davidson, L. (2006). Culture and clinical practice: Recommendations for working with Puerto Ricans and other Latinas(os) in the United States. *Professional Psychology Research and Practice, 37,* 694–701.

Atkinson, D. R., Morten, G., & Sue, D. W. (1989). A minority identity development model. In D. R. Atkinson, G. Morten, & D. W. Sue (Eds.). *Counseling American minorities* (pp. 35–47). Dubuque, IA: W. C. Brown.

Barrett, D. B., Kurian, G. T., Johnson, T. M. (2001). *World Christian encyclopedia* (2nd ed.). New York: Oxford University Press.

Berk, L. E. (1998). *Development through the lifespan*. Upper Saddle River, New Jersey: Prentice Hall.

Berry, J. W. (1980). Acculturation as varieties of adaptation. In A. M. Padilla (Ed.), *Acculturation: Theory, models and some new findings* (pp. 9–25). Boulder, CO: Westview Press.

Berry, J. W. (1986). The acculturation process and refugee behavior. In C. L. Williams & J. Westermeyer (Eds.), *Refugee mental health in resettlement countries* (pp. 25–37). Washington: Hemisphere Publishing Corporation.

Berry, J. W. (1990). Acculturation and adaptation: A general framework. In T. H. Bornermann & W. H. Holtzman (Ed.), *Mental health of immigrants and refugees* (pp. 90–102). Austin, TX: Hogg Foundation for Mental Health.

Caldwell-Colbert, A. T., Henderson-Daniel, J., & Dubley-Grant, G. R. (2003). The wisdom of years: Understanding the journey of life. In J. E. Robinson & L. C. James (Eds.), *Diversity in human interactions: The tapestry of America* (pp. 33–61). New York: Oxford University Press.

Carter, R. T., & Parks, E. E. (1996). Womanist identity and mental health. *Journal of Counseling and Development*, 74, 484–489.

Cass, V. C. (1979). Homosexual identity formation: Testing a theoretical model. *Journal of Homosexual Identity*, 4, 219–235.

Chideya, F. (1999). *The color of our future: Race in the 21st century*. New York: William Morrow & Co.

Council for Accreditation of Counseling and Related Educational Programs. (2009). *2001 standards*. Retrieved June 21, 2007, from http://www.cacrep.org/2001Standards.html.

Council for Accreditation of Counseling and Related Educational Programs. (2009). 2009 standards. Retrieved March 13, 2009, from http://www.cacrep.org/2009standards.html.

Cox, C. & Monk, A. (1993). Hispanic culture and family care of Alzheimer's patients. *Health and Social Work 18*, 92–99.

Cross, A. (1974). The black experience: Its importance in the treatment of black clients. *Child Welfare*, 53, 158–166.

Cross, W. E., Jr. (1971). The Negro-to-Black conversion experience. *Black World*, 20, 12–27.

Cross, W. E., Jr. (1978). The Thomas and Cross models of psychological nigrescence: A review. *Journal of Black Psychology*, 5, 13–31.

Cross, W. E. (1991). *Shades of black: Diversity in African-American identity*. Philadelphia: Temple University Press.

Cross, W. E., Jr. (1995). The psychology of nigrescence: Revising the Cross model. In J. G. Ponterotto, J. M. Casas, L. A. Suzuki, & C. M. Alexander (Eds.). *Handbook of multicultural counseling* (pp. 93–122). Thousand Oaks, CA: Sage.

Davison, E. H. (2004). What counselors can do to facilitate successful aging. In D. R. Atkinson & G. Hackett (Eds.). *Counseling Diverse Populations*. (3rd ed., pp. 217–233).

Downing, N. E., & Roush, K. L. (1985). From passive acceptance to active commitment: A model of feminist identity development for women. *The Counseling Psychologist*, 13, 695–709.

Elliott, T. R., & Mullins, L. L. (2004). Counseling families and children with disabilities. In D. R. Atkinson & G. Hackett (Eds.). *Counseling Diverse Populations*. (3rd ed., pp. 151–171). New York: McGraw-Hill.

Erikson, E. H. (1950). *Childhood and society*. New York: W. W. Norton.

Erikson, E. H. (1966). The concept of identity in race relations: Notes and queries. *Daedalus*, 95, 145–171.

Erikson, E. H. (1968). *Identity: Youth and crisis*. New York: W. W. Norton.

Fassinger, R. E., & Arseneau, J. R. (2007). I'd rather get wet than be under that umbrella: Differentiating the experiences and identities of lesbian, gay, bisexual, and transgender people. In K. J. Bieschke, R. M. Perez, & K. A. Debord (Eds.), *Handbook of counseling and psychotherapy with lesbian, gay, bisexual, and transgender clients* (2nd ed., pp. 19–49). Washington, DC: American Psychological Association.

Flaxman, E., Schwartz, W., Weiler, J., & Lahey, M. (1998). *Trends and issues in urban education*, 1998. New York: Institute for Urban and Minority Education. (ERIC Document Reproduction Service No. ED425247)

Fragoso, J. M, & Kashubeck, S. (2000). Machismo, gender role conflict, and mental health in Mexican

American men. *Psychology of Men and Masculinity*, *1*, 87–97.

Gallo, L. C., & Matthews, K. A. (2003). Understanding the association between socioeconomic status and physical health: Do negative emotions play a role? *Psychological Bulletin, 129*, 10–51.

Gates, G. J. (2006, October). *Same-sex couples and the gay, lesbian, bisexual population: New estimates from the American Community Survey.* The Williams Institute on Sexual Orientation Law and Public Policy, UCLA School of Law. Retrieved June 20, 2007, from http://www.law.ucla.edu/williamsinstitute/publications/SameSexCouplesandGLBpopACS.pdf

Haley, W. E., Robb, C., Jang, Y., & Han, B. (2003). The wisdom of years: Understanding the journey of life. In J. E. Robinson & L. C. James (Eds.), *Diversity in human interactions: The tapestry of America* (pp. 123–145). New York: Oxford University Press.

Halpin, A. W., & Croft, D. B. (1963). *The organizational climate of schools.* Chicago: University of Chicago, Midwest Administration Center.

Hays, P. (1996). Addressing the complexities of culture and gender in counseling. *Journal of Counseling and Development, 74*, 332–338.

Helms, J. E. (1990). Toward a model of White racial identity development. In J. E. Helms (Ed.), *Black and White racial identity: Theory, research, and practice* (pp. 67–80). Westport, CT: Greenwood Press.

Helms, J. E., & Cook, D. A. (1999). *Using race and culture in counseling and psychotherapy: Theory and practice.* Boston: Allyn & Bacon.

Hermans, H. J. M. (2001). The dialogical self: Toward a theory of personal and cultural positioning. *Culture & Psychology, 7*, 243–281.

Hutchins, A. M. (2006). Counseling gay men. In C. C. Lee (Ed.). *Counseling for Diversity.* (3rd ed., pp. 269–290). Alexandria, VA: American Counseling Association.

Jamil, H., Nassar-McMillan, S. C., & Lambert, R. (2006). Aftermath of the Gulf War: Mental health issues among Iraqi Gulf War veteran refugees in the United States. *Journal of Mental Health Counseling, 26*(4), 295–308.

Kim, Y. O. (1995). Cultural pluralism and Asian-Americans: Culturally sensitive social work practice. *International Social Work, 38*(1), 69–78.

Kosmin, B., A., Keysar, A., & Lerer, N. (1992). Secular education and the religious profile of contemporary black and white Americans. *Journal for the Scientific Study of Religion, 31*(4), 523–532.

Kosmin, B. A., Mayer, E., & Keysar, A. (2008). *American religious identity survey 2008.* Retrieved November 30, 2009, from http://www.americanreligionsurvey-aris.org/reports/ARIS_Report_2008.pdf.

Krieger, N., Williams, D., & Zierler, S. (1999). "Whiting out" white privilege will not advance the study of how racism harms health. *American Journal of Public Health, 89*(5), 782–785.

Kuhmerker, L. (1994). *The Kohlberg legacy for the helping professions.* Birmingham, AL: Doxa Books.

Lee, C. C. (1997). The promise and pitfalls of multicultural counseling. In C. C. Lee (Ed.), *Multicultural issues in counseling: New approaches to diversity* (2nd ed., pp. 3–13). Alexandria, VA: American Counseling Association.

Lee, W. M. L. (1999). *An introduction to multicultural counseling.* Philadelphia, PA: Accelerated Development.

Lewis, J., Arnold, M., House, R., & Toporek. (2003). Advocacy Competency Domains. American Counseling Association. Retrieved November 30, 2009 from http://www.counseling.org/Resources/.

Logan, C. R. (2006). Counseling lesbian clients. In C. C. Lee (Ed.). *Counseling for Diversity.* (3rd ed., pp. 291–302). Alexandria, VA: American Counseling Association.

Liu, W. M., & Pope-Davis, D. B. (2003). Understanding classism to effect personal change. In T. B. Smith (Ed.), *Practicing multiculturalism: Internalizing and affirming diversity in counseling and psychology* (pp. 294–310). New York: Allyn & Bacon.

Mayo, Y. (1997). Machismo, fatherhood, and the Latino family: Understanding the concept. *Journal of Multicultural Social Work, 5*(1/2), 49–61.

McCarn, S. R., & Fassinger, R. E. (1996). Revisioning sexual minority identity formation: A new model of lesbian identity and its implication for counseling and research. *Counseling Psychologist, 24*, 508–534.

McIntosh, P. (2003). White privilege: Unpacking the invisible knapsack. In S. Plous (Ed.), *Understanding prejudice and discrimination* (pp. 191–196). New York: McGraw-Hill.

McIntosh, P. (1998). White privilege: Unpacking the invisible knapsack. In M. McGoldrick (Ed.), *Revisioning family therapy: Race, culture, and gender in clinical practice* (pp. 147–152). New York: Guilford.

McNeil, J.M. (1997). Americans with disabilities: 1994–95. *US Bureau of the Census Current Population Reports*, (pp. 70–61). Washington, DC: US Government Printing Office.

Miller, P. H. (2001). *Theories of Developmental Psychology*. 4th ed. New York: Freeman.

Mostade, J. (2006). Affirmative counseling with transgendered persons. In C. C. Lee (Ed.). *Counseling for Diversity*. (3rd ed., pp. 303–318). Alexandria, VA: American Counseling Association.

Myers, L. J., Speight, S. L., Highlen, P. S., Cox, C. I., Reynolds, A. L., Adams, E. M., & Hanley, C. P. (1991). Identity development and worldview: Toward an optimal conceptualization. *Journal of Counseling and Development*, 70, 54–63.

Nassar-McMillan, S. C. (in press). *Counseling Arab Americans*. Brooks-Cole/Cengage.

Nassar-McMillan, S. C., & Algozzine, B. (2001). Improving outcome and future practices: Family-oriented programs and services. In D. J. O'Shea, L. J. O'Shea, B., Algozzine, & D. J. Hammite, (Eds.). *Families and teachers: Collaborative orientations, responsive practices* (pp. 273–292). Boston: Allyn and Bacon.

Nassar-McMillan, S. C., Karvonen, M., & Young, C. (2006). Multicultural competencies and teacher stress: Implications for teacher preparation, practice, and retention. In R. G. Lambert and C. J. McCarthy (Eds.), *Understanding Teacher Stress in an Age of Accountability* (pp. 87–104). Greenwich, CT: Information Age Publishing.

Nassar-McMillan, S. C., McFall-Roberts, E. J., Flowers, C., & Garrett, M. T. (2006). Ebony and ivory: Relationship between African American adolescent females' skin color and ratings of peers and self. *Journal of Humanistic and Educational Development*, 45, 79–94.

Oppedal, B., Røysamb, E., & Sam, D. L. (2004). The effect of acculturation and social support on change in mental health among young immigrants. *International Journal of Behavioral Development*, 28, 481–494.

Ottavi, T. M., Pope-Davis, D. B., & Dings, J. G. (1994). Relationship between white racial identity attitudes and self-reported multicultural counseling competencies. *Journal of Counseling Psychology*, 41, 149–154.

Pedersen, P. B. (1991). Multiculturalism as a generic approach to counseling. *Journal of Counseling and Development*, 70(1), 6–12.

Phinney, J. S. (2006). When we talk about American ethnic groups, what do we mean? *American Psychologist*, 51(9), 918–927.

Pope-Davis, D. B., & Coleman, H. L. K. (Eds.) (2001). *The intersection of race, class, and gender in multicultural counseling*. Thousand Oaks, CA: Sage Publications.

Reeves, P. M. (1999). Psychological development: Becoming a person. *New Directions for Adult and Continuing Education*, 84, 19–27.

Richards, P. S., Keller, R., & Smith, T.B. (2004). Religious and spiritual diversity in counseling and psychotherapy. In T. B. Smith (Ed.) *Practicing Multiculturalism*, (pp. 276–293). Boston: Pearson.

Robinson, T. L. (1999). The intersections of identity. In A. Garrod, J. V. Ward, T. L. Robinson, & R. Kilkenny (Eds.), *Souls looking back: Life stories of growing up Black*. New York: Routledge.

Robinson, T. L. (2005). *Multiple identities in counseling: The convergence of race, ethnicity, and gender*. Upper Saddle River, NJ: Pearson Prentice Hall.

Ross-Gordon, J. M. (1999). Gender and development. In C. Clark and R. Caffarella, *Update on Adult Development, New Directions for Adult and Continuing Education*. San Francisco: Jossey-Bass.

Sabogal, F., Marin, G., Otero-Sabogal, R., Marin, B., et al. (1987). Hispanic familism and acculturation: What changes and what doesn't? *Hispanic Journal of Behavioral Sciences*, 9(4), 397–412.

Saginak, K. A., & Saginak, M. A. (2005). Balancing work and family: Equity, gender, and marital satisfaction. *The Family Journal: Counseling and Therapy for Couples and Families*, 13, 162–166.

Samhan H. H. (1999). Not quite White: Race classification and the Arab American experience. In M. W. Suleiman (Ed.), *Arabs in America: Building a new future*. (pp. 209–226). Philadelphia: Temple University Press.

Savage, T. A., & Harley, D. A. (2005). African American lesbian, gay, and bisexual persons. In D. A. Harley & J. M. Dillard (Eds.), *Contemporary mental health issues among African Americans* (pp. 91–105). Alexandria, VA: American Counseling Association.

Sue, D. W., Arredondo, P., & McDavis, R. J. (1992). Multicultural counseling competencies and standards: A call to the profession. *Journal of Counseling and Development*, 70, 477–486.

Sue, D. W., & Sue, D. (1990). *Counseling the culturally different: Theory and practice* (2nd ed.). New York: Wiley.

Sue, S., & Sue, D. W. (1973). *Chinese-American personality and mental health*. In S. Sue & N. N. Wagner (Eds.), Asian Americans: Psychological perspectives (pp. 111–124). Palo Alto, CA: Science and Behavior Books, Inc.

Sullivan, Shannon. 2006. *Revealing whiteness: The unconscious habits of racial privilege*. Bloomington: Indiana University Press.

Troiden, R. R. (1989). The formation of homosexual identities. *Journal of Homosexualtity*, *17*, 43–73.

U.S. Census Bureau. (2003). *Married-couple and unmarried-partner households*. Retrieved June 21, 2007, from http://www.census.gov/prod/2003pubs/censr-5.pdf.

U.S. Census Bureau. (2001). *United States Census 2000*. Washington, DC: Government Printing Office.

U.S. Census Bureau. (2004, August 26). *Income stable, poverty up, numbers of Americans with and without health insurance rise, Census Bureau reports*. Retrieved June 6, 2007, from http://www.census.gov/Press-Release/www/releases/archives/income_wealth/.

U.S. Census Bureau. (2006a). *Poverty: 2005 highlights*. Retrieved June 20, 2007, from http://www.census.gov/hhes/www/poverty/poverty05/pov05hi.html.

U.S. Census Bureau. (2006b). *Poverty 2005*. Retrieved June 20, 2007, from http://www.census.gov/hhes/www/poverty/poverty05/table5.html.

U.S. Census Bureau. (2007). *USA: People quick facts*. Retrieved June 20, 2007, from http://quickfacts.census.gov/qfd/states/00000.html.

Willey, M. M., & Herskovits, M. J. (1927). Psychology and culture. *The Psychology Bulletin*, *24*(5), 253–283.

Zuckerman, M. (1990). Some dubious premises in research and theory on racial differences. *American Psychologist*, *45*, 1297–1303.

CHAPTER 6

Using Assessment in Counseling

LEARNING OBJECTIVES

After reading this chapter, you should be able to

- recount the history of testing in counseling;

- discuss the issues involved in selecting and evaluating tests that meet the purpose for which they are intended and that are appropriate for special populations and culturally diverse clientele;

- discuss the basic issues related to test selection, administration, scoring, and interpretation in counseling practice;

- understand the need to be sensitive to the major pitfalls of test use such as inappropriate choice of tests, nonstandardized administration, interpretations that are sensitive to the limitations of scores, and poor communication of test findings—all based in a multicultural perspective;

- outline the basics of test administration, interpretation of results, and integration of test data into counseling sessions; and

- describe the major ethical and legal issues that impact the testing process.

CHAPTER OUTLINE

INTRODUCTION

Tests are used extensively in counseling and serve many functions such as screening, selection, diagnostic evaluation, progress evaluation, and placement decisions. They are administered in a variety of settings, including schools/colleges, mental health clinics, businesses, and government (e.g., civil service or the military). Tests can be used to increase our self-understanding, ascertain a certain level of competence (e.g., licensure and certification exams), identify abilities and talents (e.g., musical or mechanical), or learn about human behavior (research). All of us have had some experience with a test. The word *test* can be defined as an instrument designed to measure or quantify things, from your first grade spelling test to the Graduate Record Exam (GRE) you took before entering your master's degree program. Many other tests measure human characteristics and behaviors (e.g., personality tests).

The American Counseling Association (ACA) has a division that specifically addresses the uses of tests in counseling—the Association for Assessment in Counseling and Education (AACE). Counselors use the information gained from tests as one part of a total assessment process. *Assessment* is defined as "a process that integrates test information with information from other sources (e.g., information from the individual's social, educational, employment, or psychological history)" (American Educational Research Association, American Psychological Association, & National Council on Measurement in Education [AERA/APA/NCME], 1999, p. 3). Conducting a thorough assessment that includes the use of test data helps counselors better understand students/clients and make decisions that are in their best interests.

This chapter focuses on the testing component of the assessment process by providing basic information on the history of the testing movement, psychometrics, classification, and major categorization of tests currently used in counseling. The last sections highlight the need for counselors to ethically administer, interpret, and integrate test information into the counseling process, always with the purpose of advocating for students/clients that they serve.

A BRIEF HISTORY OF TESTING IN COUNSELING

The use of tests to evaluate individuals has a long and controversial history. References to understanding individual differences can be found in the writings of the Greek philosophers Plato and Aristotle. The ancient Chinese, as far back as 2200 B.C., administered civil service examinations to government officials to determine their qualifications for various positions. The naturalist Charles Darwin's writings on the origins of species stimulated the thinking of many scientists, including those in the emerging science of psychology. Historians most often place the specific beginning of psychological testing in the late 1800s, when Wihelm Wundt of Germany and Sir Francis Galton of Great Britain earnestly began scientific investigations of individual differences. Many of you may remember Wundt from an introductory psychology courses. He is credited with founding the first psychological laboratory and was interested in measuring mental processes. Galton, a cousin to Charles Darwin, was dedicated to measuring intellect, albeit by means of evaluating a person's reaction time and sensory discrimination. Needless to say, Galton's efforts proved to be fruitless; still his work advanced the standardization of testing procedures.

An American, James McKeen Cattell, who studied under Wundt and Galton, devoted his career to the study of individual differences. Cattell, in 1890, is credited with coining the term *mental test* to describe a series of tasks he developed in his Columbia University laboratory that refined and added to Galton's work. Cattell had several students who went on to influence American testing in their own right, such as E. L. Thorndike (learning theory and achievement testing) and E. K. Strong (interest testing).

The first modern intelligence test was developed in 1905 by Alfred Binet, who was a French psychologist, and his associate Theodore Simon, who was a French medical doctor. The men were charged with identifying children who seemed unable to benefit from regular classroom instruction. The resulting Binet-Simon *intelligence test* attempted to gauge a child's ability to judge, understand, and reason. The term *mental age* was coined with the 1908 revision and was meant to "quantify" a child's overall performance on the test. The last revision to the Binet-Simon intelligence test, which expanded its use to adults, was made in 1911 after Binet's death. An American professor, Lewis M. Terman at Stanford University, undertook in 1916 a major revision of the Binet-Simon intelligence test. The resulting scale was named the Stanford-Binet Intelligence Test, with versions of the test still widely used today.

Arthur Otis, a student of Terman's, in collaboration with Robert Yerkes, is credited with having his work on the development of group-administered intelligence tests leading directly to the construction of the World War I Army Alpha test (for literate recruits) and Army Beta test (for illiterate recruits). After World War I, the College Entrance Examination Board (CEEB) constructed a scholastic aptitude test for use in college admissions. Sound familiar? You are correct in your thinking that the current SAT (Scholastic Aptitude Test) and GRE had their beginnings in this 1925 CEEB decision.

Industrialization, career development, and educational accountability all additionally spurred the development of the testing movement. One specific example is the National Defense Education Act (NDEA) of 1958, which was passed in response to the "race for space" with the Soviet Union. American students were seen as falling behind Soviet students in the area of science. The NDEA provided funding for testing to identify exceptional students and to encourage their continued study in the sciences.

The field of testing has grown exponentially since then, with hundreds of tests being commercially produced and distributed. Standardized testing, especially of academic achievement, has spread around the world. From the 1970s through the current day, computers have increasingly been used for designing tests, providing alternative ways for testees to complete tests (perhaps you took the computer-version of the GRE), and for generating test interpretation through standardized test reports.

A more recent impact on standardized achievement testing has come from the No Child Left Behind (NCLB) Act of 2001, which set standards and an assessment system for measuring the progress of students achievement in reading and math and holds states accountable for their students meeting the standards (U.S. Department of Education, 2001). NCLB enacts *standard-based education reform* (formerly known as outcome-based education), which asserts that establishing measurable goals can improve outcomes for all students. The key for us in this chapter is to realize that standardized achievement tests must be given to millions of students to assess their progress in reading and math. Student achievement must be measured annually in Grades 3 through 8 and at least once during high school. Federal funding for schools is linked to each state's ability to embrace this legislation. There are well-formed arguments for and against NCLB that are beyond the scope of this chapter. Currently, 39 states have set their own standards because NCLB does not establish a national achievement standard, but leaves the local control of schools to each state (U.S. Department of Education, 2001).

Active Learning Exercise **6.1**

From your perspective, what particular historical event seems to have had the most significant impact on testing practices? What are the underlying reasons you have for choosing the event you did? Share your thoughts with others. How do their perspectives differ from yours?

TEST PSYCHOMETRICS

A test can be a very powerful and useful tool when used correctly, though it can be useless and misleading if it is used incorrectly or yields inaccurate information. Counselors need to make informed decisions about which test to select and how best to interpret test results. Technical aspects referred to as *test psychometrics* provide information on the accuracy of the information provided by tests. Counselors, in order to evaluate the psychometrics of a test, must learn about the method used to develop the test and evidence of reliability and validity for interpreting test results. These concepts are addressed in the following three sections.

Test Construction Methods

There are several methods used to develop tests. Some tests are constructed using empirical methods. One such method known as *criterion keying* examines the responses on test items between two groups of people. One such well-known test is the Minnesota Multiphasic Personality Inventory (MMPI), which was constructed comparing psychiatric patients to a control group of people on responses to 550 test items. A second type of empirical method is *item clustering*, which uses a statistical procedure such as factor analysis or cluster analysis that groups together questions within the item pool that are correlated/related with one another. A nonempirical method for constructing tests is *rational/theoretical scale construction*. Test developers using this method create items based on logical and theoretical knowledge of the construct under investigation (e.g., a psychological attribute such as depression, introversion, or anxiety). Some test developers using this method also incorporate statistical analyses to evaluate the quality of the test items.

Reliability

A major requirement of a high-quality test is adequate reliability. *Reliability* is the extent to which we are measuring some attribute in a systematic and therefore repeatable way. *Consistency* is often a term used when discussing reliability. A test is said to be reliable if, for example, the test scores remain consistent over repeated administrations to the same individual under identical conditions. *Unreliable* would be repeated administrations of the same test providing very different results. Of course, "true scores" for individuals can never really be known as their test scores are actually estimates of some attribute. Every person's score reflects some error because no test can truly capture a construct in its entirety, and each individual has some variability when responding to test items. This error is known as *standard error of measurement* and is used when interpreting test results.

The three common ways to assess reliability are test-retest, alternative/parallel forms, and internal consistency reliability. The resulting number from testing reliably through any of these methods is called a *reliability coefficient*. In general, desirable reliability coefficients should range from about .85 and above with 1.0 maximum.

1. *Test-retest reliability* (also thought of as test stability) evaluates the stability of test scores over time. The same test is given to the same individuals under the same testing conditions over some period of time typically two weeks to 60 days. The reliability coefficient in this case is called the coefficient of stability and is calculated as a relationship (correlation) between time-1 administration scores and time-2 administration scores.

2. *Alternative/parallel forms reliability* requires that two equivalent forms of the test be developed and administered to the same individuals. This form of reliability analysis assesses the degree to which the two different forms of the test yield similar results. The reliability coefficient in this case is called the coefficient of equivalence and is calculated as a relationship (correlation) between scores on the alternative forms of the test.

3. *Internal consistency reliability* can be calculated through various methods. One option is to use Spearman's split-half method, which compares scores from two halves of the same test for the same individual. This form of reliability analysis assesses the degree to which the two sections of the same test yield similar results. The reliability of the entire test can then be calculated using the Spearman-Brown formula. Reliability can also be assessed using the Kuder-Richardson method (KR-20; Kuder & Richardson, 1937), which provides an additional way for dividing items on a test into two halves and is used when test items are scored as 0 or 1. The final option for evaluating internal consistency reliability is Cronbach's alpha coefficient (Cronbach, 1951), which is the general formula used when items have different scoring weights assigned to different responses such as a Likert scale response (1–5), where 1 equals "least like me" and 5 equals "most like me."

Validity

Validity is another important requirement of a high-quality test. *Validity* is the degree to which a test is measuring what it is proposed to measure. *Accuracy* is often a term used when describing validity. An important point to make here is that a test can provide reliable scores (provide the same results each time), but not valid scores (accurate representation of an attribute like depression). A depression inventory might repeatedly yield a score of 10 with each administration to a client indicating low level of depression (reliability), yet the client may actually be clinically depressed (validity). Another example commonly used to explain this concept is the bathroom scale—each morning a person steps on the scale and her weight registers 145 lbs (reliability), yet her true weight (validity) is 140 lbs. Her scale is 5 lbs off. Like the bathroom scale, a test can be reliable but not valid. Tests must provide both valid and reliable scores in order for counselors to be confident in the results.

Test validation is the procedure used to determine the degree of accuracy/validity of test scores. There are several types of validity: *content*, *criterion-related*, and *construct*.

Content validity (also called face validity) addresses whether or not the test items elicit responses (e.g., knowledge, skill sets, behaviors) that they were designed to assess. Content validity is most often applied to achievement, aptitude, and interest tests. The analysis of content validity is done through "expert raters" in the subject matter under study and is an essential first step in validating a test.

Criterion-related validity refers to the extent to which people's test scores are associated with ratings or other measures of performance that are called criteria. The two types of criterion-related validity are *concurrent* and *predictive validity*. Concurrent validity is established when the criterion measure is available at the same time as the test scores. For example, concurrent validity would be established when a counselor's diagnosis of depression for a client concurs with the same client's score on a depression inventory. Predictive validity focuses on how well test scores predict a preestablished outcome measure of performance (criterion). For example, you currently have available your GRE test scores, but will not have the criterion measure of your final grade point average in graduate school for a few more years.

Construct validity most directly addresses the question of whether a test measures what it is purported to measure, yet it is the most abstract/general of all validity types and is not determined in one single way or by one investigation. It would be helpful to more fully define the word *construct* before we move into this discussion. A construct is an entity that cannot directly be measured but is literally constructed. We infer a construct from other things such as the sample of behavior obtained by a test. In general, construct validation uses information from all sources of validity and is never actually completed, but is continually changing as new data is acquired. Establishing construct validity involves a process based on other sources that are similar and different from the construct. A test should have *convergent validity* (relationships with other measures of the same construct) with similar tests and *discriminant validity* (lack of relationship with different constructs) with dissimilar tests. A depression test, for example, should provide results similar to another depression inventory, but dissimilar to a test measuring anxiety.

Norms and Scores

Test scores of individuals are interpreted relative to other people who are called the *normative sample*. We begin with raw scores and then use the normative sample to make comparisons. This process places an individual's score in a larger context and provides counselors with more information from which they can interpret the results. *Norms* then come from administering the test to a large group of people who are representative of the target test population. Raw scores are converted to "derived scores," the most common among them being percentile rank or standard scores.

Percentile rank simply refers to the proportion of people in the standardization sample whose scores fall below an individual's raw score. You may already be familiar with percentile ranks as many standardized achievement–type tests that you have encountered in your academic career report results in percentiles. Your parents may have learned when you were in the fourth grade that your reading level was at the 90th percentile, meaning that 90 percent of the normative sample fell below your reading ability.

Standard scores are derived by adjusting raw scores through a simple linear transformation. These transitions are conducted so that test scores can be communicated in a standardized manner. For example, the GRE has a standard score mean of 500 and a standard deviation of 100. When you received your GRE quantitative score, you could immediately know how well you had done on that section of the test relative to the normative group.

Additionally, we may at times find it necessary to combine clients/students' scores on different tests to obtain their average achievement or to compare their standing on two or more tests. Statistically, we cannot simply compare or average scores from different tests, so we change the raw scores to standard scores in order to make the scores from different tests directly comparable. This process is called *normalized standard scores*.

Active Learning Exercise **6.2**

Make a short list of some of the tests that you've taken in your lifetime. Now make a column next to the list and write in what you know about the psychometrics of those tests. For how many tests on your list were you able to provide psychometric information? Maybe the GRE or the SAT/ACT (American College Testing Assessment)? How might you find out if the most important tests on your list are psychometrically sound, especially since major decisions like admissions to graduate school are made every day for untold numbers of individuals?

CLASSIFICATION OF TESTS

Tests can be classified in many ways. Classification of tests has its own jargon/terminology, which is based on the content of the tests, method of development, the construct they were designed to measure, and/or how they are to be administered or scored (Aiken & Groth-Marnat, 2006). Common classification terms are listed here.

- *Standardized/formal vs. nonstandardized/informal.* Standardized tests have systematic guidelines for administration, timing, and scoring that ensure the procedures will be comparable across test administrators and examinees. Nonstandardized tests have no prescribed structure so the testing process varies among people and across time. Test psychometrics that were discussed earlier refer only to standardized tests.
- *Individual vs. group tests.* Individual tests are designed to be administered to only one examinee at a time, while group tests are designed to be simultaneously administered to a group of people. Group tests provide efficiency of administration, while individual tests garner rich data about the examinee.
- *Objective vs. subjective tests.* Objective tests are scored based on an established format that has correct answers identified such as true/false or multiple-choice questions. Subjective tests (e.g., essay exams, open-ended

questions) necessitate that the test administrator judges the correctness of the each answer.

- *Speed vs. power tests.* Speed tests usually have a large number of simple items that must be answered in a given amount of time. Power tests have no time limit and fewer items with varying levels of difficulty.
- *Verbal vs. nonverbal tests.* Verbal tests rely on language use either orally or written (paper/pencil tests). Nonverbal tests are more performance based in that students/clients use their spatial or visual processing skills instead of their verbal skills (e.g., choosing matching designs or manipulation of objects). Controversy does surround the use of verbal tests with some students/clients based on issues such as cultural language differences, English as a second language, and/or learning disabilities.
- *Norm-referenced vs. criterion-referenced tests.* Examinees in norm-referenced tests are compared to the normative sample and can be compared on a number of different traits such as age, biological sex, occupation, and so forth. Criterion-referenced tests compare an individual's score with the predetermined standard (criterion) such as expected grade-level reading ability.
- *Cognitive vs. affective tests.* Cognitive tests measure mental processes while affective tests measure all noncognitive aspects of a person such as attitudes, values, interests, or personality.

MAJOR TEST CATEGORIES

Tests are also classified according to their primary purpose. The most common categories of tests that counselors are regularly called upon to administer and/or interpret are intelligence, aptitude, achievement, interest/career-related, and personality. These categories can be seen as having some overlap. For example, intelligence, aptitude, and achievement tests all assess an individual's performance on similar issues (e.g., verbal, numerical, and reasoning abilities). Intelligence can even be viewed as a type of aptitude test designed to measure aptitude for academic/occupational work that relies on verbal ability and reasoning (Aiken, 2002). Major test categories have enough unique qualities and uses to be discussed individually.

Intelligence Tests

The term *intelligence* is commonly used today, yet it was unknown 100 years ago. The concept of intelligence is actually quite controversial, with professionals debating issues such as the impact of nature (our inherited genetics) versus nurture (our environment), the cultural biases inherent in the concept of intelligence, and even the definition of the word itself. Sir Francis Galton actually reintroduced the ancient Latin term *intelligence*, which he defined as individual differences in mental abilities. Binet and Simon, who really created the first practical intelligence test, used a definition that emphasized judgment and common sense, postulating that intelligence is the ability to judge well, reason well, and comprehend well. The quest for a workable definition has been a long one with current professionals proposing that quite possibly we should use an alternative term such as "general mental ability, scholastic ability, or academic ability" (Aiken & Groth-Marnat, 2006, p. 113).

There are a host of theories of intelligence that are the basis for a various intelligence tests. Intelligence tests can be individually or group administered. You may recognize the Wechsler Intelligence Test (individual test) or the Otis-Lennon School Ability Test (group test) as an IQ test administered to you at school. Intelligence tests predict broad academic achievement and are often used in schools to assist placement of students into various educational programs (e.g., special education or honors programs).

Aptitude Tests

Aptitude tests are used to predict a person's performance in a narrow range of skills and abilities. An aptitude is defined as the ability to perform a task or type of skill. An aptitude test is designed to measure how much a person may gain from future training/experience (Aiken, 2002). Several aptitude tests are so familiar to college students that they are identifiable by their acronyms—SAT or ACT—and graduate students will recognize the GRE. These aptitude tests are all commonly used admission tests that measure scholastic ability providing one type of data for predicting college success. Aptitude testing can be divided into two categories—multiaptitude batteries and special-abilities tests.

Multiaptitude batteries are comprised of a variety of tests that measure a number of different aptitudes. One example, the Armed Service Vocational Assessment Battery, is often administered to high school students. Multiaptitude batteries are tools that counselors use to identify student/client aptitudes and match those skills with potential careers.

Special-ability tests range from mechanical and clerical (dexterity tests or computer programmer tests) to music and artistic tests. These measures of special abilities have long been used in career counseling to identify a person's potential ability in some specific area. Employers can use test scores to assist in making placement decisions in the workplace.

Achievement Tests

Achievement tests most commonly used in schools assess student academic performance in mastering educational objectives. These tests measure outcomes of various structured learning activities. Achievement tests are categorized as teacher-made or standardized, individual or group administered, and norm-referenced or criterion-referenced. They can be used to evaluate single or multiple skills (single subject tests or test batteries) and as screening or diagnostic tools. These tests measure one or more content areas such as math computation and problems solving, basic reading skills and comprehension, writing ability, and/or listening comprehension. You might be familiar with the TerraNova-2 or the Iowa Test of Basic Skills that are often group administered in schools.

Achievement testing in the public schools is also applied to special education, with results being used by counselors to advocate for students with special needs. Some achievement tests that help to identify students with special needs are the Woodcock-Johnson Test of Achievement and the Wechsler Individual Achievement Test. There are also adult achievement tests that you may recognize, including the GED (Test of General Education Development), which is the equivalent of a high school degree, and the NCE (National Counselor Examination), which is the test that many states use to license professional counselors.

Interest/Career-Related Inventories

Interest can be defined as a person's preferences for activities and objects. Interests are often categorized in three ways: expressed, manifest, and inventoried (Whiston, 2005). *Expressed* interests are identified by what students/clients tell us they are interested in, such as sports, computers, or animals. *Manifest* interests need to be inferred by observing what students/clients do with their time. The focus for this section, of course, is *inventoried* interests. Inventoried interests use tests administered to individuals with the sole purpose of identifying particular interests/preferences in many areas such as music, art, or athletics. Interest inventories are used in various settings such as schools, colleges, and the workplace by career counselors, vocational rehabilitation counselors, human resource people, and industrial consultants.

Our interests begin to emerge early in life, but are unstable and not reliable when used for early decision-making about a career. Think back to your elementary school days. What did you say you wanted to be when you grow up? Was "counselor" one of your choices? Our patterns of interest become much more specific, realistic, and stable by senior high school so, at that juncture, counselors can have relative confidence in a student/client's results on an interest inventory.

Items for many interest inventories are in the form of a checklist or forced-choice format. For example, you might be asked to choose between gardening and reading. Student/client responses to these items can be an important component in the career planning process since the inventory measures occupation-related likes and dislikes. The inventories help clients become more aware of their current areas of interest. Counselors can use the results from an inventory within a counseling session to assist clients in making informed decisions about career choices.

An interesting online resource that can also increase awareness is the O*NET occupational database that lists thousands of occupational titles. One component of this resource is the O*NET Work Importance Profiler, which helps people decide which work needs are most important to them in terms of occupations. The work values are delineated into six categories: Achievement, Independence, Recognition, Relationships, Support, and Working Conditions. A person's results are comprised of a profile that provides information about work values, thereby increasing career awareness, and links them to the list of occupational titles (U.S. Department of Labor, 2007).

There are many published interest inventories; we will briefly focus on a few of the commonly administered instruments. Measuring career interests first began in a standardized manner with the Strong Vocational Interest

Blank (SVIB) in 1927. The SVIB was developed by E. K. Strong, whom you'll remember as a student of James McKeen Cattell's at Columbia University. The "Strong" has gone through many revisions since the 1920s and is a very popular interest inventory. The Self-Directed Search (SDS), another well-known interest inventory, was developed by John Holland.

Both the Strong and the SDS are based on Holland's theory of vocational choice which specifies six major types of people and environments known as the RIASEC model—Realistic (R), Investigative (I), Artistic (A), Social (S), Enterprising (E), or Conventional (C) (Holland, 1997). Holland's theory proposes that a satisfying interaction of person and environment can create situations that allow people to use their abilities, problem-solve effectively, and express their values. A student/client's SDS score is comprised of a three-letter RIASEC summary code, which is used to explore the list of over 1,300 occupations found in the Occupational Code Finder. The Occupational Code Finder is a supplement to the SDS and corresponds to codes found in the *Dictionary of Occupational Titles*.

Personality Tests

The construct of personality has a wide variety of definitions. Basically, personality describes the character of emotion, thought, and behavior patterns unique to each individual. For example, we might say of a counselor-in-training that "it is in his [or her] nature to help others." Counselors use personality tests to assist clients in understanding their patterns of emotions, thoughts, and behaviors. This increased understanding assists clients in thinking more broadly about how they operate in their personal and professional world. Many clients, counselors, and researchers find "personality" a fascinating subject.

There are several perspectives/models of personality, including trait-factor, phenomenological, psychoanalytic/psychodynamic, and situational/social learning models (Aiken & Groth-Marnat, 2006).

Personality Models

The *trait-factor model* is a dominant force in personality research. The model proposes that human behavior can be ordered and measured along dimensions called traits and that individuals can be characterized by these stable traits that are prime determinants of our behavior. Traits that are used to describe people might be extrovert and introvert, open-minded and close-minded, agreeable and hostile, conscientiousness and rebellious, or neurotic and emotionally stable (Costa & McCrae, 1990). The Myers-Briggs Type Indicator (MBTI) and the NEO Personality Inventory are two of the best known measures developed from the trait-factor model.

The *phenomenological model* focuses on an individual's subjective perceptions of the world. The model emphasizes person factors such as the student/client's interpretation of their experiences and the meaning applied to those interpretations. The interpretation and meaning can be viewed as a person's "internal beliefs," which are considered to be fairly stable. An individual's internal beliefs and view of self are thought to be the main determinants of behavior. Several well-known measures developed from the phenomenological model are the Tennessee Self-Concept Scale and the Coopersmith Self-Esteem Inventories.

The *psychoanalytic/psychodynamic model* proposes that personality is made up of the id, ego, and superego. These terms cue you into the fact that the influence for this model of personality comes from Sigmund Freud as well as past and contemporary psychodynamic theorists. The model is seen as instinct driven with unconscious processes that are stable across situations dominating our behaviors. The MMPI and Rorschach Inkblot Test are two well-known measures that were developed from the psychodynamic model.

The *situation model* suggests that personality is defined in terms of a person's overt behaviors that are learned. Social learning theory provides the basis for this model. Influential social learning theorists, such as Bandura, Rotter, and Lewin, propose that all behavior is learned in a social context with some behaviors being reinforced and others extinguished through our social interactions. A well-known measure developed from this model is the Rotter's Locus of Control Scale.

Objective and Projective Personality Tests

Personality tests are divided into two main categories—objective and projective. *Objective personality assessments* are structured tests that rely on the student/client's self-report. This type of assessment procedure has examinees respond to various forms of a written statement. For example, the examinee could be asked to answer yes/true or no/false to a statement like, "I rarely feel happy"; or asked to choose between two words that fit them best, such as *scheduled* or *unplanned*; or respond to an item like, "When a task needs done, do you like to help organize the effort or let others organize in their own way?" These personality instruments are called objective because they are structured and are interpreted in comparison with a normative group. Objective personality instruments are relatively easy to administer, score, and interpret. A few well-known examples of objective personality tests include the MMPI, the MBTI, the Beck Depression Inventory, and the Eating Disorder Inventory.

Projective personality assessments are unstructured and provide ambiguous stimuli with few response guidelines. Sentence completion is one type of projective personality test. Examinees are asked to complete sentence fragments such as "I only wish my father had …" The infamous Rorschach provides a picture of an inkblot and examinees are asked to describe what they see. Other projective tests such as the Thematic Apperception Test for adults or the Children's Apperception Test provide pictures of people in ambiguous situations from which examinees are asked to tell a complete story about what is going on in the scene. At other times, examinees are asked to create the picture and the story as with the Draw-a-Person or the House-Tree-Person tests. Typically, extensive training is needed to competently administer, score, and interpret projective personality tests.

TEST ADMINISTRATION AND INTERPRETATION OF RESULTS

Counselors are interested in obtaining meaningful and accurate data about clients so electing the appropriate test is critical to the assessment process. Specific selection comes from knowing the purpose of the test (e.g., mental health diagnosis), the appropriateness of the test format for your particular student/client (i.e., reading level), and how the results will be used (e.g., classroom placement level or therapeutic treatment plan). Whenever possible, choose tests that contain items that best measure the construct (depression, achievement, interests) of interest, are psychometrically sound (validity and reliability), and have appropriate norm data that match your client (age, gender, ethnicity/race, and so forth). Most tests typically require that test administrators have completed a level of training/education before giving, scoring, and interpreting an instrument for an examinee. Training/education levels can vary across different types of tests. Training for counselors to administer intelligence tests can be an entire course by itself, while training for professional counselors to administer a depression inventory might be as simple as reading the test manual. Guidelines for the entire process of testing from training to interpretation are outlined in the ACA's *Code of Ethics* (ACA, 2005) and the *Standards for Educational and Psychological Testing* (AERA/APA/NCME, 1999).

Test administration should always be standardized and strictly align with guidelines put forth in the test manual. Any issues that might impact examinees' scores should be minimized and/or eliminated. These issues are called confounding factors such as environmental factors (e.g., lighting, noise, temperature), examinee factors (e.g., fatigue, anxiety, motivation, mental disorders), and/or examiner factors (e.g., competence in administering tests, demeanor).

After administering, counselors score the test and interpret the results for students/clients. Communication of test interpretation to examinees is done within the therapeutic relationship. Test results must be given in context from all you know about your clients, their goals, and available resources to reach those goals. Richard Hazler (n.d.) offers the following suggestions for interpreting test results to clients in an efficient and productive manner:

1. Put clients at ease and discuss results in the language of the client.
2. Take time to find what individual clients are really seeking in being counseled. What do they hope to learn from the test?
3. Relate the results to something the client has said, a question asked, or a choice that was made.
4. Provide information slowly and not all at once.
5. Begin interpreting those areas that highlight strengths that reinforce what clients already know about themselves. This gives clients credit for knowing himself or herself.
6. Provide time, opportunity, and permission for expression of client attitudes and their understanding of the meaning, and to ask questions about each result or area of results.
7. Help clients see the relationship of measured factors to their real-life experiences (successes and failures, training, family, leisure activities, work, and so forth).

8. Help clients face evidence of both strengths and weakness in their scores, background, situation, and abilities, and to recognize that to do otherwise is unfair to themselves.

9. Discuss clients' comparative position on the test to other groups in general terms (e.g., upper or lower third) rather than specific numerical scores. This is particularly true for heavily value-laden scores like IQ or often misunderstood scores like grade equivalent.

10. Emphasize patterns (e.g., overall scores, historical patterns) of scores, particularly when those are more important than individual scores.

11. Give reasonable consideration to potential sources of score error.

INTEGRATING TEST DATA INTO COUNSELING

The counseling process can be divided into four steps: (1) assessing student/clients' problems, (2) conceptualizing and defining their problems, (3) selecting and implementing appropriate treatments, and (4) evaluating counseling effectiveness (Whiston, 2005). Counselors can integrate testing into each of these four phases of the counseling process. Test data provide beneficial information that can help guide counselors throughout the course of treatment.

When assessing student/clients' problems, counselors will use an intake interview to understand the issues from the client's perspective. The counselor's initial understanding can be further investigated through the use of a standardized test(s). A hypothetical client, for example, could tell the counselor that he or she is feeling jittery, has difficulty concentration, worries a lot, and feels overwhelmed by the smallest issues. The counselor, suspecting that the client is suffering from an anxiety disorder, can choose to administer a test such as the Beck Anxiety Inventory (BAI). The BAI data assist the counselor in the second phase of counseling as supplemental information for gauging the scope of the client's reported problems. Test data can help the counselor rule-in or rule-out certain diagnoses by providing details (e.g., severity, frequency, duration, etc.) of client symptomology.

Once client issues are assessed and defined, counselors provide appropriate treatment to enhance the client's daily functioning. Counselors, in collaboration with clients, develop a treatment plan that establishes goals for counseling. Test data can be integrated into the treatment plan. The BAI, for example, could again be administered to the client after several weeks of counseling. The counselor would use the original BAI score (baseline score) as a comparison to the client's current score midway through the course of treatment. These score comparisons can be one piece of information that help the counselor assess how treatment is progressing. The use of test data in this way is referred to as *formative assessment*.

The final phase of counseling utilizes *summative/outcome assessment* to gauge the effectiveness of counseling in assisting the client toward fuller functioning. The BAI could once again be administered to the client, with scores compared from baseline through final counseling session. The test scores are viewed as objective data that supports the counselor's clinical evaluation of overall treatment effectiveness.

ETHICAL AND LEGAL ISSUES IN TESTING

The effective use of testing in counseling is subject to both ethical and legal issues.

Ethical Issues

The purpose of testing is to gather relevant information about an individual. To ethically use tests in counseling, counselors gather this information in a manner that achieves the goals set forth by clients and counselors. Ethical counselors are unbiased, objective, and act in the best interests of their clients. It is important that counselors use multiple assessment methods to gain the fullest possible picture of clients and their needs. Test results should *never* be used in isolation, but always within the full context of clients' lives. For example, students should never be placed in special education classes based solely on IQ test scores, or clients should never be hospitalized based only on the results of a test that assesses level of suicidality. Remember no test provides a "true/exact" score and that each test has some level of standard error of measurement. The psychometrics of every test must be taken into consideration if tests are to be used ethically.

Counselors are guided by the ACA's *Code of Ethics* (ACA, 2005), which provides standards for professional behavior. Specific standards have been developed to address diversity issues in testing—the *Standards for Multicultural Assessment* (AACE, 2003). Along with these standards, several moral principles are deemed important for counselors. Kitchener in her seminal work proposed five basic principles (1984):

1. *Autonomy.* Clients have the right to independence and to make rational decision for themselves. In testing situations, clients should be fully informed about the purpose of the test and how test results will be used (i.e., who will see test scores), and they should formally provide their informed consent before tests are administered.
2. *Nonmaleficence.* Counselors should "do no harm." Choosing appropriate tests for appropriate reasons and protecting clients' confidentiality and privacy reduces the chances of doing harm.
3. *Beneficence.* Counselors should "do good and contribute to clients' welfare." Test results are used to advocate for clients to receive appropriate services.
4. *Justice.* Counselors should conduct themselves with "fair treatment for all clients" regardless of race, age, gender, mental/physical disability, socioeconomic status, and so forth.
5. *Fidelity.* Counselors should maintain loyalty and faithfulness in their counseling relationships with clients. It is important to always honor commitments to clients.

These five principles along with the standards help to ensure that counselors are trained, competent test users and use appropriate assessment techniques to benefit their clients.

Legal Issues

Several laws that also guide counselors in terms of testing are important to mention.

- *The Family Education Rights and Privacy Act* is a federal law that protects the privacy of students' records and gives parents the right to review all educational records collected by the school including group/individual tests results.

- *The No Child Left Behind Act* is another education-based law that was addressed earlier. This controversial act encourages higher standards for education and student performance, which are evaluated through the use of group tests throughout students' school years. There can be tremendous pressure to do well on these assessments because NCLB has increased the standards of accountability for states, school districts, schools, teachers, and students. There currently is continued debate on the effectiveness and desirability of NCLB testing.

- *The Individuals With Disabilities Education Act* (IDEA) is a law ensuring services to children with disabilities. IDEA directs how states and public agencies provide early intervention, special education, and related services to children and their families.

- *Section 504 of the Rehabilitation Act of 1973* protects qualified individuals from discrimination based on their disability. The disability can be a physical or mental impairment that substantially limits one or more major life activities. The law applies to any employers and organizations that receive funding from any federal department or agency and forbids any exclusion of individuals with a disability from equal opportunity to received program benefits and services.

- *The Individuals With Disabilities Education Improvement Act* provides guidelines for assessing, identifying, placing, and instructing students with handicapping conditions in the least restrictive environment. Eligible students have an Individual Education Plans (IEP) that outlines goals and appropriate services to be provided. A multidisciplinary team, after gaining parental consent for testing and placement, develop the IEP.

- *Americans With Disabilities Act* (ADA) mandates that reasonable accommodations be made for persons who have impaired functioning. These accommodations also include adaptations for tests and assessments. The key is to fairly assess individuals with disabilities (e.g., give extra time allotted to take the test), while at the same time maintaining the psychometric integrity (reliability/validity) of the test.

There is much more information on testing than can be provided in one brief chapter. The Additional Resources section below provides a few easily accessible Web sites that are useful resources on testing practices. Counselors in various settings can find information from resources such as the ACA's *Code of Ethics* (ACA, 2005) relative to testing practices, competencies for assessment of diverse individuals, and information on specific published tests.

Active Learning Exercise **6.3**

Picture yourself working with a new client. Who is this client? What are his or her presenting problems? How might you be able to help this individual toward better functioning? What steps will you take to integrate testing into your client's counseling process? How will you ensure that the test results will improve your client's life and not become a detractor increasing their plight? Would you want a counselor to administer this test to you if you were having the same problems as your client? How would you want your test results to be used by others?

CONCLUSION

A significant amount of information has been covered in this succinct chapter, which highlighted the use of tests as a part of the overall assessment process. You have gained information on the history of the testing movement, psychometrics, classification, and major categorization of tests currently used in counseling. An important additional component enhanced your understanding about counselors' solemn responsibility to ethically administer, interpret, and integrate test outcome data as one source of information into the counseling process. The last word I would like to leave you with is *advocate*—remember to use the testing process and outcome data to *advocate* for all the students/clients you serve.

CHAPTER REVIEW

1. The use of tests in counseling has a long and sometimes controversial history. Some type of assessment is regularly used in counseling to make decisions about students/clients.
2. Competent counselors are trained to understand (a) measurement issues, (b) the manner in which tests are classified, (c) the major categories of tests as well as their primary uses, and (d) appropriate interpretation of results to clients.
3. Counselors use tests ethically by adhering to the profession's *Code of Ethics and*

Standards of Practice, Standards for Multicultural Assessment, and basic moral principles.
4. Knowing the laws that impact decisions on the "who, what, where, when, and why" of testing is vitally important for all counselors. It is imperative that counselors use tests as only one source of information to be considered as they advocate for the best possible outcomes for their clients.

REVIEW QUESTIONS

1. Describe the value of assessment for our clients.
2. Describe the inherent danger of assessment for our clients.
3. What three major historical events have impacted the course of testing?
4. How do you know that a test is reliable?
5. How do you know if a test is valid?

6. Can a test be valid if it is not reliable?
7. What type of tests help clients learn about their preferences for activities and objects?
8. Describe the standards that assist counselors in ethically administering, interpreting, and integrating tests into counseling sessions.

ADDITIONAL RESOURCES

- American Counseling Association (http://www.counseling.org)
- Association for Assessment in Counseling and Education (http://aac.ncat.edu)
  - Code of Fair Testing Practices in Education
  - Ethics in Assessment Standards for Multicultural Assessment
  - Pre-Employment Testing and the ADA Responsibilities of Users of Standardized Tests
  - Competencies in Assessment and Evaluation for School Counselors

- Standards for Qualifications for Test Users
- Test Taker Rights and Responsibilities
- American Psychological Association (http://apa.org)
- Joint Committee on Testing Practices http://www.apa.org/science/jctpweb.html
- Fair Access Coalition on Testing (http://www.fairaccess.org)
- Buros Institute of Mental Measurement (http://www.unl.edu/buros)
- Association of Test Publishers Q&A http://www.testpublishers.org/faq.htm

REFERENCES

Aiken, L. R. (2002). *Psychological testing and assessment* (11th ed.). Boston: Pearson.

Aiken, L. R., & Groth-Marnat, G. (2006). *Psychological testing and assessment* (12th ed.). Boston: Pearson.

American Counseling Association. (2005). *Code of ethics*. Alexandria, VA: Author.

American Educational Research Association, American Psychological Association, & National Council on Measurement in Education. (1999). *Standards for educational and psychological testing* (3rd ed.). Washington, DC: American Psychological Association.

Association for Assessment in Counseling and Education. (2003). *Standards for multicultural assessment*. Alexandria, VA: Author.

Costa, R. T., Jr., & McCrae, R. R. (1990). Personality disorders and the five-factor model. *Journal of Personality Disorders, 4,* 362–371.

Cronbach, L. J. (1951). Coefficient alpha and the internal structure of tests. *Psychometrika, 16,* 297–334.

Hazler, R. J. (n.d.). Interpreting test results to clients. Unpublished manuscript.

Holland, J. L. (1997). *Making vocational choices: A theory of careers* (3rd ed.). Odessa, FL: Psychological Assessment Resources.

Kitchener, K. S. (1984). Intuition, critical evaluation and ethical principles: The foundation for ethical decisions in counseling psychology. *Counseling Psychologist, 12,* 43–55.

Kuder, G., & Richardson, M. (1937). The theory of estimation of test reliability. *Psychometrika, 2,* 151–160.

U.S. Department of Education. (2001). *No child left behind*. Retrieved May 15, 2009, from http://www.ed.gov/nclb/landing.jhtml.

U.S. Department of Labor. (1991). *Dictionary of Occupational Titles*. Retrieved November 15, 2009, from http://www.oalj.dol.gov/libdot.htm.

U.S. Department of Labor. (2007). *O*NET Work Importance Profiler*. Retrieved June 30, 2007, from www.onetcenter.org/WIP.html.

Whiston, S. C. (2005). *Principles and applications of assessment in counseling* (2nd ed.). Belmont, CA: Thomson Brooks/Cole.

CHAPTER 7

The Role of Research in Counseling

LEARNING OBJECTIVES

After reading this chapter, you should be able to

- understand how research is conceptualized in counseling and the social sciences;
- describe the relationships between research and theory;
- understand how research in counseling differs from research in other fields in the social sciences;
- recognize diversity and multicultural issues and contexts in counseling research;
- explain divergent philosophical approaches to research;
- understand research problems and perspectives on research;
- list the differences and consistencies between quantitative and qualitative approaches to research;
- understand the important concepts and practices in quantitative and qualitative research; and
- discuss the influence of the American Counseling Association's *Code of Ethics* on research.

CHAPTER OUTLINE

INTRODUCTION

The word *research* is one that has different meanings across various settings, including education. For example, most students in the 12th grade are required to do a *research paper*. The student chooses a topic; finds articles, books, and other materials relevant to the topic; and writes a paper based on these resources. This activity fits with the popular conceptualization of research and with the dictionary definition of research. It does not fit, however, with the common academic conceptualization of research in counseling and the social sciences. In these fields, research involves the collection of data. For example, if your 12th-grade teacher required you to collect data (e.g., interview data, data from measurement instruments, or recorded observation data) and analyze it, you would then be doing research—according to the more scientific-empirical and professional definition used in counseling and the social sciences.

Knowledge in any field of study is created through research. Research methods vary greatly across various fields, but there are commonalities across fields and methods. Researchers seek to understand relationships among phenomena and causes of phenomena. For example, a medical researcher investigates the environmental influences on the incidence of a disease, whereas a social science researcher investigates the environmental influences on voting behavior. Researchers seek to describe processes and the functioning of systems. For example, a biochemist investigates how a drug affects the circulatory system, whereas the school counselor studies the impact of school policies on the school system. Researchers collect and analyze data in order to generate theories or test existing theories. For example, the electrical engineer performs an experiment to test some tenet of electrical theory, whereas the mental health counselor conducts an experimental study to test the efficacy of some theory-driven counseling intervention. Researchers work to develop products. For example, the materials scientist seeks to find a more effective asphalt for roads, whereas a counselor works to construct a better intervention for students with a particular disability. In short, researchers in all fields make efforts at observing, describing, understanding, explaining, and developing phenomena.

Research in counseling has the highest degree of similarity to research in other social science fields. In fact, much of the research in the social sciences (e.g., sociology, social psychology, education, developmental psychology, organizational psychology) is useful to counselors and counseling. Inversely, much of the research in counseling informs other social science fields. Researchers in counseling and researchers in other social sciences often use the same theories and methods in the design of their research. For example, the *status attainment model* (Sewell, Haller, & Portes, 1969), a theoretical model of educational and occupational attainment, was developed by researchers in the field of sociology. This model has been used by researchers in school psychology (e.g., Keith & Lichtman, 1994), education (Hanson, 1994; Hossler & Stage, 1992), and career development counseling (e.g., McWhirter, Hackett, & Bandalos, 1998; Trusty, Plata, & Salazar, 2003).

What distinguishes research in the counseling field from research in other fields is that counseling research, in general, has a more applied nature. That is, research in counseling focuses on interventions, on the experiences of counselors and clients, and on ways that clients and students can be more effectively served. Whereas some research in other social science fields may be applied in nature, the major focus is not toward practice and serving clients. Rather, the focus is on developing and testing theory. Counseling researchers, in contrast, focus more on research at a practical level, the counseling-practice level and client-needs level: How can my research be designed to find the most effective treatment for clients experiencing addictions? What variables are important to the positive growth of women who experience domestic violence? What are the critical junctures in the coming out process for lesbian, gay, and bisexual clients? How can parents best help their adolescent children in their educational development? These are important questions, and research can—at least to some degree—answer all of them.

Although theory development and theory testing are not the major focus of counseling research, theory is important. Theory guides counseling practice (see Chapter 1, "Theoretical and Historical Foundations of the Counseling Profession"), and often, research that tests theory also has implications for counseling practice. Theories (e.g., counseling theories, developmental theories, theories of personality) provide structure and direction for counseling research. Additionally, when research is designed around theory, the research becomes more connected to and informative to our knowledge bases.

Research from counseling and the broader social sciences has built our knowledge bases over the last 100 years. These knowledge bases are by no means static. Much is known about counseling, but much is unknown. There are many gaps in our knowledge bases, and researchers attempt to bridge those gaps. Researchers add to the knowledge bases daily by developing new theories, models, and approaches, or by applying known models to various populations or settings. The need for knowledge in counseling is constantly changing, with new knowledge gaps arising frequently. As our economy and society changes, new challenges arise for counselors. For example, one change that has had a large impact on counselors and researchers over the last few decades is the increasing diversity of populations, and an increasing recognition that counseling has not served diverse populations effectively.

MULTICULTURAL AND DIVERSITY ISSUES IN RESEARCH

One valid criticism of counseling theory and methods is that much of the theory and practice of counseling was developed through research using mostly White, Western, college-student, cultural, and socioeconomic mainstream samples of participants. Thus, much of the knowledge in counseling may not be relevant to populations outside the mainstream. This point has been made with regard to counseling theory, research, and practice in general (e.g., Ponterotto, 1998) and to career development theory, research, and practice in particular (e.g., Arbona, 1996).

Until the latter decades of the 20th century, the perspective of counseling was *monolithic* (Jackson, 1995). That is, counseling was based on a single view of the world, the Anglo-European view. Ivey (1995) termed this the *naïve Eurocentric approach*, and Sue and Sue (1999) referred to this worldview as *ethnocentric monoculturalism*. Counseling, according to Jackson (1995) and Ivey (1995), is shifting to a more pluralistic or multicultural perspective, a perspective that is more flexible in addressing the needs of those outside the cultural mainstream. This multicultural perspective involves focusing on the commonalities as well as differences across cultures and groups, and within cultures and groups. This perspective involves seeing our clients and ourselves as cultural beings (Ivey, Ivey, & Simek-Morgan, 1993; Ramirez, 1999). This perspective also involves developing theories and models relevant to groups outside the mainstream, and research is the means for developing multicultural knowledge (Ponterotto, 1998, 2002, 2005).

Over the last four decades there has been a marked increase in the number of published studies that focus on groups outside the socioeconomic and cultural mainstream. New divisions of the American Counseling Association (ACA) have established journals focusing on diversity issues (e.g., *Journal of Multicultural Counseling and Development, Journal of LGBT Issues in Counseling*), and multicultural issues have gained increased attention in other ACA journals.

Active Learning Exercise **7.1**

Compile a list of possible challenges or difficulties in doing research with diverse groups of people, particularly those outside the mainstream of Western culture.

RESEARCH PERSPECTIVES IN COUNSELING

There are two general perspectives in counseling and social science research. The quantitative perspective has dominated counseling research across the history of the field. The qualitative perspective, however, has gained in use across the last few decades (Ponterotto, 2005). The most obvious difference between quantitative and qualitative research approaches is in the nature of the data. The data of quantitative research are numbers, whereas the data of qualitative research are mostly words. Qualitative data may also come in the forms of visual observations or audiovisual materials. Differences between the two, however, go much deeper than the nature of data. There are also marked differences among various qualitative approaches, and among some quantitative approaches. Qualitative research approaches originated in the fields of anthropology, sociology, and history—more subjective and interpretive fields. Quantitative approaches originated in agriculture and related disciplines—naturally more objective and scientific fields.

When qualitative research began to gain recognition and use in counseling and the social sciences in the latter decades of the 20th century, qualitative perspectives were often described in contrast to quantitative perspectives. Authors used the language and concepts of the more prominent quantitative tradition to define and describe qualitative research (e.g., Merrill, 1985; Stainback & Stainback, 1984). Comparisons of quantitative and qualitative approaches are rarely simple and perfect because the two are qualitatively different from one another. In the last several years, qualitative researchers have developed language consistent with qualitative perspectives, and now more authors (e.g., Morrow, 2005; Silverstein, Auerbach, & Levant, 2006) are illuminating the philosophical and conceptual characteristics of qualitative approaches by using this new language.

Although direct comparisons of qualitative and quantitative approaches are not always tenable, comparisons do aid in understanding the differing characteristics of the two. Because both qualitative and quantitative approaches are described in this chapter, I will make qualitative-quantitative comparisons.

Philosophical Variables and Research Perspectives

Creswell (2007) described five philosophical variables that influence perspectives on research:

1. *Ontology*, study of the nature of reality
2. *Epistemology*, study of the nature of knowledge
3. *Axiology*, study of the nature of values
4. *Rhetoric*, the language used in research
5. *Methodology*, a set of practices followed by the researcher

These variables form quantitative and qualitative research perspectives, and they influence choices of particular research techniques within both quantitative and qualitative research paradigms.

Ontology

Ontology is concerned with the nature of being and the nature of reality. Creswell (2007) notes that qualitative approaches necessarily embrace the idea of multiple realities. Reality is held in the eye (mind) of the perceiver because perceptions of reality can only be formed through the filters of our senses. Glesne (1999) maintains that research participants' realities are constructed in relation to their particular social worlds, and reality cannot be separated from the perceiver. Through the qualitative research process, reality is co-constructed between the researcher and the research participant.

The philosophy of quantitative research is based on the ontological assumption of a relatively stable reality. Reality can be separated from the perceiver and observable knowledge can be defined. Social, environmental, and individual-psychological variables can be quantified and accounted for in studies. Knowledge is generated through objective measurement of variables.

From the quantitative ontological perspective, the researcher is objectively detached from the research participants, exercising careful controls so as to not bias the results in any way. From the qualitative ontological perspective, the researcher is deeply involved with the research participants, seeking to learn participants' realities and co-construct realities with them.

Epistemology

Epistemology is the study of the nature of knowledge and the grounds for knowledge. Ideas about the nature of knowledge inherently connect to ideas about the nature of reality. Researchers from both quantitative and qualitative perspectives seek to generate knowledge by observing or interacting with some reality.

Qualitative researchers believe that knowledge can be gained by close and prolonged contact with the participant in the natural environment of the participant. Creswell (2007) notes that the logic process in qualitative research is inductive. That is, knowledge proceeds from the ground up, or from the researcher-participant interactions to a comprehensive set of themes or abstractions (from the particular to the general). In this process, knowledge is formed interactively and collaboratively. Even the research questions themselves may change as the researcher interacts with the participants.

In contrast, quantitative perspectives are more objective and deductive in epistemological perspective, and the research categories are determined beforehand. The quantitative researcher begins with fixed research questions and a fixed research design. The logic for the study is determined by review of empirical research and theory. This general knowledge guides deduction. Deduction flows from the general to the particular. Although both quantitative and qualitative approaches involve deductive and inductive inferences, they differ epistemologically in the process of knowledge generation. That is, induction guides the logic or reasoning process in qualitative research, whereas deduction guides the process in quantitative research.

Axiology

Axiology is the study of the nature of values and value judgments. From the qualitative perspective, all research stems from the values of the researcher, theory, or research paradigm, and the social and cultural norms influencing the researcher and participants. Many social science researchers in the quantitative paradigm would agree with this assertion. Where qualitative and quantitative perspectives differ, however, is in how values are used and manifested in the process of research. From the quantitative perspective, researchers seek to minimize the influence of their own values in conducting the study and in presenting the results. They seek to be objective and scientific. Quantitative researchers' values are implicit in the empirical and theoretical formulations on which they base their research, in the variables they quantify, and in the research designs they employ. Qualitative researchers, in contrast, are explicit in their values, being reflexive (open, forthcoming) in how their values guide their studies. Because the researcher is the main active instrument in the research, researcher values are axiomatic in qualitative research.

The interpretive character of qualitative research illuminates the salience of axiology (Marshall & Rossman, 2006). If reality is perceived only through the researcher's senses, then values undoubtedly influence perceptions of that reality. Values not only determine how interactions are interpreted but also when attention is activated and where it is directed. The values of participants are also salient, and particularly when qualitative models stress the importance of participant-researcher social interaction.

Rhetoric

The rhetorical philosophical variable addresses the style of writing and use of language—in writing studies and in describing studies, methods, or phenomena. The rhetoric of the qualitative perspective is personal and literary. For example, a researcher writing a qualitative journal article might use metaphors extensively (Creswell, 2007). In scientific writing, metaphors are discouraged (see American Psychological Association [APA], 2001; note that the APA *Publication Manual* is the style guide that is followed by most counseling journals).

Much writing in qualitative studies is of a storytelling nature. Narrative studies in particular focus on the stories that participants tell. Narrative studies are sometimes biographical or autobiographical, and they are often structured around common literary forms. Other types of qualitative research studies (e.g., phenomenology, ethnography) are literary in character.

In the quantitative research tradition, the language is scientific and objective, and the use of literary forms and techniques is discouraged. The form and content for reports of research is explicitly prescribed in the quantitative paradigm (see APA, 2001).

Methodology

A methodology is a coherent set of activities, rules, or practices followed by the researcher. The philosophical variable methodology is a general, overarching one. That is, ontology, epistemology, axiology, and rhetoric drive methodology. Researchers' philosophical perceptions of reality and knowledge, their values, and their perceptions of language shape the methods they use.

Induction is the framework for generating and organizing knowledge in most qualitative methods. Thus, methods and research designs often emerge as qualitative studies are being conducted. This practice is generally referred to as *emergent design*. That is, as researchers become insiders in environments, their methods may be changed to accommodate or refine the emerging knowledge. For example, a qualitative researcher may begin a study with a set of broad, open-ended interview questions. As the researcher learns from the participants, new areas of interest emerge, and the researcher engages the participants in an additional round of interviews or observations.

Quantitative studies, in contrast, are designed before data are collected. Some quantitative studies are exploratory in nature, but even in exploratory studies, the variables are determined beforehand. Most often, quantitative studies are designed a priori (beforehand) and based on existing empirical evidence and theory.

How researchers perceive the character of the philosophical variables and how they weight the variables relative to one another determine the research methodology chosen. Also, the philosophical variables might not place a particular study neatly within one methodology or another, but may suggest a blend of qualitative methods, or a blend of qualitative and quantitative methods (a *mixed-methods* approach).

A general comparison of quantitative and qualitative research approaches is presented in Table 7.1. Quantitative and qualitative traditions stand in stark contrast to one another, as seen in the cells of this table.

These differences are functionally real in the conduct of research; however, the differences are not as pure or perfect as they might seem at first glance. Numbers and frequencies do sometimes have a role qualitative research. In some qualitative research methodologies, the researcher reports the frequency

TABLE **7.1**

Comparison of Quantitative and Qualitative Research Traditions

	Quantitative	Qualitative
Nature of data	Numbers, frequencies, percentages, scores on instruments, numerical ratings	Words, people's stories, visual observations, audiovisual materials
Ontology	Single stable reality, reality exists outside the perceiver, reality can be represented by discrete quantified variables	Multiple realities, reality exists in the mind of the perceiver, researcher-participant co-constructed reality
Epistemology	Deductive, research categories determined beforehand, researcher detached from participants	Inductive, knowledge gained through interaction with participants, research categories emerge
Axiology	Researcher values implicit, role of values minimized	Researcher values explicit, role of values maximized
Rhetoric	Impersonal, scientific, quantitative concepts and terminology used	Personal, literary, qualitative concepts and terminology used
Methodology	A priori designs, categories determined beforehand	Emergent designs, categories generated from the data

of occurrences of words or phrases, or the numbers or percentages of participants who had responses that support particular themes. Some qualitative methodologies use underlying quantitative processes (e.g., computer software programs) for data analysis. Quantitative researchers also use data typically associated with qualitative traditions (e.g., visual observations, people's stories), but these are typically quantified in some way. With regard to ontology and epistemology, some quantitative research methods and analysis techniques are inductive (e.g., factor analysis, cluster analysis).

Research Problems and Research Perspectives

Counselors and researchers will naturally gravitate toward one research perspective or the other depending on their own experiences and the ways they perceive the world. If counselors, however, only read qualitative research, or only read quantitative research, they will be missing a large portion of our knowledge bases. Research from both quantitative and qualitative perspectives contributes to what we know about counseling and clients. In fact, if a research finding is supported by both quantitative and qualitative studies, the finding is made stronger.

As researchers decide on which method to use for a study, they should be driven more by the particular research problem than by their own philosophy or preferences. The research problem (the first step in the *scientific method* process) defines the gaps in knowledge bases and describes the issue, concern, or need to be addressed (Creswell, 2005). Qualitative methods have advantages in particular areas of research problems, as do quantitative methods.

Quantitative studies are indicated when established constructs are used or when objective data are accessible or available. For example, if a researcher wants to investigate the influence of clients' cognitive coping skills on anxiety, there are established theories and measurement instruments that can be used in designing the study. If a school counselor wants to study the school climate in the middle school, there are several established school climate measures from which to choose. There are theories, measures, and established quantitative research methods for many of the variables important to mental health counseling (e.g., depression, anxiety, personality dimensions), career counseling (e.g., interests, values, career adaptability), addictions counseling (e.g., substance use, attitudes, risk assessments), rehabilitation counseling (e.g., physical functioning, living skills, cognitive assessments), and school counseling (e.g., achievement, aptitude, learning styles).

In general, qualitative methods are warranted when little is known about a research area or problem. When there is no existing theory or measurement instruments to guide a quantitative study, interviews with research participants may lay the groundwork for theory or at least determine more defined research problems for subsequent qualitative or quantitative studies. Many phenomena in counseling are best studied qualitatively. For example, if the researcher's interest is in the phenomenological experiences of clients in counseling, there is an established qualitative research method, phenomenology, that can be applied. As knowledge develops from qualitative studies, quantitative studies may be used to verify or support the qualitative findings.

The character of research problems is salient. For example, if the researcher wants to investigate the lived experiences of a particular group of people, defined by experience or culture, a qualitative study is likely needed. If a researcher can describe the research problem in terms of variables, a quantitative study is likely needed. If the phenomena to be studied are highly subjective in character, a qualitative study is indicated. If the phenomena are either objective or can be validly objectified, a quantitative study is probably best.

As consumers of research, counselors should be knowledgeable of various quantitative and qualitative methods so they can use research to inform their practice of counseling. As counselor trainees, you will likely learn that researchers often fall into philosophically rigid camps, frequently purporting that their "knowledge" is the only true knowledge. I encourage counselor trainees to take a flexible and pragmatic approach in using counseling and social sciences research literature and in learning about the field of counseling. My belief is that a flexible approach will increase your flexibility in serving diverse clients.

It seems naturally logical that complex problems are best solved by approaching them from multiple perspectives. A pragmatic approach seems particularly applicable to many research problems in counseling. Ponterotto and Grieger (1999) described the merging of qualitative and quantitative perspectives as similar to being bilingual and bicultural. The pragmatic approach to research begs the questions, Is it useful or advisable to ignore methods and data because they are not consistent with a particular researcher's ideology? Should research be driven by philosophy and ideology or by research problems and data?

Active Learning Exercise **7.2**

Start this exercise by identifying a knowledge gap in our knowledge base (i.e., a research problem). This should be a knowledge gap in your area of interest or emphasis. Provide a rationale for using either quantitative or qualitative methods, or both, to address your research problem.

QUANTITATIVE APPROACHES TO RESEARCH

Quantitative research methods are used in the vast majority of research studies published in counseling and psychology journals (Nilsson, Love, Taylor, & Slusher, 2007; Ponterroto, 2005). Quantitative research articles in counseling focus on a variety of topics. For example, Nilsson et al. performed a content analysis of quantitative research articles recently published in the *Journal of Counseling & Development*. They found that the most frequent research topics were the following:

- Career and academic development
- Multicultural issues
- Symptoms and disorders
- The counseling process
- Interventions and treatments

- Counselor training and supervision
- Gender issues

There are numerous quantitative research methods. It is beyond the scope of this chapter to describe any of the methods in detail. Thus, I will focus on general principles and engage in general discussion of prominent quantitative research issues, including measurement, sampling, and research design.

Measurement and Variables

A variable is simply any phenomenon that is able to vary (i.e., it has at least two categories or levels). Measures are the means through which variables are delineated in quantitative research. Measures may be formal assessment instruments; they may be seemingly straightforward ways of categorizing groups of people; or they may be complex ways of quantifying behaviors, perceptions, responses, or other phenomena. The number of possible measures in the world and beyond is infinite.

In quantitative research, the importance of measurement cannot be overstated. Measurement influences almost every aspect of the research process. If a research study is not built upon sound measures, the research results will necessarily not be sound. When particular research findings are challenged (and often rightfully so), the point of challenge is frequently how the variables used in the research were measured. For example, samples of people from various populations are frequently polled on their attitudes and perceptions regarding political matters. Responses of people to polls likely depend on whether the question was asked in the negative or positive, the context of the question among preceding questions, the wording of the question, and how possible response categories are defined. Poll results are frequently challenged on how polling questions were posed.

Measures directly influence the results of research. Most research involves examining relationships or differences based on multiple variables. If a single measure is not precise or genuine, then how that particular variable relates to other variables is not precise or genuine. An analogy is travel over distances. If a spacecraft leaves the earth and if a single measurement of trajectory is off by a fraction of an inch, the path will be off by a great distance as the craft leaves our atmosphere, and off by an even greater distance as it reaches orbital height. Likewise, if we are, for example, building an empirical model of help-seeking for groups outside the mainstream of Western culture and if our measure of social mistrust is not precise or genuine, then our results could easily mislead us toward an erroneous conclusion about this population and help-seeking behavior.

Sampling

In quantitative research, the population to be studied is first defined. For example, a population might be defined as U.S. women ages 21 to 35, or as counseling clients presenting with career concerns, or as middle school students categorized as victims of bullying. The units in populations are not always individual people. Analysis units might be defined as dyads (e.g., couples, counselor-client dyads), or counseling groups, or schools, or mental health counseling facilities. Populations are not necessarily people, but in counseling and the social sciences, populations are most often a collection of people; in samples, the person is commonly the unit of analysis.

After a population is defined, the researcher seeks to obtain a representative sample of the population as research participants. Participants are measured along a set of variables, analyses of data are conducted using inferential statistics, and the researcher generalizes (infers) findings from the sample studied to the population it represents. Researchers use samples because it is expensive and otherwise difficult to access and measure every member of an entire population.

Simple random samples are those in which every member of a given population has an equal chance, or equal probability, of being selected. These samples are sometimes called *strict probability samples*, and this is the gold standard in quantitative research. In fact, inferential statistics operate on the assumption that samples are simple random samples. In the practical research context, simple random samples are often very difficult to achieve. It is rare that all people selected will volunteer to participate in the research and that all volunteers will respond on all measurement instruments.

Stratified sampling involves selecting a sample from subgroups (strata) of the population to ensure that subgroups in the sample are representative of the subgroups in the population. Typically, stratified sampling is simple random sampling from the strata of the population.

A stratification variable is one that is important to the context of the study. For example, a school counselor is researching students' awareness of cultural differences in a culturally diverse school. In the context of this particular study, it is necessary that the sample be proportionally representative of the racial-ethnic composition of the school. That is, if Mexican Americans comprise 30 percent of the school population, Mexican Americans should comprise 30 percent of the sample; and likewise with other represented racial-ethnic groups.

Cluster samples are used in large-scale studies. Cluster sampling is most useful when the population is large and distributed over a wide geographical area. Researchers performing national studies (e.g., National Center for Education Statistics) often use complex sampling techniques to obtain representative samples. For example, schools might first be sampled and then students within schools are sampled. What results is clearly not a simple random sample. Researchers, however, use statistical techniques to estimate and correct for the sampling error inherent in complex sampling designs.

Convenience samples are simply samples of convenience. All convenience samples are biased by their nature. Unfortunately, most samples in the counseling and social sciences literature are convenience samples. For example, in the content analysis of the counseling journal by Nilsson et al. (2007), random sampling techniques were used in only 12 percent of the quantitative research articles. Nilsson et al. also noted a seeming overrepresentation of general college student samples and underrepresentation of clinical samples. The most frequently occurring type of convenience sample that I have seen in the literature is "student volunteers in an introductory psychology course in a large Midwestern university." One major problem with convenience samples is the lack of generalizability. How much is the rest of the world like the world of students at large universities in the Midwest? Is there sampling bias in who comes to a psychology class and seeks extra credit for participating in research?

Research Design

There are numerous research designs used in counseling and the social sciences. Research designs are frameworks that researchers follow in addressing research problems, answering research questions, and testing hypotheses. Quantitative research designs are determined prior to conducting the study. In various quantitative designs, the terminology used and the procedures that are followed are largely based on scientific tradition.

Research designs can be classified into two general groups, experimental designs and nonexperimental designs. All quantitative research designs that involve studying the efficacy of an intervention or treatment are classified as experimental. Those studies that do not involve a treatment or intervention are classified in the broad category of nonexperimental. For example, if researchers provide different interventions to treatment and control groups and compare outcomes, then the study is experimental. On the other hand, if researchers investigate the relationships between participants' scores or ratings on variables to other scores or ratings, the studies are nonexperimental.

Experimental studies are best for supporting or demonstrating cause (e.g., the counseling intervention experienced by the treatment group resulted in, or caused, better outcomes for the treatment group as compared to the control group). The most prominent issues regarding experimental studies, therefore, are those that surround cause, and the most effective experimental designs are those that make the strongest case for causal relationships between treatment and outcome. Researchers use the terminology *careful controls* when speaking of experimental studies, and careful controls are those that account for issues surrounding cause. When researchers apply careful controls to experimental studies, they can often validly conclude that outcomes were caused by the intervention or treatment. Careful controls include, for example, randomly assigning participants to treatment or control groups and controlling for the effects of experimenters on the participants.

There are several types of nonexperimental quantitative studies. Three common major categories are (1) descriptive designs, (2) causal-comparative designs, and (3) correlational designs. Descriptive designs have the purpose of describing phenomena only. Researchers may take measurements or report frequencies on more than one variable; but in most descriptive studies, variables are examined one at a time (i.e., the focus in not on relationships among variables). Variables are investigated in more a descriptive sense than in a theory-testing sense or causal sense or predictive sense.

The purpose of causal-comparative designs is to examine how subgroups within the study differ (e.g., a mean-difference approach, a comparison of averages). Causal-comparative studies compare two or more groups on one or more outcome variables. The grouping variables in causal-comparative studies are typically status variables (non-manipulatable variables like ethnicity or language) or other variables that naturally precede the outcome variable in time. Causal-comparative designs are also called ex post facto designs. Causal-comparative research designs are used in lieu of experimental designs because it is often not possible or ethical to manipulate variables (e.g., withhold a needed treatment for the control group).

The purpose of correlational research designs is to discover relationships and patterns of relationships among variables. Causal-comparative and correlational designs have many qualities and issues in common. The major advantage of correlational designs over causal-comparative designs is that the former better accommodates larger numbers of variables; therefore, correlational studies are more comprehensive. Although experimental designs are the best for determining causal relationships, well-designed correlational and causal-comparative studies can either support or disconfirm causal linkages. Correlational and causal-comparative studies are often used to test theory, and all theories purport causal relationships. If the results of the study show relationships specified in the theoretical formulations, the results then support those causal linkages. If the results are not as the theory predicted, the results disconfirm the theory. Note that the words *support* or *disconfirm* are tentative in nature, particularly in the positive direction (i.e., *support*). Words such as *prove* are not used to describe nonexperimental research results.

Active Learning Exercise **7.3**

In this exercise, you will formulate a research problem aimed at addressing some knowledge gap around the comparative effectiveness of two interventions for a particular population or group of people. Design an experimental study with a treatment group (a new intervention) and a control group (the usual intervention). Discuss how your research could (a) add to our knowledge base and (b) help the group in question.

QUALITATIVE APPROACHES TO RESEARCH

Qualitative approaches to research are more subjective and interpretive than quantitative approaches, relying on data derived primarily from interviews and observations rather than numerical data.

Qualitative Methods

Qualitative researchers in counseling and the social sciences most often use interviews of participants as the source of data. In qualitative research, *purposeful sampling* is used. Researchers purposefully select participants that are information rich—the participants most likely to bear the information sought. Qualitative samples are typically much smaller than samples in quantitative research. A case study may use a sample of one person, or a grounded theory study may employ a sample of 6 to 10 participants. In qualitative studies, selection of participants may continue until a data saturation point is reached. Interviews, for example, may continue until no new data are forthcoming.

There are many qualitative methods and research designs. Some of the most commonly used are the following:

- Ethnographic study
- Case study
- Grounded theory study
- Phenomenological study

Ethnographic studies are used to gain knowledge about some culture-sharing group. In ethnography, researchers interview and observe participants and investigate documents or other products. Researchers seek to understand some group of people from an insider perspective.

Case studies provide in-depth description of the experiences of a person, a group, or other entity. Case studies often focus on a set of issues encountered by the participant(s). In counseling, case studies are often the description of a single counseling client and the experiences of the client within and outside the process of counseling.

In grounded theory studies, researchers seek to build a theory from the ground up. Grounded theory studies are indicated when little is known about the research problem, and thus the grounded theory inductive process is useful. Researchers discover themes in participants' experiences, and these themes form the basis for theory.

Phenomenological studies seek to understand the common lived experiences of a group of participants. The researcher's goal is to understand the essence of the experience from the perspectives of the participants.

Qualitative researchers do not claim generalizability of findings in a quantitative sense (generalization from the sample to the population). Instead, they focus on *transferability*—the degree to which findings transfer to some other case or some other setting. A counselor, for example, reads a case study and decides how the findings from the case transfer to the counselor's own clients or work setting. Also, qualitative findings sometimes generalize from the sample to the theory (e.g., grounded theory research).

Active Learning Exercise **7.4**

In this exercise, you will formulate a research problem aimed at addressing some knowledge gap around a particular group with whom you are familiar. Frame your research problem within one of the four common qualitative methods. Discuss how your research could (a) add to our knowledge base and (b) help the group in question.

Research Worldviews

A *worldview* is a set of beliefs and values through which people operate. Ponterotto and Grieger (1999) described worldviews as culturally and socialization-based perspectives. Research worldviews are formed around philosophical variables, particularly ontology and epistemology. Creswell (2007) described four general worldviews connected to qualitative—and some-times quantitative—research: (1) postpositivism, (2) social constructivism, (3) advocacy/participatory, and (4) pragmatism.

Postpositivism

The postpositivist worldview embraces the current common, scientific approach to research. The assumptions of postpositivist qualitative research are similar to the assumptions of current quantitative research. It is assumed that there is a relatively stable and objective reality, and reality can exist outside the perceptions of the research participant. Haverkamp and Young (2007) note that postpositivism differs from its predecessor, positivism, in that reality cannot be assessed perfectly. Therefore, convergence of findings across numerous studies using various methods is needed to produce dependable knowledge.

Postpositivist research is likely linked to existing or emerging theory. The purpose of studies is often testing the viability of some theoretical formulation or model. Thus, postpositivist research is largely concerned with supporting or disconfirming cause-and-effect relationships, and it is deductive in charac-ter. The researcher typically makes methodological decisions beforehand, accomplishing the study through a series of logical steps.

Social Constructivism

The social constructivism worldview posits that people construct their reali-ties through social interactions with others. There are multiple, equally valid realities, and knowledge is co-constructed among researchers and participants (Haverkamp & Young, 2007). Reality cannot be observed directly; thus, real-ity must be interpreted to produce knowledge. Social constructivism is often termed the *interpretivist worldview*. This worldview stands in sharp contrast with the postpositivist worldview.

Social constructivism is non-reductionistic and inductive in character. The researcher is focused on the complexities and multiple meanings of partici-pants' experiences. Researchers ask open-ended questions, seeking to learn participants' views in social, cultural, and historical contexts. The processes of social interactions are important to researchers. Rather than operating from an a priori theory, as in the postpositivist worldview, social constructi-vists inductively generate a pattern of meanings from their interactions with participants.

From this worldview, researchers recognize the salience of their own values to the interpretive process, and they position themselves within the study (Cresswell, 2007). That is, researchers exercise reflexivity, paying close attention to how their own values influence their interpretations. Because of the complexities of social processes and the strong influences of researcher and participant values, researchers typically need prolonged contact with partici-pants to develop adequate depth of co-constructions. The social constructivist worldview is strongly reflected in phenomenological studies and grounded the-ory studies and, to a variable extent, in narrative studies, ethnography, and case studies.

Advocacy/Participatory Worldview

Researchers operating from an advocacy/participatory worldview often reject postpositivism because the theories and research frameworks used by postpositivists were not generated from research with marginalized groups and do not fit for these groups. Advocacy/participatory researchers might argue that social constructivist researchers do not focus enough on producing positive gains for their participants and the groups they represent (Cresswell, 2007).

From the advocacy/participatory worldview, the purposes of research are to (a) advocate for changing oppressive social structures and (b) empower participants and groups to effectively advocate for themselves. The research is focused on action toward changing institutions, service systems, policies, or any practices or events that affect participants' lives. Researchers seek to "give a voice" to the participants or the groups they represent.

Researchers holding to an advocacy/participatory worldview believe that a common, relatively consistent reality exists. This reality embodies historical, cultural, economic, social, and political influences that serve to marginalize groups of people. Haverkamp and Young (2007) noted that the researcher's role is both interactive and proactive. The researcher interacts with participants to understand their social and cultural milieu, and the researcher and participants take actions to address inequities. The research effort typically ends with the development of an action agenda.

Pragmatism

As the name of this research worldview implies, there is no alignment with any one particular ontology or epistemology. Pragmatists believe that the world is complex, and no unified philosophy explains all phenomena or perhaps even one phenomenon. Instead of accepting one philosophy and rejecting others, pragmatists embrace various approaches to research, including quantitative ones. From the pragmatic worldview, reality exists both within the mind and independent of the mind.

Pragmatists devote minimal attention to philosophical abstractions, being more interested in what works and believing that various qualitative and quantitative methodologies can be useful for answering questions and solving problems. Thus, researchers are free to choose an array of research techniques and methods that fit their purposes.

Pragmatists use *mixed methods* in research, and this term often identifies a pragmatic worldview. Ponterroto (2002) noted the strengths of qualitative and mixed methods in multicultural counseling research. Brannen (2005) described the dynamics in mixed-methods research designs. Mixed methods can provide *corroboration*. That is, when different approaches converge on a common answer or solution, research findings are strengthened. Mixed methods might also provide *elaboration* when one method extends or amplifies the findings from another method. Findings from mixed methods could also produce *complementarity* when findings are different across methods yet they provide useful insights. Findings across methods might also produce *contradiction*. Contradictions, however, often provide useful information.

Table 7.2 presents a comparison of salient features of various qualitative (and sometimes quantitative) research worldviews.

TABLE **7.2**
Basic Features of Research Worldviews

Worldview	Major Focus	Ontology	Epistemology
Postpositivism	Scientific verification of theory	Relatively stable, objective reality	Convergence of findings produces dependable knowledge
Social constructivism	Participants' social experiences	Realities constructed through human interactions	Interpretive and inductive, knowledge arises from interactions
Advocacy/ participatory	Positive gains for participants and groups	Relatively stable reality	Knowledge emerges from participants' historical and cultural experience
Pragmatism	Eclectic use of methods, what works	Flexible, reality exists both within and outside the mind	Knowledge is generated from various sources with various methods

---

Active Learning Exercise **7.5**

Choose one of the four research worldviews that is most consistent with your own personal worldview. Develop a rationale for why this worldview generates useful knowledge in your field of interest or emphasis. Next, select one of the other research worldviews and provide a *valid* rationale why it can contribute to the knowledge base in your area of interest or emphasis.

ETHICS IN RESEARCH

The *ACA Code of Ethics* (ACA, 2005) addresses research in counseling in several sections. Sections with particular focus on research are Section B.7 (Research and Training), Section E (Evaluation, Assessment, and Interpretation), and Section G (Research and Publication).

Section B covers confidentiality, privileged communication, and the privacy of clients in many areas. Section B.7 focuses mainly on confidentiality of information gained through research, informed consent for research participants, and following institutional guidelines and relevant laws in conducting research. For example, B.7.b addresses the importance of adherence to governmental and institutional policies in conducting research. B.7.c and B.7.d stress the salience of confidentiality and research participants' privacy rights.

Section E addresses the use of assessment instruments for research or other purposes. Particular statements in this section address research issues such as client welfare and rights, counselor competence in interpreting instruments, validity of measurement, and multicultural-diversity dimensions in measurement and research. For example, E.2.a relates that counselors do not overstep the bounds of their knowledge when using assessment instruments.

Section G speaks to many issues in counseling research, including confidentiality, respect for diverse groups of people, minimizing research bias, protection of the rights of research participants, accurate reporting of research results, and publication practices. In this section, researchers are encouraged to take cultural variables into account in their research studies (e.g., G.1.g).

All counselors, counselor trainees, and counselor educators should be knowledgeable of the *ACA Code of Ethics* in research and other areas. Counseling professionals and trainees should note the introduction to Section C, Professional Responsibility. In this section, the *Code of Ethics* maintains that counselors should employ counseling practices that are supported by research.

CONCLUSION

It is hoped that those new to the field of counseling will utilize the knowledge that research offers. Research informs professional counseling practitioners in many areas, including (a) what variables are important to clients' functioning; (b) the extent to which counseling theories, techniques, and interventions are effective; (c) what measures of variables are useful; and (d) the subjective experiences of persons or groups. In short, research helps counselors better serve clients and groups of people.

It is further hoped that those new to the field of counseling become researchers, or generators of knowledge in our field. Quantitative and qualitative research offer many tools with which counselors-researchers can generate new knowledge. Much is known in the field of counseling, but much is not known, and clients' lives and society are ever changing. A dynamic world demands vigorous and adaptable practitioners and researchers.

CHAPTER REVIEW

1. Research is the means by which knowledge about counseling is generated. Research methods in counseling are similar to methods in other social science fields, and the knowledge bases in counseling and the broader social sciences often inform one another. Research in counseling, in contrast to much social sciences research, is applied in nature, focusing on the practical application of findings.

2. Counseling theory, practice, and research have often been criticized because they were formed around mainstream populations. The field of counseling has come to recognize this shortcoming, and researchers have been moving toward a greater focus on diverse populations.

3. Two broad research perspectives exist in counseling and the social sciences, namely, quantitative and qualitative. Although most published research in counseling is quantitative, qualitative approaches are gaining in use. The philosophical variables of ontology, epistemology, axiology, rhetoric, and methodology form researcher perspectives both within and between quantitative and qualitative approaches. Research problems, rather than ideology, should drive the approaches that researchers take. Counselors can benefit from understanding various approaches to research because various perspectives offer knowledge around counseling.

4. Quantitative researchers design their studies before they begin them. Their designs are based on existing theory and empirical evidence. They define a population to be studied, draw a sample from the population,

administer measurements and otherwise collect data, analyze data, and generalize findings from the sample to the population. Studies are designated as experimental if the effectiveness of a treatment or intervention is investigated. If no active treatment or intervention is used in the study, it is non-experimental. Researchers exercise careful controls in conducting their studies, and they seek to be objective and unbiased. Quantitative researchers in the field of counseling focus on a variety of research topics.

5. Qualitative researchers use inductive processes to design their studies. Researchers themselves are active instruments in the research process, seeking to understand the subjective experiences of participants by co-constructing reality with participants. They use a variety of methods, and various methods have divergent purposes. The purpose may be to understand a social milieu from the insider's perspective, or the goal may be to develop an action plan aimed at eliminating discriminatory practices.

6. Researchers in counseling are increasingly fostering a pragmatic or mixed-methods approach to generating knowledge. Mixed methods provide researchers flexibility in solving complex problems. A mixture of quantitative and qualitative methods can approach a research problem from multiple perspectives, thus having potential to corroborate or elaborate research findings.

7. The *ACA Code of Ethics*, in numerous sections, speaks directly to research and the conduct of research in counseling. Researchers, counselors, and counselor trainees should be knowledgeable of the ACA code. The *Code of Ethics* represents the explicit values of our field, and it is recognized that counseling practice should be informed by and supported by research.

REVIEW QUESTIONS

1. How does the common, layperson concept of research differ from the professional counseling concept of research?
2. Discuss how research has been or can be used as an instrument of discrimination and oppression toward marginalized groups of people.
3. Compare and contrast quantitative and qualitative approaches to research in terms of ontology, epistemology, axiology, rhetoric, and methods.
4. How is measurement foundational to effective quantitative research?
5. In using quantitative knowledge (e.g., to inform your counseling practice), why is it important to know the sampling methods the researcher used?
6. Why are experimental studies best at supporting or demonstrating the existence of causal relationships?
7. What are the advantages of inductive research approaches and deductive research approaches?
8. How do research worldviews relate to general (not only research) multicultural counseling competence?
9. With regard to research, what are the major principles set forth in the *ACA Code of Ethics*?

ADDITIONAL RESOURCES

• Domestic Violence and Sexual Assault Data Resource Center (data on domestic violence by state; http://www.jrsainfo.org/dvsa-drc/index.html)

• Drug and Alcohol Services Information System, U.S. Department of Health and Human Services. (http://www.jrsainfo.org/dvsa-drc/index.html)

- The Education Trust—Data Tools and Presentations: Closing Opportunity and Achievement Gaps Pre–K Through College. (http://www2.edtrust.org/EdTrust/Data+Tools+and+Presentations)
- The National Center for Education Statistics (NCES; many types of data on U.S. schools and colleges, students, and families; http://nces.ed.gov/)
- NCES Data Tools (http://nces.ed.gov/datatools/)
- National Institute of Mental Health (http://www.nimh.nih.gov/index.shtml)
- National Longitudinal Study of Adolescent Health (data and resources on adolescent health; http://www.cpc.unc.edu/projects/addhealth)
- National Rehabilitation Information Center (abstracts of many studies on rehabilitation; http://www.naric.com/research/rehab/advanced.cfm)
- School Matters (data on U.S. K–12 schools; http://www.schoolmatters.com/schools.aspx/q/page=hm?gclid=CODLwNul9poCFRYpFQodQy4bdg)
- U.S. Bureau of Labor Statistics, U.S. Department of Labor (http://www.bls.gov/)
- U.S. Census Bureau, U.S. Department of Commerce (http://www.census.gov/)

REFERENCES

American Counseling Association. (2005). *ACA code of ethics*. Retrieved March 15, 2008, from http://www.counseling.org/Files/FD.ashx?guid=ab7c1272-71c4-46cf-848c-f98489937dda.

American Psychological Association. (2001). *Publication manual of the American Psychological Association* (5th ed.). Washington, DC: Author.

Arbona, C. (1996). Career theory and practice in a multicultural context. In M. L. Savickas & W. B. Walsh (Eds.), *Handbook of career counseling theory and practice* (pp. 45–54). Palo Alto, CA: Davies-Black.

Brannen, J. (2005). Mixing methods: The entry of qualitative and quantitative approaches into the research process. *International Journal of Social Research Methodology, 8*, 173–184.

Creswell, J. W. (2005). *Educational research: Planning, conducting, and evaluating quantitative and qualitative research* (2nd ed.). Upper Saddle River, NJ: Pearson Education.

Creswell, J. W. (2007). *Qualitative inquiry & research design* (2nd ed.). Thousand Oaks, CA: Sage.

Glesne, C. (1999). *Becoming qualitative researchers: An introduction* (2nd ed.). New York: Longman.

Hanson, S. L. (1994). Lost talent: Unrealized educational aspirations and expectations among U.S. youths. *Sociology of Education, 67*, 159–183.

Haverkamp, B. E., & Young, R. A. (2007). Paradigms, purpose, and the role of literature: Formulating a rationale for qualitative investigations. *The Counseling Psychologist, 35*, 265–294.

Hossler, D., & Stage F. K. (1992). Family and high school experience influences on the postsecondary educational plans of ninth-grade students. *American Educational Research Journal, 29*, 425–451.

Ivey, A. E. (1995). Psychotherapy as liberation. In J. G. Ponterotto, J. M. Casas, L. A. Suzuki, & C. M. Alexander (Eds.), *Handbook of multicultural counseling* (pp. 53–72). Thousand Oaks, CA: Sage.

Ivey, A. E., Ivey, M. B., & Simek-Morgan, L. (1993). *Counseling and psychotherapy: A multicultural perspective* (3rd ed.). Boston: Allyn & Bacon.

Jackson, M. L. (1995). Multicultural counseling: Historical perspectives. In J. G. Ponterotto, J. M. Casas, L. A. Suzuki, & C. M. Alexander (Eds.), *Handbook of multicultural counseling* (pp. 3–16). Thousand Oaks, CA: Sage.

Keith, P. B., & Lichtman, M. V. (1994). Does parental involvement influence the academic achievement of Mexican-American eighth graders? Results from the National Education Longitudinal Study. *School Psychology Quarterly, 9*, 256–272.

Marshall, C., & Rossman, G. B. (2006). *Designing qualitative research* (4th ed.). Thousand Oaks, CA: Sage.

McWhirter, E. H., Hackett, G., & Bandalos, D. L. (1998). A causal model of the educational plans and career expectations of Mexican American high school girls. *Journal of Counseling Psychology, 45*, 166–181.

Merrill, S. C. (1985). Qualitative methods in occupational therapy research: An application. *Occupational Therapy Journal of Research, 5,* 209–222.

Morrow, S. L. (2005). Quality and trustworthiness in qualitative research in counseling psychology. *Journal of Counseling Psychology, 52,* 250–260.

Nilsson, J. E., Love, K. M., Taylor, K. J., & Slusher, A. L. (2007). A content and sample analysis of quantitative articles published in the *Journal of Counseling & Development* between 1991 and 2000. *Journal of Counseling & Development, 85,* 357–363.

Ponterotto, J. G. (1998). Charting a course for research in multicultural counseling training. *The Counseling Psychologist, 26,* 43–68.

Ponterotto, J. G. (2002). Qualitative research methods: The fifth force in psychology. *The Counseling Psychologist, 30,* 394–406.

Ponterotto, J. G. (2005). Qualitative research in counseling psychology: A primer on research paradigms and philosophy of science. *Journal of Counseling Psychology, 52,* 126–136.

Ponterotto, J. G., & Grieger, I. (1999). Merging qualitative and quantitative perspectives in a research

identity. In M. Kopala & L. A. Suzuki (Eds.), *Using qualitative methods in psychology* (pp. 49–62). Thousand Oaks, CA: Sage.

Ramirez, M., III (1999). *Multicultural psychotherapy: An approach to individual and cultural differences* (2nd ed.). Boston: Allyn & Bacon.

Sewell, W. H., Haller, A. O., & Portes, A. (1969). The educational and early occupational attainment process. *American Sociological Review, 34,* 82–92.

Silverstein, L. B., Auerbach, C. F., & Levant, R. F. (2006). Using qualitative research to strengthen clinical practice. *Professional Psychology: Research and Practice, 37,* 351–358.

Stainback, S., & Stainback, W. (1984). Broadening the research perspectives in special education. *Exceptional Children, 50,* 400–408.

Sue, D. W., & Sue, D. (1999). *Counseling the culturally different: Theory and Practice* (3rd ed.). New York: John Wiley & Sons.

Trusty, J., Plata, M., & Salazar, C. F. (2003). Modeling Mexican Americans' educational expectations: Longitudinal effects of variables across adolescence. *Journal of Adolescent Research, 18,* 131–153.

Professional Counseling Settings

CHAPTER 8

Counseling in School Settings

LEARNING OBJECTIVES

After reading this chapter, you should be able to

- explain the key historical events and influences that have shaped the school counseling profession;

- list the four main components of the *ASCA National Model*;

- identify how leadership, advocacy, collaboration and teaming, and systemic change are essential for effective school counseling;

- recognize the importance of accountability in a school counseling program;

- describe the components of a comprehensive developmental school counseling program and explain the importance of developmentally appropriate planning;

- recognize the effectiveness of school counseling programs;

- understand some of the special issues that school counselors will encounter; and

- explain the role of the school counselor in promoting student achievement.

CHAPTER OUTLINE

INTRODUCTION

This chapter provides a brief yet comprehensive overview of the school counseling profession, including historical events that shaped the profession; introduction to the *ASCA* (American School Counselor Association) *National Standards* and *ASCA National Model*; a focus on accountability, advocacy, and systemic change; special issues in school counseling (e.g., crises, at-risk populations, multicultural competence, clinical issues, and students with special education needs); and some challenges that face the current and future generations of professional school counselors. Throughout the chapter, real-life perspectives are shared by experienced professional school counselors, and the clear message is given that continuing educational reform has resulted in the need for school counseling programs to be data driven and for school counselors to be accountable for the outcomes of their counseling initiatives and activities.

A BRIEF HISTORY OF SCHOOL COUNSELING

Although the school counseling profession has only existed for roughly a century, the field has periodically undergone rapid evolution due to myriad social, political, and economic forces and events that have driven the need for reform in the schools. The creation of school counseling itself clearly illustrates how events of the time have influenced and shaped the profession. Starting in the late 19th and early 20th centuries, the United States was experiencing multiple paradigm shifts in education and related fields as it moved from an agricultural society to a primarily industrial society during the Industrial Revolution. In addition, massive waves of immigrants settled in the United States during this period, attracted by new economic opportunities. These occurrences, as well as other significant changes, established progressive social agendas (e.g., human migration, child labor, human dignity, the need to match individuals to an expanding workforce) to the forefront of the nation's social and political discourse. Thus, educational reform at the turn of the 20th century was initiated to address these concerns, and a significant result was the creation of vocational guidance counseling programs in schools.

During the first several decades of the 20th century, teachers were often appointed as vocational counselors despite receiving no formal training. Likewise, no formal organizational structure was yet devised to regulate or even guide a vocational counselor's duties or responsibilities (Gysbers & Henderson, 2001). As the 20th century progressed, pioneers such as Frank Parsons, Jessie Davis, and Eli Weaver, as well as various institutions and national policies, helped to revolutionize the field to fit the needs and philosophies of the time. Often considered the creator of vocational guidance, Frank Parsons was an engineer turned social reformer who adapted a formal system of occupational decision-making (Niles & Harris-Bowlsbey, 2005). In particular, Parsons believed that adolescents and young adults should receive guidance and support in order to choose a vocation. Parson's system, known as the trait-and-factor model, stressed the use of formalized assessments to identify abilities, values, and interests in youth by counselors or practitioners.

Traditional vocational guidance counseling gradually began to move in the direction of a more formal framework known as pupil personnel work. Toward the mid-20th century vocational guidance was still a high priority in schools, but psychological and testing concerns were also beginning to be addressed as the country experienced events such as the Great Depression and World Wars I and II. During the 1940s and beyond, the school counseling profession was further influenced by the works of Carl Rogers and his client-centered counseling approach in which relationship building and collaboration were stressed between the client and the counselor. But it was not until the late 1950s that the school counseling profession in the United States finally came into its own, in response to a perceived national crisis.

The National Defense Education Act

Several key events occurred in the 1950s that were arguably the most influential in the history of the development of the school counseling profession. During the 1950s, the United States and its allies were in the midst of the Cold War with the Soviet Union. The fields of science, engineering, mathematics, and technology were pushed to the forefront in both countries in order to rapidly develop wartime technologies. The general consensus in the United States was that the country lost the Cold War when the Soviet Union launched *Sputnik* in 1957, the first human-made satellite to orbit the Earth. Many parties blamed this loss on an educational system that they believed was not adequately preparing American youth in the math and sciences areas nearly as well as the Soviets. Due to these perceived deficits, the National Defense Education Act (NDEA) was passed in 1958.

This important piece of legislature called for promising secondary students to be identified and encouraged to pursue "hard sciences" in high school and beyond. Guidance counselors were chosen as the professionals to undertake the tasks of testing, identifying, and providing support to these students. In order to fulfill these goals, the NDEA provided several essential provisions. Title V-A apportioned funding to schools that had presented formalized proposals to employ professional school counselors and provide the necessary resources for counseling programs (Herr & Erford, 2011). Title V-B of the NDEA designated funding for higher education institutions to prepare new professional school counselors or to advance the knowledge and skills of existing counselors. In order to receive these funds institutions had to provide program proposals or offer specialized programs. Subsequent amendments to the NDEA expanded the focus and funding to include elementary school counselors and other educational institutions such as community colleges. But it was almost four decades after the launch of Sputnik before school counselors began to coalesce around professional standards and an agreed upon systemic model.

The *ASCA National Standards*

In the three decades following the implementation of the NDEA, several other pieces of federal legislation and educational reform movements helped to refine the school counseling profession. Some prominent examples include the Career Education Incentive Act of 1976, the Carl D. Perkins Vocational Education Act of 1984, and the Elementary School Counseling Demonstration Act of 1995. Despite such important legislation, it was not until 1997, when the ASCA published *Sharing the Vision: The National Standards for School Counseling Programs* (Campbell & Dahir, 1997), that the profession promoted a unified, comprehensive, and developmental foundation that school counseling programs and services nationwide could be based upon.

The *ASCA National Standards* offered a unified focus and provided consistent language to all professional school counselors (Dahir, 2001). It identified the skills, knowledge, and attitudes that students should acquire through proactive and preventive school counseling. These student content standards were organized around three primary domain areas: academic, career, and personal/social (Campbell & Dahir, 1997). Overall, nine national standards were provided, three in each content area. These standards promoted academic achievement and supported success for all students. By using these standards and the associated competencies, professional school counselors were able to clarify counseling and guidance roles that focused on the needs of students. The standards exemplify how the profession continues to evolve and serve as a source of excitement for many counseling professionals. For example, Dr. Lynn Linde (the president of the American Counseling Association for 2009–2010) notes the following:

A Reflection upon School Counseling over the Past 25 Years

In many ways professional school counseling has changed significantly over the past 25 years, but the core of what we do has remained the same. Professional school counseling has always been, and continues to be, a wonderful, challenging, and rewarding profession. Counselors are in such a unique position in schools. Each child sees the world differently, and counselors are the professionals who help students negotiate their world, grow and develop, and advocate for students when they need assistance. Counselors facilitate the development of human potential through their relationships with students and the programs and services they provide. They are for ALL students, not just for an identified few. The underlying mission of school counseling has not changed, but some of the challenges counselors face have.

Schools, as a microcosm of society, reflect the changes in the world around us. As the world, and therefore schools, has changed, so must professional school counselors in order to continue to provide appropriate, relevant, and ethical services for all students. The list of changes during the past 25 years is almost overwhelming. The structure of families has changed; counselors cannot assume that students live at home with their parents. Schools enroll many more students from blended, multigenerational, single-parent, same-sex parent, foster/kinship care, and non-traditional families than ever before. Our schools have also become more diverse, regardless of where one practices. Many students come to school speaking no English, even those students who were born in this country. Professional school counselors have had to become familiar with many ethnicities and cultures and develop culturally sensitive counseling practices. Technology has changed the world, the way we do things, and has increased students' access to information, as well as presenting challenges to keeping inappropriate information from students.

There have been some changes in the issues and problems confronting students. It seems as if more students are coming to school with greater mental health needs and less access to services and interventions. While counselors have always dealt with friendship issues, child abuse, depression and suicidal behavior, substance abuse, sexual behavior and pregnancy issues, the list seems to continue to grow. Anger management, eating disorders, self mutilation, bullying and harassment, cyber bullying, sexual orientation, and changing families are some of the more recent additional issues with which professional school counselors assist students. Crisis planning and violence prevention are cornerstone activities in all schools and ones in which the school counselor has a critical role in addressing the emotional safety of students. Twenty-five years ago violence was viewed as something that happened in other schools; now there is a growing recognition that it could happen anywhere, that no school is immune.

(continued)

A Reflection upon School Counseling over the Past 25 Years *(continued)*

The accountability movement in schools has affected counselors as well. School counseling has moved from a collection of services that the counselor wanted to and was requested to provide to a comprehensive, developmental program that is outcome-based, guided by systematic needs assessment, and regularly evaluated. While this is a positive change as all students receive comprehensive and coordinated services, it has become more of a challenge for counselors to find the time during the academic day to deliver their program. There seem to be more laws, policies, and procedures that impact counseling practice, although much of what we do remains in the gray area. A related change seems minor: we now call ourselves "professional school counselors," rather than "guidance counselors" as we did prior to 1990. But the name change reflects the growing credentialing and professionalism of school counselors. And lastly, there is now an expectation that every school, PreK–12, will be staffed with professional school counselors. Professional school counselors are no longer viewed as nice to have if the system can afford them, but rather needed and often required professionals whose services are valued and seen as integral to the academic success of students.

Dr. Lynn Linde, Director of Clinical Programs in School Counseling at Loyola University Maryland, 2009–2010 President of the American Counseling Association, former Guidance Supervisor in the Baltimore City Public School System, and former Branch Chief of Pupil Services at the Maryland State Department of Education

The *ASCA National Model*

While the *ASCA National Standards* provided much-needed direction to a profession still developing a cohesive identity, it did not propose specific methods of delivery or counseling activities. The standards merely encouraged curricular consistency as programs were adjusted to support individual school system missions. Thus, the *ASCA National Model* (ASCA, 2005) was developed in 2003 to provide a comprehensive framework that addressed *how* professional school counselors could meet the national school counseling standards and goals. It also stressed the use of data to make decisions and the evaluation of those decisions in terms of student achievement and success (Sabella, 2006). The *ASCA National Model* was innovative in that it challenged professional school counselors to move away from the traditional focus on specific students to a more all-inclusive, program-centered focus. To accomplish this, the model's framework centered around four central elements: program foundation, delivery, management, and accountability.

Program foundation provided the backbone for student expectations and counselor services. It included assumptions, beliefs, philosophies, and mission statements. Some of the key assumptions concerning school counseling programs given as examples (ASCA, 2005, p. 28) included the following:

- Reaches every student
- Is comprehensive in scope

- Is preventative in design
- Is developmental in nature
- Is an integral part of a total educational program for student success
- Selects measurable student competencies based on local need in the areas of academic, career and personal/social domains
- Has a delivery system that includes school guidance curriculum, individual planning, responsive services and system support

Program foundations also included the *ASCA National Standards* (i.e., goals), domains (i.e., developmental areas), competencies (i.e., expectations), and indicators (i.e., knowledge, abilities, or skills).

 The next part of the *ASCA National Model* outlined how professional school counselors could implement and deliver their programs to students. An effective *delivery system* should include individual student planning, responsive services (e.g., consultation, individual and group counseling, crisis counseling, peer facilitation), system support and management, and an emphasis on curriculum. Interestingly, in previous decades, a guidance program was almost totally geared toward providing planning and responsive services to selected students with identified problems or in need of specific services (e.g., college counseling). The *ASCA National Model* recognizes that direct service delivery is only one component of a comprehensive program, and that every student deserves to receive school counseling services.

Once the foundations and a delivery system for a school counseling program have been established, a *management system* should be developed. Attention should be placed upon management agreements, use of data, action plans, and use of time. Because thorough school counseling programs are data driven, the use of data is especially important in order to monitor student progress and evaluate counseling programs. For example, school achievement data can be disaggregated by race and socioeconomic status to identify achievement gaps. Also, enrollments in rigorous courses meant to prepare students for college success can be disaggregated to insure that all students, regardless of gender, race, disability, or English language usage proficiency, are given access to rigorous curricula. Data helps school counselors to identify systemic barriers to student success and to close achievement, access, and attainment gaps.

The final component of the *ASCA National Model*, *accountability*, allows professional school counselors to determine that their programs are making a difference for students. Accountability can be measured through performance standards, results reports, and program audits. This data allows school counselors to determine the impact over time of their programs and share the results with stakeholders (e.g., students, parents, teachers, administrators). Thus, the accountability system gives professional school counselors the opportunity to serve as advocates and supporters for every student's academic achievement and competency mastery.

The *ASCA National Model* (ASCA, 2005) also looked beyond program foundation, delivery, management, and accountability to other necessary aspects of school counseling programs. Leadership, advocacy, collaboration and teaming, and systemic change were four themes that were incorporated into the framework. These themes had been emphasized during the late 20th century by educational reformers and visionary organizations such as Education Trust's Transforming School Counseling Initiative as early as 1996. This initiative recognized that school counselors were valuable agents of change in eliminating achievement, access, attainment, and funding disparities between specific populations such as gender, socioeconomic, English language learners, disability, and racial subpopulations. In order to eradicate achievement, access, attainment, and funding disparities, the initiative stressed data-driven school counseling programs and services, as well as issues such as leadership, advocacy, and social justice.

Professional school counselors can demonstrate effective *leadership* by creating comprehensive counseling programs and providing services that facilitate academic success in all students. As shown in the past, school counselors should be moving beyond being secondary service providers to becoming active advocates and leaders of their counseling programs (Dollarhide, 2003). Professional school counselors can provide leadership in various formats such as adhering to the *ASCA National Model* or hosting interdisciplinary summits focusing on promoting academic success and lifelong learning (SchwallieGiddis, ter Maat, & Pak, 2003). Consequently professional school counselors can serve as leaders not only within the school, but within the community and state as well.

Advocacy for students can be viewed as the identification of needs and the successive work to meet those needs. Professional school counselors promote and support the goals of the school and their programs, as well as overcome potential barriers to students' academic success and individual growth. In some cases, this may mean the school counselors must challenge preexisting systems and ideologies. Bemak & Chung (2005, 2008) propose strategies for empowering professional school counselors as advocates for their students by addressing counselor training at the preservice, in-service, and supervision levels.

The third theme incorporated into the framework of the *ASCA National Model* involves *collaboration and teaming*. Professional school counselors must work with various stakeholders not just within the school, but among the school system, parents, and community at large. Such collaborations should focus on developing, implementing, and evaluating programs and services that promote academic success and counseling goals. In the school, collaborations are typically characterized by joint goal setting/planning and knowledge sharing, focused on the needs of individual students (Green & Keys, 2001). By working with stakeholders and related agencies and resources, professional school counselors can create genuinely comprehensive counseling programs.

Systemic change, the fourth and final theme, is achieved when schoolwide change occurs in services, policies, procedures, and expectations. This change is based upon data-driven programming that allows for the identification of areas that need improvement. The overall goal of systemic change is the academic success of all students. By following the framework of the *ASCA National Model* and applying the themes of leadership, advocacy, and collaboration, professional school counselors are in a position of exacting positive systemic change in the schools.

Active Learning Exercise **8.1**

Peruse the ASCA website (http://www.schoolcounselor.org/). Search for and familiarize yourself with information on current hot topics in school counseling and education. Identify two to three hot topics. Consider how the issues you encounter differ from the days when you were in elementary, middle, or high school.

School Counseling from a Supervisor's Perspective

The greatest challenge of supervising school counselors is helping them build an identity as courageous change agents with a moral and professional obligation to pave an equitable path for all students. The need to function as a leader and change agent is the most significant movement I have seen in the school counseling profession during the last ten years. This is difficult as professional school counselors have been dutifully trained to resolve conflicts and listen to others rather than create conflicts and challenge systems. Further, traditional training programs focus heavily on counseling and clinical skills and offer little formal training in negotiating systems and systemic change. This means that school counselors are well equipped to counsel individual students but often ill prepared to affect systemic change. I believe that highly effective school counselors, true leaders, must dedicate their life's journey to finding their own voice, demonstrating the courage to use their voice, and taking risks for the good of others. This of course is something that cannot be fully taught in the classroom, but it is essential to the success of a school counselor.

As a supervisor I grapple with how to reinforce and support the courageous action required for school counselors to step up and behave as true leaders in their work. Further, teaching school counselors the art of leadership and underscoring the importance of courage, ethics, and balance is an exciting challenge and part of my personal journey as a leader. It is exhilarating to watch school counselors fully develop both personally and professionally and feel the satisfaction of affecting the larger system through their actions and efforts. Professional school counselors who embrace their role as educational leaders are among the most energetic and effective change agents in educational institutions. They take risks by altering past practices and focusing clear attention to systemic interventions. Their work opens doors for students and lifts barriers that have historically limited opportunities for many students. I believe that school counselors can play a major role in school reform and will change what is written in future history books about public education. Constantly seeking ways to teach, mentor, and support school counselors as they find their voice is in fact the most challenging and exciting part of my role as a supervisor of school counselors!

Gayle M. Cicero, M.Ed., LCPC, Coordinator of School Counseling, Anne Arundel County Public Schools, Maryland

COMPREHENSIVE DEVELOPMENTAL SCHOOL COUNSELING

If a school counseling program does not currently exist in a school, one of the first tasks of a new school counselor is to create a *comprehensive developmental school counseling program*. Professional school counselors will typically base school counseling programs upon a school's School Improvement Plan, the *ASCA National Standards*, and the demonstrated needs of the school and students as determined through data collection and analysis. Moore-Thomas (2009a) notes that a school counseling program is considered comprehensive when it is integrated into the mission of the school, supplements existing programs, provides an extensive range of services, and uses a team approach, including collaboration and consultation. Furthermore, a developmental school counseling program incorporates foundational developmental theories (e.g., Erikson's psychosocial theory, Piaget's cognitive developmental theory) so that services and counselor efforts are appropriate for students of all developmental levels.

Gysbers and Henderson (2006) created an inclusive, step-by-step model for developing and managing a comprehensive developmental school counseling program. Consisting of five distinct phases (planning, designing, implementing, evaluating, and enhancing), the model provides a theoretical foundation, detailed procedures, and methods, and specifies required personnel and resources. The first phase involves *planning*. One of the first steps in the planning phase is getting organized. This includes understanding conditions for change, appreciating potential challenges, developing trust, providing leadership, and establishing work groups and committees. Next, a professional school counselor should focus on the specific elements of the program. Elements such as content, organization frameworks, and resources are necessary. Suggested allocation of counselor time is also outlined in the Gysbers and Henderson model. Conducting a methodical evaluation of the current program is the final step of the planning phase. When conducting a methodological evaluation, a professional school counselor should identify current activities and resources, gather relevant information on the students and community, establish the populations served, and obtain perceptions on the current program.

The second phase outlined by Gysbers and Henderson (2006) is *designing* the comprehensive school counseling program. When designing a program, professional school counselors should define the basic structure of the program, identify student competencies, establish policy support, and define parameters and priorities. School counselors should also outline a plan for the transition to the new program including a comprehensive timeframe. In this plan changes should be specified, leadership expanded, and program improvements explored. One must keep in mind the climate of the school and needs of the population.

Implementing the newly designed program is the next phase for professional school counselors. The first order of business is to make the transition to the new program. Some of the tasks involved in a successful transition are developing the appropriate resources, focusing on any special projects, facilitating changes, and employing public relations activities. It is important that the program leader recognizes his or her responsibilities and roles in the transition process. The second step in the implementation phase is managing the program. Changes should be made to improve effective activities and replace non-guidance tasks.

At this point in the process, with the planning and designing of the program finished and the implementation proceeding as planned, the counselor must monitor improvement plans and the overall program implementation. Encouragement and reinforcement should be provided and adjustments made as necessary. Finally, counselor competency must be assessed and continuously enhanced. This can be done by identifying resources, implementing a counselor performance improvement system, encouraging professional development among school staff, improving competence, and clarifying roles. The implementing phase of developing a comprehensive developmental school counseling program will require constant monitoring and attention. However, such due vigilance will aid in the transition to and implementation of an effective program.

Gysbers and Henderson's (2006) fourth phase is the *evaluating* stage. Several different evaluations should take place during this phase. One type of evaluation is for school counselor performance and consists of different components such as goal attainment or self-evaluation. Program evaluation is another type of evaluation. It examines the written counseling program and determines if the actual implementation of the program matches. Finally, a results evaluation can provide invaluable data concerning the outcomes of counseling programs and services. A main goal of any type of evaluation is to collect and interpret data so that informed decisions can be made about program improvement. It is also important to remember that evaluation is not a one-time process. A successful school counseling program requires regular monitoring and evaluation to make sure it is meeting the needs of the current school population.

The fifth and final stage is *enhancing* the school counseling program based upon the data collected during the evaluation phase. Gysbers and Henderson (2006) outline a comprehensive program redesign process that includes how often the program should be revised, who should be involved, and what steps need to be taken. If and when a counseling program needs to be replanned, qualitative and quantitative evaluation data and updated needs information should be used. From this data new design decisions can be determined and then implemented.

Gysbers and Henderson's (2006) model concisely demonstrates the comprehensive aspect of a school counseling program. But what about the developmental component of the program? Gysbers and Henderson used a life career development theoretical perspective as a foundation for their model. They defined life career development as "self-development over the life span through the integration of the roles, settings, and events in a person's life" (p. 49). Regardless of the specific developmental theory used, an underlying belief of a well-designed school counseling program should be that school counseling needs to incorporate a lifespan approach to student growth and development.

MacDonald and Sink (1999) identified seven global issues or assumptions accepted by most developmental theorists. These include patterns, uniqueness, culture, social tasks, holistic considerations, acceleration, and transitions.

McDonald and Sink also listed specific developmental characteristics that could be found within the domains outlined by the *ASCA National Standards*: cognitive, personal-social, citizenship, and career. These developmental assumptions and characteristics should be reflected within comprehensive developmental school counseling programs. At the same time, counselors working in urban environments or with at-risk students should pay close attention to contextual factors that may hinder healthy development not addressed in traditional developmental theories (Green & Keys, 2001). Overall, an effective developmental program is one that is both preventive and proactive and helps students acquire skills, abilities, awareness, and knowledge that are essential for mastery of typical developmental tasks (Borders & Drury, 1992).

A Day in the Life of a School Counselor

"My Mom's Having a Vasectomy!" Never a Dull Moment for Elementary School Counselors

Being the only counselor for four schools can be overwhelming at times and I believe that having a passion for what I do is what keeps me going. When making a career choice, it was clear to me that I wanted to be in an elementary school setting. The innocence of the children, the thought that the students are young enough that what I do can make a big difference for years to come, and the endless creativity that I foresaw are just some of the reasons why I chose to work with this age group.

There are many things that can work against your best efforts to remain passionate about your work, such as a difficult parent, pessimistic teachers, feeling like what you're doing doesn't matter, not allowing yourself to make mistakes, or work place politics. If I find myself giving any of these issues too much attention, I remind myself that I chose this career to make a difference in the lives of children and I try to think about the things I love about this job, like putting a smile on a child's face, providing a ray of hope in a child's life, hearing from a parent or teacher about the progress seen in one of my students, and listening to a child when he or she feels like no one else cares. I also try to remember some of the humorous things that the children have told me or done. One story that always brings a smile to my face is when one of my fifth graders, who always tries to impress me by using big words, told me that his mother had gotten a vasectomy. I know his mother relatively well and knew that she would physically not be able to have this procedure performed on her as she was pregnant the last time that I saw her, and by extension, was female. After some further questioning, I realized that he meant that his mother had given birth to his younger sibling by having a caesarean section.

Some of the best advice about working with this age group was given to me by my supervisor. I was feeling discouraged about a group of girls that I had been working with for over a year. To me, it seemed like any progress that the girls made was short lived. My supervisor shared with me that when children are in elementary school, counselors are planting lots of seeds. I have thought about that statement a lot, and when I am feeling discouraged about my work with a young child, I remember that change sometimes takes a long time, and that we don't always see the changes that students will make. In some cases, the

issues that students have are not resolved until they are older and have moved on to another school. When the issues are resolved, I would like to think that at least one of the seeds that I planted made a difference in this student's life.

Katie Young, M.Ed., Itinerant Counselor, Montgomery County Intermediate Unit, Non Public School Services Division, Pennsylvania

---

Active Learning Exercise **8.2**

Offering counseling services to students in schools presents the school counselor with myriad ethical and legal challenges. Visit the ASCA Web site at http://www.schoolcounselor.org/content.asp?contentid=173 and peruse ASCA's *Ethical Standards for School Counselors*. As you read the ethical standards, think about potential circumstances that may arise while working with school-aged children apply the standards to these dilemma.

ACCOUNTABILITY AND DATA-DRIVEN SCHOOL COUNSELING

As seen through the history of school counseling, the establishment of the *ASCA National Standards* and *ASCA National Model*, and the development of comprehensive developmental school counseling programs, there are several key themes present. One essential component professional school counselors should be aware of is the need for data-driven school counseling and, consequently, counselor accountability. Dahir and Stone (2003, p. 215) report that accountability requires "systematically collecting, analyzing, and using critical data elements to understand the current achievement story for students, and to begin to strategize, impact, and document how the school counseling program contributes towards supporting student success."

The concept of accountability is not a new phenomenon. Since its inception, the profession of school counseling has involved accountability, although it has meant different things over the past century. Gysbers (2004) provides a brief history of the evolution of accountability in comprehensive counseling programs. In the 1920s accountability focused on creating standards by which a program could be considered complete. Counselor training was a central issue in the 1940s. By the 1960s, the accountability movement had fully emerged. Based upon reform movements and important legislation it was obvious at that time that school counselors had to report objectives that were measurable and correlated with educational goals. Over time, as educational funding was reduced, the pressure for professional school counselors to show their importance to the academic achievement of students increased.

The No Child Left Behind (NCLB) Act of 2001 was created in order to eliminate the achievement gap between minority and disadvantaged students and their constituents. Educational equity, access, and success for all students were stressed. NCLB also accentuated the importance of accountability and results evaluation for school systems and staff (Dahir & Stone, 2003). Traditionally, professional school counselors were not held accountable to the same standards as principals or teachers, but if current school counselors strive to be leaders and key players in students' academic success, then they must be held just as accountable as other professional educators. Thus, professional school counselors must view the student as their primary client and design their programs in terms of measurable results (Johnson & Johnson, 2003). Whiston (1996) believed that without the appropriate data, school counselors would be susceptible to outside local sources that lack the knowledge of counselors' responsibilities and thus might question the necessity of counseling services.

Being accountable then means that professional school counselors take responsibility for their programs and the resulting outcomes—whether those outcomes are positive or negative. In determining accountability for school counselors, Myrick (2003) notes that three key questions should be addressed: (1) Does the school counselor have a written program that includes standards and goals? (2) What are the activities or interventions being used to tackle the outlined standards and needs? and (3) Is there evidence that demonstrates that the program, activities, and interventions are making a positive difference in students? This required empirical evidence has highlighted the need for school counseling programs to be data driven. For professional school counselors to continue services and programs, they must focus their efforts on providing specific and understandable data that demonstrates the benefits of their work (Erford, 2011; Otwell & Mullis, 1997). C. B. Stone and Dahir (2007) provide an accountability model for focusing the work of school counselors using the acronym MEASURE: Mission, Element, Analyze, Stakeholders Unite, Reanalyze, and Educate. This model culminates in a SPARC (School Counseling Program Accountability Report Card), which communicates the outcomes, results, and achievements of the school counseling program on an annual basis.

Even before comprehensive programs are planned, professional school counselors must define their desired outcomes in specific, measurable, operational terms. Isaacs (2003) notes that accountability is a concept that includes data collection, decision-making, measurement, and evaluation. This requires counselors to move beyond traditional roles and have a sufficient knowledge of research methodology techniques to collect, analyze, and evaluate data with which informed counseling decisions can be made. At the heart of accountability lie several key elements: needs assessments, program evaluation, service assessment, outcome studies, and performance appraisal, which are the familiar components of any comprehensive school counseling program. Before these components of accountability are discussed, the School Counseling Program Advisory Committee, a necessary aspect of a school counseling program, needs to be addressed.

School Counseling Program Advisory Committee

While professional school counselors should serve as leaders and are responsible for their programs and services, they should not try to undertake everything on their own. Erford (2011) discusses the necessity, composition, and role of the School Counseling Program Advisory Committee (SCPAC). When deciding upon the members of the SCPAC, it is important to consider influence. Choosing influential committee members should make accomplishing future program changes easier and provide a ready contingent of potential resources. The school principal is an essential potential member to consider, along with prominent and influential teachers and parents. The final members of the committee should be a school resource person and community or business leaders. Once the SCPAC is established, it should assemble at least twice a year depending upon the current program needs. The chief role of the SCPAC is to make recommendations, review results and data, and locate potential sources of funding for the school counseling program. Since the SCPAC has tremendous political and practical potential, professional school counselors should make its establishment a top priority.

A Day in the Life of a School Counselor	**For an Elementary School Counselor, It's Not Just Buttered Toast and Personal Hygiene**

When I asked my second grade students at the beginning of this school year to write down what I do as the school counselor, their responses ranged from "She teaches friendship" and "She helps people with problems" to "We play lots of games" and "We made a band aid person and [learned] not to call people names!" Other students wrote, "She told us not to talk to strangers"; "Mrs. Bryant helps people if they are sad or mad"; "[We talk about] what we want to be when we grow up"; and "A guidance counselor is a person who helps you get rid of bullies."

My second graders summarized much of what *they see me do* as a school counselor: teach classroom lessons, facilitate groups, and conduct individual counseling to deal with bullying, anger management, family changes, conflict resolution, paying attention, etc. But an elementary school counselor wears many hats within the school. Teaching about friendship and helping students solve problems are only two of them.

I'm a member of many different teams within the school, so my day typically begins with a meeting before the students arrive. The meeting may be held to write an IEP, to discuss a student who is not performing up to par academically, or to resolve a student's ongoing behavior problems. Throughout the day, I have a handful of other scheduled activities: classroom lessons, groups, individual counseling time, additional meetings, or consultation time with teachers/parents. But aside from these activities, the rest of my day is spent fulfilling many additional and quite different responsibilities within the school setting. Following are a few roles I'm frequently asked to assume.

I am a comforter for the kindergarten student who comes to school in tears because he wants to stay home. Only after dad leaves and I pull him into my office, do I discover that he is being picked on during recess by a fellow classmate. I tell him I will talk to the teacher, and she will make sure he is not bothered at recess anymore. Finally, I convince him to let me walk him to the classroom.

I am a mediator for a group of second grade girls who are friends one minute and enemies the next. In the world of 7-year-olds, it seems that the

(continued)

A Day in the Life of a School Counselor *(continued)*

only way they know how to say "No" to someone is to say, "I don't want to be your friend anymore" instead of the more accurate, "I really want to play with Sarah today. We can play tomorrow at recess." I spend a lot of time working with my students on "I Messages" to help them express their feelings.

I am a problem solver in the eyes of the boy who tells his teacher all day that he needs to meet with me about a problem. When he finally comes to my office, he says, "I have a problem." As I probe deeper, I learn that he doesn't like the buttered toast his mother serves him for breakfast. When I ask him what I can do to help, he tells me that he lives in Douglassville (because of slightly impaired speech, at first I thought he said something about Dr. Phil) and I should come to his house and make him something else for breakfast. Instead, I call his mother and talk to her about the toast problem. She assures me that she will no longer make toast for breakfast. While this isn't a typical "guidance" problem, I am glad he knows to come to me for help!

I am the public school's version of the "Super Nanny." Frequently, I receive phone calls from distraught parents about a child who doesn't listen or who spends a tearful two hours tackling homework. I listen to their situation and provide a book for parents to read, suggest an egg timer to make homework seem like a game, or explain the amazing power of sticker charts to help children in primary grades learn independence and complete tasks at home, among other tricks of the trade.

I was startled to find that one student expected me to be a personal hygiene specialist ... a job I wasn't quite ready for. Last year a very young kindergartener who couldn't quite get my name right called to me from the bathroom, "Mr. Brian, you wipe me?!?" I told him to stay there and quickly found the school nurse for reinforcement!

I am a grief counselor for a student whose cat died over the weekend. I listen to her tell funny stories about her cat, including the time her cat jumped onto the grill and almost set herself on fire. As she talks, the girl draws a picture of her cat during the grill episode. Although she came in crying, the girl leaves my office laughing about good memories.

Finally, I am a coordinator of many things. I plan the "Kindergarten Bus Ride," an activity which lets incoming students check out the school and also allows us to screen their academic/behavior skills. I organize our Child Study Team which helps identify students who are struggling academically, behaviorally, or with speech. From there, I manage special education referral paperwork for all new evaluations.

As a school counselor, every day is unpredictable, and I often feel like a chameleon, waiting to change into whatever I need to be for the day. But for someone like me, who thrives on change and new challenges, being an elementary counselor keeps me on my toes. I look forward to the adventure each day holds.

Emily M. Bryant, M.Ed., Elementary School Counselor at Amity Primary Center (K–2), Daniel Boone School District in Douglassville, Pennsylvania

Needs Assessment

The SCPAC ordinarily facilitates and evaluates program *needs assessment* and program evaluation. There are two primary purposes of a needs assessment (Erford, 2011). The first is that a needs assessment allows professional school counselors to recognize the needs of various subpopulations within the school. These subpopulations are not just limited to students, but include parents, teachers, administrators, and the community at large as well. The second purpose is to determine priorities that can aid in the construction of counseling programs or improve upon the quality of an existing program. In order to fulfill these purposes, needs assessments can be data driven or perceptions based. Data-driven needs assessment examines actual needs and begins with an analysis of school-based performance data. When exploring performance data, there are two concepts school counselors should consider. *Aggregated data* consists of results that are all lumped together to present grade level or school-wide results. On the other hand, *disaggregated data* means results have been broken down by subpopulations so that performance differences can be analyzed. From both types of data different conclusions can be drawn that can help drive counseling programs and school improvement plans.

By contrast, a perceptions-based needs assessment is perception and content driven. A perceptions-based needs assessment consists of the perceived needs of stakeholders that can be attended to through a comprehensive developmental school counseling program. Regardless of the format being conducted, the frequency of a needs assessment is cyclical and should be directed by accurate assessment. Erford (2011) proposes a six-year assessment cycle for established programs based upon the three ASCA domains of academic, career, and personal/social development. If the needs assessment is conducted accurately, it should be straightforward to translate the results into goals. Professional school counselors should remember to prioritize needs, match needs with the goals of the *ASCA National Standards*, and operationalize these goals through the use of learning objectives.

Program Evaluation

A well-implemented program evaluation (i.e., program audit) can determine if there is a written program document and if the school counseling program is being implemented properly. L. A. Stone and Bradley (1994) propose that the six main purposes of evaluation are to (1) measure the effectiveness of the counseling program and related activities; (2) collect data that can be used to direct future program modifications; (3) determine the degree of support and acceptance of the program; (4) collect data to enhance staff evaluations; (5) investigate the program budget against future needs; and (6) obtain data that can be reported to the general public. Given that program evaluations can provide a multitude of useful data, it can be helpful to start small and build upon successes. Hence, program evaluation can help professional school counselors examine student progress, determine the need for change, challenge counselor processes, and reveal barriers to student achievement (Johnson & Johnson, 2003).

Service Assessment

Service assessments are basically documentations of how and on what professional school counselors spend their time. These assessments are typically requested by supervisors or school boards and can be quite impressive when aggregated. Service assessments typically come in two types: event-topic counts and time logs. Event-topic counts provide documentation of how frequently the professional school counselor contacts or provides services to individuals and the topics discussed. Time logs record the amount of time spent in both counseling and non-counseling activities by the school counselor. Service assessments can provide a large amount of information, but unfortunately they do not give data on the quality or effectiveness of the school counselor and the counseling program.

A Day in the Life of a School Counselor

Middle School Counseling: It's the Little Things That Matter the Most

Choosing to go to graduate school to be trained as a professional school counselor seemed natural to me. I have always been the person that people seek out to talk about their problems, whether personal or professional. I did not know at the time that I would have such a rewarding and satisfying career.

Students in middle school have a skewed idea of what a counselor does and I often hear, "Am I in trouble?" when they walk in my office. As a middle school counselor, I help students, parents, and staff with many different issues. Some are very serious and we take the time to work the situations through. Some are normal middle school issues: problems with friends or teachers, divorce, grief, organization of time and academics, etc. These are my favorites and where I seem to make the greatest impact.

I love to talk with students. I love the hugs that I get. I love to hear students say, "Thanks for helping me." The students know that I am in their corner, even if they make poor choices—when they need someone the most. The middle school years are a difficult, transitional time for students and if I can touch just one student's life in a positive way, then I have made an impact.

I laugh. I cry. Daily, I celebrate successes of my students, parents, and colleagues. My administrators and staff value my role as a professional school counselor. I hear students repeat what we practiced in my office to the friend they were having a problem with. I am a teacher, a mentor, and a support to students. The staff seeks me out when they need help with a student. Parents call and ask, "Can you help me? I just don't know what to do with my child." I often find that they just need to talk things out ... they generally already have the answer.

I appreciate the ups and downs of the work. Sure, some days are more difficult and exhausting than others, but the relationships I have formed with the students, families, and staff make an important difference each and every day.

Ashley Harig, M.Ed, NCE, Middle School Counselor, Patuxent Valley Middle School, Howard County Public School System, Howard County, Maryland

Outcome Studies

Outcome studies, also referred to as *results evaluations*, analyze the effectiveness and quality of school counseling programs. They show if and how individuals are different after receiving counseling services or activities. Outcome studies require that professional school counselors measure outcomes through research-type, empirically based studies. Since outcome evaluations should be an integrated and continuous process for program improvement, current professional school counselors should be familiar with proper research and assessment techniques. A central feature of outcome studies is that the results can and should be reported. The SCPAC can be useful in preparing an executive summary and comprehensive report of outcome results that should be periodically released to stakeholders.

Performance Appraisal

A final feature of accountability is *performance appraisals*. With the emphasis on data-driven school counseling, professional school counselors are now accountable for results rather than merely completing tasks. The ability of the school counselor to design, implement, manage, and evaluate successful school counseling programs can be a difficult concept to measure and appraise. Principals, supervisors, and school staff can still evaluate counselor performance through the use of performance appraisals. These appraisals are usually composed of various rating systems. For examples of different school counselor performance appraisals see Erford (2011). As mentioned previously, the *ASCA National Model* also provides performance standards including subcomponents for school counselor evaluation. Despite the evaluation format used, the focus of performance appraisals should be on the advancement of higher levels of counselor skills.

Given all of the components of data-driven school counseling and accountability practice, there may be resistance from both the school counselor and staff. The process of accountability can be time-consuming and detailed, so professional school counselors should start off slowly and tackle problems one at a time if possible. Isaacs (2003) recommends working with school staff resistant to changes in programming by interacting with them individually and concentrating on issues that are essential to them through data collection and analysis. Resistance from school counselors occurs for several different reasons, including lack of time, knowledge, or skills; fear of failure; difficulties in measuring results; and confronting oneself (Myrick, 2003). It is important to realize that professional school counselors do not always have to be successful and must be willing to take risks when being held accountable (Otwell & Mullis, 1997). With careful planning and adequate knowledge, data-driven school counseling can be a powerful tool and resource for professional school counselors.

A Day in the Life of a School Counselor	### A Typical Day for a Middle School Counselor

A Day in the Life of a School Counselor

A Typical Day for a Middle School Counselor

I am convinced that an adolescent is not much different than my two-year-old. Both are lovable, egocentric, need lots of rest, and amazingly brilliant when it comes to manipulating a situation to get what they want. They both seem frequently to be on an emotional roller coaster and are capable of turning on

(continued)

A Day in the Life of a School Counselor *(continued)*

you with little or no warning. Fortunately, you can reason with an adolescent (most of the time) and that is what makes working with them everyday so rewarding.

The best thing about being a middle school counselor is that there really is not a typical day. Typical responsibilities include individual and group counseling, consultation with parents and teachers, facilitating 504 meetings, scheduling, articulating with elementary or high school counselors and teachers, crisis intervention, and yes, I do have lunch duty and other duties that an administrator might toss my way. However, even when you think that you have your day scheduled, and have things figured out, the best laid intentions frequently get tossed into the circular file. That being said, if you like a job where you can honestly say that you are never bored, learn something new every day, and make a difference to a child during a very challenging stage of life, then this is the job for you!

Working with the adolescent population forces you to be honest with yourself and others. Teens and preteens are incredibly perceptive and able to see through the facades that adults seem to be good at putting up. Working with adolescents allows you to remember what it was like to look in the mirror as a youngster and be unsure of yourself and uncomfortable in your own skin. It encourages you to be patient, understanding and empathic. It invites you to laugh, have fun and enjoy life for what it is on a daily basis. The job of a middle school counselor is challenging, gratifying and incredibly important. You can't put a price on the life of a child or a comment like, "Thanks for believing in me when I could not believe in myself."

Beth Lucas, Middle School Counselor, Lime Kiln Middle School, Howard County Public School System, Maryland

OUTCOME RESEARCH IN SCHOOL COUNSELING

Despite the current trends and importance of accountability and data-driven school counseling, there is still a limited amount of outcome research available for professional school counselors produced through single case empirical studies, known commonly as *clinical trials*. When reviewing outcome literature, there are two common methods used to aggregate multiple clinical trials into more comprehensive analyses: qualitative research reviews and meta-analysis. A *qualitative research review* is a rational, analytical review of research trends based upon literature analysis (Sexton, 1996). While sometimes criticized as subjective, qualitative reviews typically are systematic and consist of clearly defined variables. Because they are research based, qualitative reviews should provide an appropriate representation of the current literature. By contrast, meta-analytic studies are quantitative by nature. Erford (2008) notes that a *meta-analysis* is an aggregation of multiple clinical trials on a given topic using a single metric (i.e., an effect size) in order to reduce the limitations of individual studies. Meta-analyses produce an effect size that is an estimation of the strength of a targeted intervention when compared with a control group. Effect sizes can range from no difference to large differences.

So what has outcome research revealed about school counseling effectiveness? The good news is that, overall, the majority of studies and reviews have reported that school counseling interventions and services have a positive effect on students (Gerrity & DeLucia-Waack, 2007; Lapan, Gysbers, & Sun, 1997; Prout & Prout, 1998; Whiston, 2011; Whiston & Sexton, 1998). It has also been reported that almost all school counselors surveyed collected accountability information in some type of format. In doing so, counselors used a variety of data collection methods including tabulation, rating scales, time analyses, case studies, and interviews. Once the data had been collected, professional school counselors reported sharing their data through the use of formal reports, teacher and school newsletters, and community newspapers; data was also shared with local school boards. Thus, professional school counselors in the past and present have been compliant with accountability efforts based upon various models and approaches.

Borders and Drury (1992) conducted a qualitative research review on comprehensive school counseling programs and discovered several key findings. Professional school counselors who worked in schools that were rated excellent by students tended to provide more direct services than school counselors who worked in schools that were rated as average or below average. Several studies reported that the academic performance, behaviors, and attitudes of students who received counseling services were improved when compared to those students who did not receive services. Borders and Drury noted that numerous studies have shown that group counseling interventions in schools can significantly improve school attendance, self-esteem, classroom behaviors, academic achievement and persistence, and attitudes toward others and school. Various levels of positive empirical support have also been given for classroom guidance, consultation, and coordination efforts by professional school counselors.

Eder and Whiston (2006) provide a more recent review of primarily meta-analytical studies on psychotherapy outcome research conducted with students. As with previous studies, the researchers reported that intervention groups scored higher than control groups on various positive outcome measures. In particular, counseling services and interventions had a significant effect on problem-solving and observed behaviors. Counselor factors were also found to play a role in intervention effectiveness, with counselors who possessed higher levels of formal training providing more effective counseling. However, this finding was found to be more complex in subsequent studies. Eder and Whiston's review also reported that several studies noted greater positive effects with behavioral interventions.

While the general consensus appears to be that the majority of school counseling services and programs are beneficial to students, there have been several areas in school counseling–related outcome research that have been inconclusive. Whiston (2011) reported that outcome research has thus far been inconclusive on certain client factors. Some studies have indicated that elementary-aged students showed the greatest gains, while others report older students benefited most from counseling interventions.

Numerous outcome research studies have been conducted on the type of treatment modality as well. Gerrity and DeLucia-Waack (2007) reported moderate support for the effectiveness of both counseling (remediation) and psychoeducational (preventive) groups. This was found for groups that were both short in session time and the number of overall sessions. In particular, moderate effect sizes were found for interventions that addressed eating disorders, bullying and anger management, child sexual abuse prevention, and social competency, but not for pregnancy prevention programs. Other research studies found varying levels of support for the effectiveness of other treatment modalities, including social skills training, career planning, peer mediation, and responsive services (Erford & Wallace, 2010; Whiston, 2011; Whiston & Sexton, 1998).

Despite the various outcome studies and analyses, one must keep several factors in mind. Outcome research concerning school counseling tends to use descriptive studies or self-report (Sexton, 1996). Therefore, there may be methodological or validity concerns. In addition numerous inconsistencies exist within the literature. As a result, caution should be taken when interpreting and using school counseling outcome research. Erford and Wallace (2009) recommend four implications of outcome research for school counselors: (1) be active consumers of school counseling outcome research; (2) keep grounded in the principal conditions of effectual helping; (3) consider individual students and contexts; and (4) implement action research through one's own programs.

A Day in the Life of a School Counselor	**There Are No Typical Days in the Life of a High School Counselor** "Not to worry Mrs. Smith, I will contact all of Jimmy's teachers and be sure to have them e-mail Jimmy with his assignments. Please tell him to get well and we will see him soon." (First Bell) It is 7:42 A.M. and I'm three phone calls, 15 emails, and two cups of coffee into my day. While on the phone a line has formed outside my door. Two students are anxiously waiting to tell me where they've been accepted to college and one panicked parent must see me immediately because AP registration has passed and her daughter has forgotten to sign up. The most wonderful thing about being a high school counselor is that there truly is no typical day. Each hour, each day, and each year are completely different. High school counseling is not a slow paced environment, but rather it is ever-changing and requires the vigor and energy of a very special person. As with any career, counseling has its ups and downs, but as a high school counselor there are redeeming qualities in even the worst moments. Over the past few years I have been fortunate to have worked with amazing students and they continue to inspire me. High school counseling is cyclical and a counselor can expect that responsibilities will be similar from year to year. The first few weeks of school are an absolute mad house. Lines of students wait outside my door. "Can I take sculpture instead of photography? Psych AP instead of honors? I absolutely cannot have this teacher again! Uh …, I forgot to go to summer school." In the midst of this our secretary might say, "We have a new student. Can you do a registration at 2 P.M.?"

A high school counselor's office is always a revolving door. One learns to expect a drop-by parent, a crying student, or an angry teacher at any given time. All the while, it is understood that I will write 60–65 college recommendations each year, most of which will be written prior to the increasing November 1 deadlines. This might sound daunting or tedious to some, but for me it has been enthralling. I have the opportunity to learn so much about these wonderful young people. How else will a college know that Sherry will receive her Girl Scout's Gold Award for collecting instruments for children in underprivileged school districts? Or learn that one of my students has an obsession with Rubik's Cubes and can complete this task in less than 60 seconds?

Of course things around the counseling office are not always ideal. At Ridgewood counselors play a major a role in scheduling and testing, but I truly see this as an opportunity. It is through the scheduling process that I have gotten to know most of the near 240 students on my caseload. And it is because of this interaction that my students will stop by between periods or seek me out when life gets tough. We are the core liaisons in the building, forming connections between students, parents, teachers, and administrators. We are an integral part of the school environment.

(Last Bell) 2:58 P.M., the phone rings. "Hello, Lauren Klein." "Hi Lauren, it's Kelly from _____ College. I got your email and I wanted to let you know first that Sammy has been accepted and we could not be more excited for him to be a part of our college community!" Phone calls like these are wonderful, but it will be the look on the face of the student that makes everything worth it.

When I think about the career path I've chosen, I could not be happier. Each day is less predictable than the last and it is this uncertainty that makes high school counseling so wonderful. Although I might not know what my day will be like tomorrow, I know that I will have the opportunity to make a difference in an adolescent's life. And there is nothing better than that!

Lauren Klein, M.Ed., Professional School Counselor, Ridgewood High School, Ridgewood, New Jersey

SPECIAL TOPICS IN SCHOOL COUNSELING

A professional school counselor will encounter numerous challenges when addressing the needs of all students in the school setting. Following are introductions to special topics in school counseling: peer mediation, crisis intervention, at-risk populations, multicultural competence, clinical issues, and students with special educational needs.

Peer Mediation

Conflict and violence in schools has been receiving increased attention over the years. School violence not only refers to physical altercations, but also interpersonal conflicts such as teasing and rumors (i.e., relational aggression), bullying, and harassment. One way professional school counselors have been dealing with issues of school conflict and violence is through the use of peer mediation programs. *Peer mediation* is a method of conflict resolution through which two parties attempt to resolve a dispute through a neutral third party (student or adult). In peer mediation programs, professional school counselors typically serve as the coordinator of the program and are involved in training peer mediators in the basic principles and techniques of conflict resolution (Erford, Lee, Newsome, & Rock, 2011).

Sheperis and Chandler (2009) also noted that there are various stages of implementation in peer mediation programs. The first stage involves outlining the program, introducing it to the staff, and gaining support for the mediation program. The second stage consists of selecting the peer mediators and providing appropriate training. In the final stage, the peer mediation program is put into place, evaluation occurs, and changes and additional planning occur as needed. Various levels of support have been found for school-based peer mediation programs in the literature; however, additional research is still needed on a variety of factors associated with peer mediation. Given that some research has shown the effectiveness of peer mediation in reducing conflicts, peer mediation programs can be a valuable resource for professional school counselors at all levels of practice (Schellenberg, Parks-Savage, & Rehfuss, 2007).

Crisis Events in Schools

Unfortunately, throughout their careers professional school counselors are likely to encounter significant crisis events in the school. Crisis events could include the death of a student (e.g., suicide, illness, accident), natural disasters, gang-related incidents, and abuse. *Crisis work* for school counselors then can take very different forms. Steigerwald (2009) reported that crisis intervention involves quick and decisive action to provide direction and support for the student(s) in crisis. Crisis counseling may entail providing counseling or other support services for the student(s) during the crisis event or immediately after the crisis has been stabilized.

It is essential that schools have prearranged plans that can be implemented in crisis situations. While professional school counselors are an essential component of crisis work in schools, they should work as part of an interdisciplinary team to address and cope with significant crises. Numerous crisis models exist in the literature that can be useful to school counselors who are creating a new crisis plan or improving upon a currently existing plan.

At-Risk Populations

Historically, youth classified as "at-risk" were those identified as culturally or socioeconomically deprived. As time passed, it was realized that youth at risk came from all racial, ethnic, and socioeconomic backgrounds. Therefore, this population evolved to include youth who were disengaged from organizations and even society. A current definition of students at risk are youth who "lack the familial, community, cultural, institutional, and societal supports necessary to develop and grow in an environment that is safe, positive, healthy, and conducive to personal, social, cultural, intellectual, spiritual, economic, and physical development" (Erford et al., 2011).

There are several potential problems when categorizing youth at risk that can sometimes result in ineffective programming for these students. Erford et al. (2011) recommend nine responsibilities that can ensure effective interventions with students classified as at risk: (1) develop authentic partnerships, (2) facilitate collaboration, (3) maintain a multicultural focus, (4) be an agent of change, (5) empower students, (6) seek out short-term successes, (7) advocate, (8) document and disseminate outcomes, and (9) take responsibility for both successes and failures. In addition, there are several documented approaches that can be useful when working with at-risk populations, such as cognitive-behavioral therapies and brief counseling models (Holmes-Robinson, 2009). Overall, though, the goal for working with students at risk should be to identify and intervene before the students can develop a pattern of negative behaviors.

Multicultural Competence

Given the diversity of people and cultural groups within the United States, it is essential that professional school counselors practice multiculturally competent school counseling. Culture and diversity not only apply to traditional components of race and ethnicity, but sexual orientation, age groups, disability status, and gender as well (Harper, 2003). Multiculturalism, which was once only considered desirable in professional school counselors, is now mandatory. There is also an increasing awareness of the necessity for professional school counselors to understand how culture can influence the learning process for students and how students can be affected by their culture in schools (Holcomb-McCoy & Chen-Hayes, 2011).

When creating comprehensive developmental school counseling programs, school counselors must keep in mind that activities and services must be considerate of diversity and culture. Use of the *ASCA National Standards* can be helpful. Moore-Thomas (2009b) also recommends that professional school counselors improve insight and awareness of one's own culture; recognize and eliminate barriers to multicultural counseling; avoid stereotypes; understand the needs of the students and school; assume various helping roles; and promote staff development and school-wide programs. Additionally, professional school counselors should consider using preventive counseling, increasing counselor preparation and knowledge, consulting with other professionals, and using the appropriate counseling research (Harper & McFadden, 2003).

Active Learning Exercise **8.3**

The role of the school counselor has changed markedly since the 1990s. Visit the "Career/Roles" Web page of the ASCA Web site (http://www. schoolcounselor.org/content.asp?pl=325&sl=133&contentid=133) and orient yourself to the role of the professional school counselor at the elementary, middle, and secondary school levels, as well as the certification issues around becoming a school counselor.

Clinical Issues

Given the increase of clinical issues displayed by children and adolescents during recent years, professional school counselors must have basic knowledge and awareness of the vast array of clinical disorders that are present among school-aged students. Clinical disorders and issues include a wide variety of mental, emotional, and physical disorders that can occur in K–12 students such as attention-deficit/hyperactivity disorder, drug and alcohol problems, eating disorders, mood and anxiety disorders, mental retardation, and pervasive developmental disorders. A full review of the different clinical issues professional school counselors may encounter in school settings is beyond the scope of this chapter, but there are certain basic elements and guidelines for school counselors to follow.

Kaffenberger (2011) provides several key insights for helping students with clinical disorders. First, professional school counselors must fully comprehend both normal and atypical development in children and adolescents. It is noted that the professional school counselor is often the school-based professional parents or teachers will contact initially concerning a clinical issue in a student. Second, as mentioned previously, school counselors should display appropriate knowledge of mental health issues. This should include a basic understanding of the diagnostic criteria for clinical disorders. Finally, school counselors can work to increase awareness of clinical issues, identify children and adolescents who are experiencing significant difficulties, recommend potential interventions and services, and make referrals to outside specialists when necessary. It is extremely important to note that professional school counselors are not expected to clinically diagnosis or treat students with profound clinical issues unless they are properly trained to do so. School counselors can and should provide secondary services to this population of students as per ethical standards and school policies.

Students with Special Educational Needs

Students with disabilities have had traditionally poorer educational outcomes and increased barriers to academic, career, and interpersonal success than other populations in school settings. They typically receive lower grades, have higher dropout rates, are retained more often, and sometimes graduate without a diploma (Rock & Leff, 2011). In order to overcome some of these negative outcomes, federal legislation has provided concise requirements to schools. There are two key pieces of legislature with which professional school counselors should be familiar. The first is the Individuals with Disabilities Education Improvement Act (IDEA) and its subsequent amendments and reauthorizations. This act required that schools recognize and provide special education services to students with disabilities. Federal funding is provided to those schools that adhere to the outlined policies and procedures. For example, schools must take an individualized approach and use multidisciplinary teams to assess and determine student needs. Professional school counselors are often a part of this team and provide related services to students with disabilities. Within multidisciplinary teams, assessments may take place to determine eligibility and an Individual Education Plan (IEP) may be implemented. IEPs are based upon the needs and developmental level of students with disabilities and outline specific outcomes. Therefore, professional school counselors should become familiar with some of the basic principles of the IEP process and the overall IDEA guidelines.

Section 504 of the Vocational Rehabilitation Act of 1973 is an important piece of civil rights legislation mandating access to environments and services not covered under special educational law. Under Section 504, schools receiving federal funding must not discriminate or exclude students with disabilities from participation in any service, activity, or program. Students with disabilities must also be provided accommodations to access educational programs. In contrast to IDEA, Section 504 does not provide funding to schools. Students with 504 plans typically remain in regular education classrooms because the act only guarantees access, not services. When working with students with 504 plans, professional school counselors can serve as advocates, make appropriate referrals, provide counseling services, and practice effective coordination and collaboration.

A Day in the Life of a School Counselor	**A Passion for High School Counseling**

A Passion for High School Counseling

I became a counselor because I wanted to give something back to the community, something of myself in an attempt to help make things better for others. I wanted to use the knowledge I had gained from my personal life experience combined with my professional training to help others overcome issues of grief and loss the way others had helped me. I thought I was well prepared as a professional. I had the highest quality education from two highly accredited institutes. I had experience working with children in elementary, middle, and high schools and experience raising a child myself. I thought I had everything I needed to be a successful and effective professional school counselor. What I have learned is that preparation is but one part. As counselors, we are never completely prepared; we are always learning, growing, and developing. The day I feel I know it all or have seen it all is the day I shall submit my application for retirement. Even as educators we are never finished learning until we die, and I believe even after.

I chose high school students because when I worked at the elementary school I seemed to catch every bug and virus that the children brought in. I felt it would be better for my own health if I worked with a slightly more hygienic age group. In working at the middle school level I found that the kids weren't ready to embark on interest inventories and college searches as the curriculum directed but they spent more time in my office with the "he said, she said" issues. After a year in the middle schools I felt I lacked patience for dealing with such issues on a daily basis. I have so much admiration and respect for the counselors who do work with the younger students but recognize that is not my area of strength. My true desire to work with teenagers in high school was drawn from my own experience in high school. For the most part I enjoyed high school but remembered going through some particularly difficult times, and my school counselor was a source of strength in helping me through what appeared at that time in my life to be some very difficult issues.

I love working with students at this age because you get to run the gamut on all kind of issues but there always seems to be a balance. There are always issues of addiction, pregnancy, abuse, and academic peril but the beauty of working in the school system is that you also get the winner of the science fair,

(continued)

A Day in the Life of a School Counselor *(continued)*

the one that got into Harvard, and the winners of the state championship. You get to watch them come in as small gangly freshmen and see them struggle and then grow, develop, plan their future, and then graduate and go off to college. If you are lucky they keep in touch and stop by to say hello and let you know how they are doing. They are real and they tell it like it is. They keep you honest and to a certain extent keep you young. You share their highs and their lows and if you do your job properly you somehow hold the balance.

Being a high school counselor is like Forrest Gump's box of chocolates. As much as you plan in your daily or weekly schedule, "you never know what cha gonna get." Sometimes it's a relief when things go as you had planned, but what I have learned is there may be more valuable professional learning when things don't go according to plan, and how you deal with that is what defines you as a professional school counselor.

Jennifer McKechnie, M.Ed., Professional School Counselor, Centennial High School, Howard County Public Schools System, Howard County, Maryland

FUTURE ISSUES IN SCHOOL COUNSELING

As one can see, the evolution of the school counseling profession and the development and roles of professional school counselors has been a complex process spanning many years. Influenced by societal changes, federal and state policies, and the establishment of core standards and systemic school counseling programs, the profession has gradually become more unified and supported by empirical research. Even still, there are multiple challenges that professional school counselors currently face. DeVoss (2009) outlines several current and future issues and challenges for school counselors. Professional school counselors must still continue to define their roles in school settings and develop effective school counseling programs and services. This may include issues of delivery systems, leadership, advocacy, and public relations. There is also debate as to whether school counselors are generalists versus specialists. This may depend greatly upon the needs and climate of the school. Another challenge school counselors must face is reasonable student-to-counselor ratios. Finally, issues such as technological competence, professional development, and school counselor preparation and training are likely to arise.

In a comprehensive look into these futuristic challenges, Herr and Erford (2011, pp. 27–29) report the following list of 10 issues that will become essential determining factors in the future of the school counseling profession:

1. The degree to which school counseling programs are systematically planned, tailored to the priorities, demographics, and characteristic of a particular school district or building; and clearly defined in terms of the results to be achieved rather than the services to be offered.
2. The degree to which school counseling programs begin in the elementary school or in the secondary school ... [is] truly ... longitudinal (K–12) and systematically planned.

3. The degree to which school counseling programs are seen as responsible for the guidance of all students or for only some subpopulations, such as those at risk.

4. The degree to which school counseling programs include teachers, other mental health specialists, community resources, parent volunteers, and families as part of the delivery system.

5. The degree to which school counseling programs are focused on precollege guidance and counseling; counseling in and for vocational education and school to work transition; counseling for academic achievement; and counseling for students with special problems such as bereavement, substance abuse, antisocial behavior, eating disorders, and family difficulties (single parents, stepparents, blended family rivalries).

6. The degree to which professional school counselors should be generalists or specialists; members of teams or independent practitioners; and proactive or reactive with regard to the needs of students, teachers, parents and administrators.

7. The degree to which professional school counselors employ psychoeducational models of guidance curricula as well as individual forms of intervention to achieve goals.

8. The degree to which the roles of professional school counselors can be sharpened and expanded while not holding counselors responsible for so many expectations that their effectiveness is diminished and the outcomes they affect are vague.

9. The degree to which professional counselors have a reasonable student load, 250 or less, so that they can know these students as individuals and provide them personal attention.

10. The degree to which professional school counselors effectively communicate their goals and results to policy makers and the media both to clarify their contributions to the mission of the school and to enhance their visibility as effective, indeed vital, components of positive student development.

How professional school counselors address these 10 key developmental issues will in large part chart the course for the future of this exciting and fulfilling profession.

CONCLUSION

This chapter highlighted the evolving field of school counseling and the services and initiatives provided by professional school counselors. At the present time, school counselors frequently implement the *ASCA National Model* (2005), strive to collect and use data, and seek to improve their focus on demonstrating the outcomes of interventions. Only through demonstration of outcomes can school counselors show their effectiveness and practice ethically. No doubt, the societal and clinical challenges, as well as situational crises, encountered by school-aged youth will lead to future innovations and directions for practice. Becoming a school counselor allows you to dedicate your life to helping young people grow and develop in healthy and happy ways. It is a great profession and a very satisfying career choice.

CHAPTER REVIEW

Much like the students they counsel, school counselors are a part of a dynamic and ever-changing field. While students today face many of the same basic issues and concerns that their peers experienced during the times of Frank Parsons or Carl Rogers, technological advances and shifting social, economic, and educational policies and reforms have created unique and challenging difficulties. Since its inception, the field has been revolutionized in order to meet the needs and demands of the times. The National Defense Education Act helped pave the way for school counselors to be a primary resource of support and service to students. More recently, the creation of the American School Counselor Association's *National Standards* and subsequent *National Model* provided a unified vision and framework for school counselors and their programs. School counseling initiatives became centered on three critical developmental domain areas (academic, career, and personal/social) and national standards supplied consistency. Professional school counselors now have a comprehensive approach, preventive in design and developmental in nature, which outlines how to achieve goals and standards. No longer the reactive service providers of the past, professional school counselors are now leaders and advocates who strive for the success and achievement of *all* students.

The *ASCA National Standards* and *ASCA National Model*, comprehensive developmental school counseling programs, and the role of accountability and data-driven school counseling are just some of the fundamental foundations that professional school counselors have developed to help them attain primary goals of healthy development and successful achievement of all students. Once these critical frameworks are in place, professional school counselors have an assortment of resources—such as needs assessments, program evaluations, and performance appraisals—to make sure their goals, programs, and initiatives are effective. School counselors can then efficiently tackle the special challenges and needs of their students, schools, and communities.

Continuing educational reform has resulted in the need for school counseling programs to be data driven and for school counselors to be accountable for the outcomes of their counseling initiatives and activities. The establishment of data-driven school counseling models aid school counselors in incorporating specific elements and themes into their programs and goals. School counseling programs are written using measurable, operational terms and evaluated. Additionally, professional school counselors are able to use a collection of data-driven tools such as needs assessments, program evaluations, and outcome studies in order to increase their effectiveness and efficiency. Just as the methodologies of school counselors had expanded, so have the issues they address. Professional school counselors must continue to define their roles and develop effective counseling programs in the face of new educational reform and societal change.

The roles and responsibilities of the professional school counselor may be constantly evolving, but it is clear that school counselors are an essential part of the educational system. As one can see from the words and thoughts of the professionals highlighted in this chapter, the evolving school environment makes the field of school counseling profoundly challenging, yet perpetually rewarding.

REVIEW QUESTIONS

1. List some of the key historical influences that have affected the school counseling profession. What recent events do you feel will have an impact on the field? Why?
2. Imagine that you are a professional school counselor who has just been hired at a new school with no existing counseling program. What elements and themes would make up your counseling program?
3. There are a variety of special topics and concerns that professional school counselors are responsible for. Select one of the topics

discussed in this chapter and describe a potential school counseling initiative you would implement to address this area.

4. What are some of the primary roles of the professional school counselor? How has this changed over the last century?

5. Discuss the role of accountability in school counseling. How can school counselors know if their counseling programs are effective?

6. Think of the three domain areas of the *ASCA National Standards*. In what ways do these areas affect student achievement?

ADDITIONAL RESOURCES

- ASCA *Ethical Standards for School Counselors* (http://www.schoolcounselor.org/content.asp?contentid=173)
- ASCA *National Model* (basic introduction; http://www.ascanationalmodel.org/)
- ASCA Careers/Roles (basic information on a school counseling career and role; http://www.schoolcounselor.org/content.asp?pl=133&contentid=133)

- The Education Trust (for information on the Transforming School Counseling Initiative—http://www2.edtrust.org/edtrust/)
- College Board (information for K–12 counselors; http://professionals.collegeboard.com/educator/k-12-counselor)
- National Board for Certified Counselors (information on becoming a National Certified School Counselor; http://www.nbcc.org/certifications/ncsc/Default.aspx)

REFERENCES

American School Counselor Association. (2005). *The ASCA national model: A framework for school counseling programs* (2nd ed.). Alexandria, VA: Author.

Bemak, F., & Chung, R. C. (2005). Advocacy as a critical role for urban school counselors: Working toward equity and social justice. *Professional School Counseling, 8,* 196–202.

Beamk, F., & Chung, R. C. (2008). New professional roles and advocacy strategies for school counselors: A multicultural/social justice perspective to move beyond the nice counselor syndrome. *Journal of Counseling and Development, 86,* 372–381.

Borders, L. D., & Drury, S. M. (1992). Comprehensive school counseling programs: A review for policy-makers and practitioners. *Journal of Counseling & Development, 70,* 487–498.

Campbell, C. A., & Dahir, C. (1997). *Sharing the vision: The national standards for school counseling programs.* Alexandria, VA: American School Counselor Association.

Dahir, C. A. (2001). The national standards for school counseling programs: Development and implementation. *Professional School Counseling, 4,* 320–327.

Dahir, C. A., & Stone, C. B. (2003). Accountability: A M.E.A.S.U.R.E. of the impact school counselors have on student achievement. *Professional School Counseling, 6,* 214–221.

DeVoss, J. A. (2009). Current and future perspectives on school counseling. In B. T. Erford (Ed.), *Professional school counseling: A handbook of theories, programs & practices* (2nd ed., pp. 25–34). Austin, TX: Pro-Ed.

Dollarhide, C. T. (2003). School counselors as program leaders: Applying leadership contexts to school counseling. *Professional School Counseling, 6,* 304–308.

Eder, K. C., & Whiston, S. C. (2006). Does psychotherapy help some students? An overview of psychotherapy outcome research. *Professional School Counseling, 9,* 337–343.

Erford, B. T. (Ed.). (2008). *Research and evaluation in counseling.* Boston: Houghton Mifflin.

Erford, B. T. (2011). Accountability. In B. T. Erford (Ed.), *Transforming the school counseling profession* (3rd ed., pp. 236–278). Columbus, OH: Pearson Merrill Prentice Hall.

Erford, B. T., Lee, V. V., Newsome, D. W., & Rock, E. (2011). Systemic approaches to counseling youth with complex and specialized problems. In B. T. Erford (Ed.), *Transforming the school counseling profession* (3rd ed., pp. 279–303). Columbus, OH: Pearson Merrill Prentice Hall.

Erford, B. T., & Wallace, L. L. (2009). Outcomes research on school counseling. In B. T. Erford (Ed.), *Professional school counseling: A handbook of theories, programs & practices* (2nd ed., pp. 35–42). Austin, TX: Pro-Ed.

Gerrity, D. A., & DeLucia-Waack, J. L. (2007). Effectiveness of groups in the schools. *The Journal for Specialists in Group Work, 32,* 97–106.

Green, A., & Keys, S. (2001). Expanding the developmental school counseling paradigm: Meeting the needs of the 21st century student. *Professional School Counseling, 5,* 84–95.

Gysbers, N. C. (2004). Comprehensive guidance and counseling programs: The evolution of accountability. *Professional School Counseling, 8,* 1–14.

Gysbers, N. C., & Henderson, P. (2001). Comprehensive guidance and counseling programs: A rich history and a bright future. *Professional School Counseling, 4,* 246–256.

Gysbers, N. C., & Henderson, P. (2006). *Developing and managing your school guidance program* (4th ed.). Alexandria, VA: American Counseling Association.

Harper, F. D. (2003). Background: Concepts and history. In F. D. Harper & J. McFadden (Eds.), *Culture and counseling: New approaches* (pp. 1–19). New York: Pearson Education.

Harper, F. D., & McFadden, J. (2003). Conclusions, trends, issues, and recommendations. In F. D. Harper & J. McFadden (Eds.), *Culture and counseling: New approaches* (pp. 379–393). New York: Pearson Education.

Herr, E. L., & Erford, B. T. (2011). Historical roots and future issues. In B. T. Erford (Ed.), *Transforming the school counseling profession* (3rd ed., pp. 13–37). Columbus, OH: Pearson Merrill Prentice Hall.

Holcomb-McCoy, C., & Chen-Hayes, S. F. (2011). Multiculturally competent school counselors: Affirming diversity by challenging oppression. In B. T. Erford (Ed.), *Transforming the school counseling profession* (3rd ed., pp. 74–97). Columbus, OH: Pearson Merrill Prentice Hall.

Holmes-Robinson, J. (2009). Helping at-risk students. In B. T. Erford (Ed.), *Professional school counseling: A handbook of theories, programs and practices* (2nd ed., pp. 735–744). Austin, TX: Pro-Ed.

Isaacs, M. L. (2003). Data-driven decision making: The engine of accountability. *Professional School Counseling, 6,* 288–295.

Johnson, S., & Johnson, C. D. (2003). Results-based guidance: A systems approach to student support programs. *Professional School Counseling, 6,* 180–184.

Kaffenberger, C. J. (2011). Helping students with mental and emotional disorders. In B. T. Erford (Ed.), *Transforming the school counseling profession* (3rd ed., pp. 351–383). Columbus, OH: Pearson Merrill Prentice Hall.

Lapan, R. T., Gysbers, N. C., & Sun, Y. (1997). The impact of more fully implemented guidance programs on the school experiences of high school students: A statewide evaluation study. *Journal of Counseling & Development, 75,* 292–302.

MacDonald, G., & Sink, C. A. (1999). A qualitative developmental analysis of comprehensive guidance programmes in schools in the United States. *British Journal of Guidance & Counseling, 27,* 415–430.

Moore-Thomas, C. (2009a). Comprehensive developmental school counseling programs. In B. T. Erford (Ed.), *Professional school counseling: A handbook of theories, programs and practices* (2nd ed., pp. 257–263). Austin, TX: Pro-Ed.

Moore-Thomas, C. (2009b). Multicultural counseling competence in school counseling. In B. T. Erford (Ed.), *Professional school counseling: A handbook of theories, programs and practices* (2nd ed., pp. 639–646). Austin, TX: Pro-Ed.

Myrick, R. D. (2003). Accountability: Counselors count. *Professional School Counseling, 6,* 174–179.

Niles, S. G., & Harris-Bowlsbey, J. (2009). *Career development interventions in the 21st century* (3rd ed.). Columbus, OH: Pearson Merrill Prentice Hall.

Otwell, P. S., & Mullis, F. (1997). Academic achievement and counselor accountability. *Elementary School Guidance & Counseling, 31,* 343–348.

Prout, S. M., & Prout, H. T. (1998). A meta-analysis of school-based studies of counseling and psychotherapy: An update. *Journal of School Psychology, 36,* 121–136.

Rock, E., & Leff, E. H. (2011). The professional school counselor and students with disabilities. In B. T. Erford (Ed.), *Transforming the school counseling profession* (3rd ed., pp. 318–350). Columbus, OH: Pearson Merrill Prentice Hall.

Sabella, R. A. (2006). The ASCA National School Counseling Research Center: A brief history and agenda. *Professional School Counseling, 9,* 412–415.

Schellenberg, R. C., Parks-Savage, A., & Rehfuss, M. (2007). Reducing levels of elementary school violence with peer mediation. *Professional School Counseling, 10,* 475–481.

Schwallie-Giddis, P., ter Maat, M., & Pak, M. (2003). Initiating leadership by introducing and implementing the *ASCA national model. Professional School Counseling, 6,* 170–173.

Sexton, T. L. (1996). The relevance of counseling outcome research: Current trends and practical implications. *Journal of Counseling & Development, 74,* 590–600.

Sheperis, C. J., & Chandler, T. D. (2009). The evolution and application of peer mediation in schools. In B. T. Erford (Ed.), *Professional school counseling: A handbook of theories, programs and practices* (2nd ed., pp. 369–377). Austin, TX: Pro-Ed.

Steigerwald, F. (2009). Crisis intervention with individuals in the schools. In B. T. Erford (Ed.), *Professional school counseling: A handbook of theories, programs and practices* (2nd ed., pp. 829–841). Austin, TX: Pro-Ed.

Stone, C. B., & Dahir, C. A. (2007). *School counselor accountability: A M.E.A.S.U.R.E. of student success* (2nd ed.). Upper Saddle River, NJ: Pearson Merrill Prentice Hall.

Stone, L. A., & Bradley, F. O. (1994). *Foundations of elementary and middle school counseling.* White Plains, NY: Longman.

Whiston, S. C. (1996). Accountability through action research: Research methods for practitioners. *Journal of Counseling & Development, 74,* 616–623.

Whiston, S. C. (2011). Outcomes research on school counseling interventions and programs. In B. T. Erford (Ed.), *Transforming the school counseling profession* (3rd ed., pp. 38–50). Columbus, OH: Pearson Merrill Prentice Hall.

Whiston, S. C., & Sexton, T. L. (1998). A review of school counseling outcome research: Implications for practice. *Journal of Counseling & Development, 76,* 412–426.

CHAPTER 9

Mental Health Counseling in Community Settings

LEARNING OBJECTIVES

After reading this chapter, you should be able to

- describe the history of mental health counseling in community settings;

- discuss community counseling, comprehensive mental health counseling, and recovery models;

- identify the variety of credentials and career options for mental health counselors practicing in community settings;

- outline the major treatment approaches—including case management, community-based counseling, crisis intervention, day treatment, advocacy, consultation, prevention programming, and educational programs—as well as the role of counselors in shaping public policy and promoting social change; and

- understand the ethical issues that are uniquely impacted by the practice of mental health counseling in community settings.

CHAPTER OUTLINE

Introduction

Historical Perspectives

Philosophical Orientation and Models

The Community Counseling Model
The Comprehensive Mental Health
   Counseling Model
The Recovery Model

Professional Development
Credentialing
Career Options

Special Topics in Mental Health Counseling in Community Settings
Direct Client Services
Indirect Client Services
Direct Community Services
Indirect Community Services

Further Considerations in Mental Health Counseling in Community Settings
Confidentiality
The Counseling Relationship
Professional Responsibility

Conclusion

CHAPTER REVIEW
REVIEW QUESTIONS
ADDITIONAL RESOURCES
REFERENCES

INTRODUCTION

Many mental health counselors work in community settings where they encounter the unique needs of individuals and families experiencing struggles associated with mental disorders and related community problems such as poverty, school dropout, and violence. Estimates suggest that 1 in 4 (25 percent) people ages 18 and older experience a diagnosable mental health problem each year, and approximately 1 in 17 (6 percent) struggle with serious mental illness (U.S. Department of Health and Human Services [USDHHS], 2008). Acute mental health concerns are also experienced by children and adolescents. Among youth, data indicates that 1 in 5 (20 percent) have a diagnosable mental health disorder and 1 in 10 (10 percent) experience serious emotional disturbances that significantly impair their ability to succeed at home, school, or in the community (Knoph, Park, & Mulye, 2008). With an unemployment rate of approximately 8 percent (U.S. Bureau of Labor Statistics, 2009), nearly 40 percent of children living in low-income families (National Center for Children in Poverty, 2007), and only 50 percent of racial minority students graduating from high school (Orfield, Losen, Wild, & Swanson, 2004), many individuals are living in communities impacted by larger social issues that may result in or exacerbate mental health problems. To address individual mental health concerns and related social problems, mental health counselors who practice in community settings provide direct and indirect services to both individuals and community populations (Lewis, Lewis, Daniels, & D'Andrea, 1998). This chapter provides an overview of the historical perspectives, philosophical orientation and models, professional development, major treatment approaches, and potential ethical issues associated with mental health practice in community settings.

HISTORICAL PERSPECTIVES

Notably, although services initially occurred in primarily academic locations, the counseling profession began in a community setting with the establishment of the Vocational Bureau of Boston in 1908 (Hershenson & Berger, 2001).

Despite roots in the community, however, the professionalization of community and mental health counseling did not occur until the 1970s following the Community Mental Health Centers Act of 1963 (Gerig, 2007). This federal legislation—created in response to inhumane treatment associated with the institutionalization of individuals with mental illness, the promise of psychopharmacology to manage symptoms outside institutional settings, empirical support for a variety of psychotherapies to treat mental disorders, and shortages of mental health professionals practicing in the public sector—provided funding for the establishment of community mental health centers across the United States. The initial act stipulated the delivery of five core services (inpatient treatment for short-term care, outpatient treatment, partial hospitalization, crisis intervention, and consultation/psycho-education services) within each center, and later amendments to the act expanded the requirements to include services to address substance use disorders and mental health concerns among children and adolescents (Gerig, 2007).

Recognizing the increased workforce needs associated with the creation of community mental health centers across the nation, counselor education programs began to develop courses and clinical experiences that directly reflected the competencies necessary for effective mental health counseling practice in community settings (Gerig, 2007). With the establishment of the Council for the Accreditation of Counseling and Related Educational Programs (CACREP) in 1981, a master's level program track in Community and Other Agency Settings (COAS) was initiated (Wilcoxon, 1990). During a revision of CACREP accreditation standards in 1988, the program track in COAS was divided into two programs: community counseling (CC) and mental health counseling (MHC) (Wilcoxon, 1990). The creation of two specialty tracks, however, related to the professional development of counselors to offer mental health services in community settings created ongoing debate within the profession about the shared and distinct professional identities of community and mental health counselors. Some argued that MHC was distinguished from CC by its more intensive graduate training standards (60 versus 48 hours), which increased the clinical focus of MHC programs by allowing time for curricula related to diagnosis, abnormal development, psychotropic medications, and plans of care (Pistole & Roberts, 2002). The creation of an American Counseling Association division called the American Mental Health Counselors Association, a journal (*Journal of Mental Health Counseling*), and a newsletter (*The Advocate*) to support professional development and identity were cited as additional factors that distinguished MHC from CC (Pistole & Roberts, 2002). The lack of professional organization for CC may have been a factor related to ongoing struggles to define the profession and differentiate it from related counseling specializations.

While articulating that CC be viewed as an orientation rather than a specific work setting, the CC specialty area continued to struggle with professional identity, with many CC program coordinators and related CACREP standards describing it as a generic training track for counselors who wished to practice outside of academic settings (Hershenson & Berger, 2001). More specific definitions of community counseling, however, were eventually offered. Community counseling, defined by Hershenson, Power, and Waldo (1996, p. 26), refers to "the application of counseling principles and practices in agency, organizational, or individual practice settings that are located in and interact with their surrounding community." Lewis et al. (1998, p. 5) later defined community counseling as "a comprehensive helping framework of intervention strategies and services that promote the personal development and well-being of all individuals and communities." With similar yet different definitions, there seemed to be additional lack of consensus within the CC specialty area about the need for additional representation on the CACREP board and/or professional organization as a division or with a related journal within the American Counseling Association (ACA).

Historical tensions surrounding attempts to distinguish CC from MHC culminated during recent revisions to the CACREP accreditation standards. The 2009 standards combine CC and MHC into one shared entry-level program, Clinical Mental Health Counseling (CMHC). The new 60-hour CMHC program track merges the philosophical orientation of CC programs (viewing the person within the context of their environment) with the clinical (diagnosis, treatment) focus of MHC programs. While the evolution of MHC in community settings has clearly been dynamic and challenging, it remains unclear how CC and MHC will develop a shared professional identity under the new CMHC program track. Those questions along with additional issues surrounding professional organization (e.g., ACA divisions, journals) will likely be answered as the 149 CC and 53 MHC programs begin to merge. Meanwhile, as you seek to define MHC in community settings, you may receive direction from the historical philosophical orientations and models common to both CC and MHC.

Active Learning Exercise **9.1**

Using the link below, visit the online exhibit titled, "The lives they left behind: Suitcases from a state hospital attic" to learn more about the institutionalization of individuals with mental illness. After viewing the exhibit, reflect on the social and cultural norms and values associated with the institutionalization of individuals with mental illness? What progress has the field made in reducing stigma and treating individuals with respect and dignity? How could mental health counselors working in the community work to improve circumstances for individuals with mental illness? Link to exhibit: http://www.suitcaseexhibit.org.

PHILOSOPHICAL ORIENTATION AND MODELS

Mental health counselors practicing in community settings recognize the reciprocal interactions between persons and their environment and work to empower both individuals and related social systems to engage in activities that promote mental health and wellness. As a result, mental health counselors working in community settings also utilize both direct and indirect approaches to promote well-being among individuals and the systems with which they interact. Several models provide a shared framework for understanding the philosophical orientation of mental health counselors who practice in community settings. The first two models (community counseling and comprehensive mental health counseling) were specifically developed by leaders in the counseling profession for MHC in community settings. The last model (recovery) presented is a more recent universal orientation to community mental health services that provides a shared framework for practice across disciplines. Mental health counselors working in community settings may find that the use of models developed by counselors are helpful for guiding profession-specific functions, while the recovery model may be useful for guiding interdisciplinary approaches.

The Community Counseling Model

Lewis et al. (1998) developed a model for mental health counselors who practice in a variety of community settings. The philosophical orientation of the model is centered on the following assumptions: (a) environmental influences can both support and impede healthy development; (b) counseling should focus on both individual and community empowerment; (c) comprehensive rather than singular approaches to treatment are more efficient; (d) the context of culture, race, and ethnicity should be reflected in the design and delivery of services; (e) promotion of mental health is more effective than treatment of mental illness; and (f) the model is applicable across settings (e.g., human services, mental health, education). The philosophical assumptions of this model help provide a framework for guiding four categories of services offered by mental health counselors in community settings.

The model suggested by Lewis et al. (1998) states that there are four distinct categories of mental health services provided in community settings (Table 9.1). The first category, *direct client services*, refers to interventions provided to clients who are experiencing mental health concerns or who have demonstrated risk for developing mental health problems. For example, a counselor working at a community mental health center may provide outpatient individual counseling services to a woman with depression, while a mental health counselor involved in a local nonprofit youth organization may provide outreach to lesbian, gay, bisexual, and transgender (LGBT) adolescents based on increased risk for suicidal ideation among this population. The second category, *indirect client services* (advocacy, consultation, linkage to other resources), may also be reflected in the work of these two counselors. The counselor working with the woman with depression may consult with the client's psychiatrist about managing side effects associated with a particular antidepressant, while the counselor outreaching to LGBT adolescents may provide linkages or referrals to a local organization that provides educational support and social activities specifically for sexual minority youth. The third category, *direct community services*, seeks to broaden the scope of intervention to systems that influence clients. Mental health counselors involved in direct community services offer educational workshops and preventive education to the larger community. The counselor who is working at the local community mental

TABLE **9.1**

The Community Counseling Model: Four Categories of Mental
Health Services (Lewis et al., 1998)

Category	Description and Examples
Direct client services	Address the immediate mental health needs of clients; examples include counseling, case management, and day treatment
Indirect client services	Address the various ecological systems (e.g., school, family, community) that influences the mental health of clients; examples include advocacy and consultation
Direct community services	Describe interventions that focus on communities rather than individuals; examples include prevention programming and educational programs
Indirect community services	Refer to services that help extend change made at the local level to larger social and cultural institutions that influence the community; examples include shaping public policy and promoting social change

health center may provide monthly educational workshops to the local community or other targeted groups (e.g., employers, schools) about identifying the signs of mental health problems and related resources; the counselor working for the nonprofit youth organization may offer sexuality-oriented programming at a local school. Finally, the fourth service category, *indirect community services*, focuses on the work of counselors in affecting public policies and systemic problems that impact clients. Writing a letter to a state representative regarding mental health parity (reimbursement that more closely reflects fees paid by third parties for physical health care) may be an example of an indirect community service provided by the counselor working in the community mental health center, while the counselor working for the nonprofit youth organization may be involved in applying for funding to support the design and delivery of suicide prevention programming for adolescents. The CC model provides a framework for mental health counselors to guide and organize their services. Lewis et al. (1998) suggest that in order for services to be considered comprehensive, mental health counselors practicing in community settings must offer services within each of the four categories.

The Comprehensive Mental Health Counseling Model

A more recent contribution (Gerig, 2007) to the available knowledge on MHC in community settings suggests that mental illness and mental health should not be conceptualized on the same continuum but rather within a two-dimensional framework that also considers the micro-, meso-, exo-, and macrosystems of clients. The author of this model suggests that it is faulty to characterize mental health as the absence of mental illness; instead, mental health is a dynamic state of being that includes physical, psychological, social, and spiritual wellness. Using this assumption, the model offers four rather than two (either mentally ill or healthy) categories of mental health/illness: (1) low mental illness/low mental health (no diagnosable mental illness and little mental wellness); (2) high mental health/low mental illness (elevated degree of mental wellness and no diagnosable mental illness); (3) high mental illness/low mental health (diagnosable mental illness and little mental wellness); and (4) high mental illness/high mental health (diagnosable mental illness and elevated mental wellness). According to this model, therefore, a person can be both mentally ill and mentally well at the same time, or someone may not be mentally ill but could also not be described as mentally well. For example, an individual diagnosed with major depressive disorder may also be physically active, be experiencing typical elevations in mood, have a strong social support network, and practice meditation daily, whereas another individual with no diagnosis may not be engaged in any regular exercise, not be addressing feelings, have few friends, and not be involved in any type of spiritual activity. This two-dimensional model provides mental health counselors practicing in community settings with theoretical direction for simultaneously assessing, conceptualizing, and addressing both mental health and mental illness.

The value of this model is further extended by Gerig's (2007) suggestion that mental health counselors practicing in community settings should not limit their assessments, conceptualizations, and interventions for mental illness and mental health to just individuals but should also extend this work to related systems. More specifically, it is recommended that mental health counselors consider and address the micro-, meso-, exo-, and macro-systems that impact clients. As conceptualized by Bronfenbrenner (1989), the microsystem addresses the development of individuals as it is relates to interpersonal relationships within specific systems (e.g., home, school, work). This system considers how interpersonal relationships within specific contexts have shaped both the individual and the setting. A mental health counselor working with a youth diagnosed with a mood disorder who is having behavioral problems at home might consider how the behavior of the adolescent prompts responses from her mother and how the responses of her mother influence the behavior of the youth. The mesosystem considers how the microsystems the individual is embedded in interact with one another. For example, the mother and the teachers of the youth described earlier might maintain frequent and positive communication that is helpful in developing consistent expectations for behaviors across environments. The exosystem considers systems that the individual does not directly interact with but that influence one or more of the systems in which they are involved. Extending the example with the youth who has been diagnosed with a mood disorder, a system that the youth is not engaged with (e.g., job market in the local community) may influence another system she interacts with (e.g., school). More specifically, the mother may not be able to find full-time employment and, as a result, work three part-time jobs that result in less time spent with her daughter and inconsistent expectations for behaviors. The lack of time available to help her child may exacerbate symptoms associated with the mood disorder and increase behavioral problems at school. The final system, the macrosystem, considers the broader social and cultural contexts and related values and expectations as they

mutually interact with the micro-, meso-, and exosystems. The culture within which the mother and adolescent are situated, for example, may not acknowledge the existence of mental health problems among adolescents, which may result in few available local mental health resources to help decrease symptoms and increase wellness.

Using both the two-dimensional conceptualization of mental illness and mental health and addressing the systems in which individuals are embedded, Gerig (2007) suggests, this comprehensive model can help direct the practice of mental health counseling in community settings in three specific ways: (1) assessment includes attention to the strengths and needs of both individuals and related ecological systems; (2) conceptualization involves consideration of direct and indirect factors that reciprocally influence the client; and (3) interventions address all ecological systems that influence the client.

The Recovery Model

As the counseling profession developed philosophical models that focused on the strengths of individuals and communities as well as the mutual influence of persons and their environments, over the past 15 years there has been a similar paradigm shift in community mental health services from a focus on pathology to the promotion of recovery (Drake, Green, Mueser, & Goldman, 2003). Unlike services based on traditional medical perspectives of mental illness that emphasize symptom reduction, services grounded in recovery focus on improving quality of life (Drake et al., 2003). Recovery, according to the USDHHS (2008, p.1) refers to "a journey of healing and transformation enabling a person with a mental health problem to live a meaningful life in a community of his or her choice while striving to achieve his or her full potential." The recovery movement, according to Drake et al. (2003), is historically embedded in the grassroots efforts of individuals with mental illness who started a community club, Fountain House, in New York that emphasized career development and building supportive interpersonal networks. The Fountain House model (which was disseminated nationally) combined with the proliferation of treatment approaches focused on building skills (e.g., social, coping, problem-solving) within normative environments (e.g., homes, communities, workplace) rather than traditional talk therapy in clinical settings, contributed to the recovery movement. Today, recovery-oriented services within community mental health settings primarily focus on assisting individuals with acute mental health problems to define and realize personal goals related to living arrangements, competitive employment, higher education, vocational training, supportive relationships with family members, and hobbies. For example, instead of focusing on helping individuals with mental illness access social security income for their disorders, recovery-oriented services may help individuals develop a plan for securing competitive employment with a national corporation. While not a counseling-specific model, many counselors practicing in community mental health settings encounter the recovery model as the philosophical orientation that guides treatment planning and service delivery across disciplines. Recovery as a philosophical orientation is illustrated in the following narrative describing a day in the life of a mental health counselor working in a community setting:

A Day in the Life of a Mental Health Counselor

The Client Knows Best

Mental health counseling in community settings can be very rewarding as you are able to work with people in a more meaningful manner. This is because consumers become empowered. It therefore becomes less about "treatment" and more about assisting with skills trainings *they request* to achieve goals *they desire*. Consumers are taught skills to manage the illness and advocate for themselves and for others. As professionals we have, at times, lived under the credence that we know best. How wrong that can be. The most knowledgeable person is the person who struggles with mental illness. I have much training, a master's degree, and a professional license, yet my knowledge pales in comparison to the knowledge held by the person with a mental illness, and the knowledge they have given freely to me. There is no person who knows about what they need and desire more than the person with the illness. I have to focus differently to see the strengths and resiliencies they possess and the source of those strengths as well. Consumers work to achieve by utilizing those strengths. I believe it is safe to say I do it because of this difference between treatment and empowerment. I also want to acknowledge a major advance in the empowerment of people with mental illness. In Georgia we work with staff who are known as Certified Peer Specialists (CPS). These are people who know what it is like to live with a mental illness, have received specialized training, and have passed a rigorous written and verbal exam. Their contributions to a person's recovery can be immense, they work in all areas of care, they are mentors, symbols of hope and strength, and examples of what recovery can be. There is no one better qualified to walk along with someone on the road to recovery, than a person who has/is experiencing that journey.

Tom Abrams, Director of Peer Supports, McIntosh Trail Community Services Board, Georgia

Active Learning Exercise **9.2**

The purpose of this set of activities is to further explore community mental health counseling models. Visit the home page of Fountain House (http://www.fountainhouse.org). As you review the Web page, look for representations of the community counseling, comprehensive mental health, and recovery models in their mission, events, services, training, and resources. After reviewing the page, reflect on how these models differ from other models of counseling you have learned about. What aspects of these models appeal to or concern you? If possible, interview counselors and clients who are involved in services that reflect these models and ask them about the challenges and benefits in practice.

PROFESSIONAL DEVELOPMENT

Traditionally, mental health counselors who practice in community settings were often graduates of CC or MHC programs. As previously discussed, however, the 2009 CACREP accreditation standards merged CC and MHC into one program area, CMHC. In addition to the eight CACREP core curricular areas, students completing academic work in CMHC receive training and supervised clinical experiences focused on the requisite knowledge and skills needed to address a variety mental health needs in community settings (CACREP, 2008). More specifically, students in CMHC will complete 60 semester or 90 quarter hours of coursework and clinical experiences that address mental health–specific topics such as evidence-based treatments, multiaxial diagnosis, administrative management of mental health programs, and biopsychosocial case conceptualization and treatment planning. In addition to coursework, students in CMHC programs are also involved in a 900-hour internship that includes a minimum of 360 direct service hours. Decisions about where students will initially practice are usually based on the availability of on-site supervision by a counselor and specialty interest areas of students (e.g., children, older adults, HIV/AIDS). These clinical experiences vary and can include supervised practice in substance abuse treatment facilities, community mental health settings, school-based mental health programs, juvenile detention centers, nonprofit agencies, and hospice programs. Students engaged in initial clinical experiences receive both individual and group supervision by faculty and on-site supervisors. New counselors seeking professional credentials will continue to receive clinical supervision after they matriculate from the program.

Credentialing

Mental health counselors practicing in community settings are often required by agencies and managed care organizations to be licensed to practice independently or working toward independent licensure through supervision and passing of the National Counselor Examination (NCE) or state-specific test. Licensure is a state-specific legal process that regulates and monitors the scope and quality of practice, while certification is a profession-specific credential that reflects a person has met the minimum standards for a profession, but it does not regulate or monitor the scope or quality of practice. Although certification is not required to practice mental health counseling in community settings, some counselors seek and maintain certification to promote their professional identity and the counseling profession. General information about counselor certification and licensure was presented in the second chapter of this book, and as a result, the following discussion is limited to additional information specific to mental health counselors.

The National Board for Certified Counselors (NBCC) offers the Certified Clinical Mental Health Counselor (CCMHC) and Master Addictions Counselor (MAC) to counselors who earned the National Certified Counselor (NCC) credential (NBCC, 2008). Perhaps because of the voluntary nature of the certification and associated costs with maintaining the credential, there are only 1,127 CCMHCs and 646 MACs, while there are over 90,000 counselors who maintain professional licensure. To be eligible for the CCMHC credential, mental health counselors must have completed 60 hours of coursework that includes curricular attention to mental health–specific topics (e.g., diagnosis, abnormal development); completed 9–15 hours of supervised clinical experiences; completed two years post-master's clinical experience that includes 3,000 direct client hours and 100 hours of clinical supervision; passed the Examination of Clinical Counseling Practice; and submitted a videotaped clinical counseling session for review in addition to holding the NCC credential. Mental health counselors interested in pursuing the MAC credential must produce evidence that they have completed 12 or more hours of coursework focused on addictions counseling, have practiced as an addictions counselor with supervision for a minimum of 20 hours per week over three years (two of the years must be post-master's), and have earned a passing score on the Examination for Master Addictions Counselors. In order to be eligible for the MAC credential, individuals must also be an NCC.

While in most cases mental health counselors do not have to seek and maintain the NCC credential for professional practice in community settings, satisfactory performance on the NCE is often one requirement for licensure as a professional counselor. There are more than 103,000 licensed professional counselors in 48 states and the District of Columbia. For reimbursement purposes, third-party payer sources such as managed care and employers often require that mental health counselors are either licensed or working toward licensure as evidenced by receiving clinical supervision and passing the NCE or state-specific test. The ACA's 2007 publication, *Licensure Requirements for Professional Counselors*, indicates that requirements for licensure vary from state to state, but in addition to examination requirements such as the NCE, typically include specific educational and supervised practice experiences. To maintain professional licensure, most states require that mental health counselors participate in continuing education. Additional information about continuing education requirement for certification and licensure can be found in Chapter 2.

Career Options

Mental health counselors practicing in community settings will encounter a wide variety of career options. Many mental health counselors primarily focus on designing and delivering prevention programs to adolescents in school or community settings, while others work in community mental health settings with individuals who have severe mental illness. Often, after a couple years of practice, mental health counselors are recruited by agencies and organizations to work in administrative roles. The work of mental health counselors in community settings is therefore varied, and counselors can work in a variety of roles throughout their careers. The following information provides examples of mental health counselors who are working in related but different roles within community settings.

Outreach and Prevention

Marisol recently graduated from a community counseling program and works for a nonprofit center for LGBT youth in North Carolina. In her role she provides outreach and prevention services focused on reducing the risk of depression and suicide among LGBT youth. Marisol provides professional development seminars to teachers at local high schools about recognizing and intervening in bullying of LGBT youth. On Saturday evenings, Marisol distributes information about signs of depression and suicidal ideation during teen night at the center she works for. Once a year, she organizes and runs a booth at the annual LGBT Pride festival that offers free wellness services (e.g., chair massage, yoga) and coupons to local providers of wellness-related activities. In addition, Marisol provides brief counseling services to LGBT youth and their families and runs a weekly support group focused on enhancing self-esteem. Marisol works closely with members of the community to plan the services she offers. Monthly, she meets with a local advisory board made of representatives from local businesses, schools, churches, mental health agencies, and youth organizations in addition to LGBT adolescents and their families to review the outcome of services provided, make necessary adjustments, identify additional community resources, and plan new programming.

Clinical Work

Randy is a counselor in the state of Florida who graduated from a MHC program. He works for a community mental health center that provides services to adults with severe mental illness (SMI). In his role as a clinician, Randy completes diagnostic assessments, treatment plans, and interventions for approximately 50 clients per month. In addition to direct client services, Randy also provides indirect services to his clients by consulting with other treatment providers such as psychiatrists and physicians and through ongoing review of client treatment plans with members of an interdisciplinary treatment team. In his five years working for this community agency, Randy has observed that because of symptoms associated with their SMI and related social issues such as unemployment and poverty, many clients are homeless. As a result, Randy has begun to apply for grants to secure supported housing for individuals with SMI. Additionally, Randy has begun to call his state representatives to inform them about the difficulties associated with finding housing for individuals with SMI and the need for additional funding for quality housing options.

Administrative Work

Jamie practiced as a child and adolescent mental health counselor for approximately five years before starting her current position as a director of a school-based mental health program that specializes in providing services to immigrant and refugee youth in California. In her administrative role, Jamie oversees program development and delivery and supervises approximately 50 staff who serve 20 schools within one district. Staffs employed within her program come from a variety of disciplinary backgrounds, including education, sociology, public administration, nursing, psychology, and social work. Jamie is responsible for completing community needs assessments, setting program goals, overseeing the design and delivery of a variety of school-based mental health services, budgeting, fundraising, and program leadership. A key part of her role is creating partnerships with other community organizations to create shared vision, common purpose, and linked resources. While many of the skills Jamie learned in her CC program have been useful in her current administrative role, she feels she could use additional training in the areas of budgeting and finance and, as a result, is taking some additional coursework in public health administration at a local college. The grant that supports the school-based mental health program she administers pays for continuing education and training opportunities for employees. The following narrative also provides a glimpse into a day in the life of a counselor who is working in an administrative role.

A Day in the Life of a Mental Health Counselor	**My Role as an Administrator** I am the Executive Director of a public behavioral health organization that provides services and supports to individuals and families with mental illness, addictive diseases, or developmental disabilities. My professional training was focused on mental health counseling in community settings and I have worked in many roles including counselor, clinical supervisor, and program manager with my degree. In my current role as an administrator, I oversee services in for about 500 individuals annually, over a seven-county area, and with a workforce of approximately 300. There is no typical day in the life of an Executive Director. One day, I may be working with program staff or consumers to ensure the quality of services provided, reviewing contracts to ensure compliance, or planning new services for the community. On another day I may be gathering data for the board, reviewing revenue and expenses, or working to utilize existing community resources to address gaps in services. Each day, I utilize many of the counseling skills I have learned from completing an assessment of community needs, consultation, program development, and program evaluation. Pam McCollum, Executive Director, Macintosh Trail Community Services Board, Georgia

TABLE 9.2
Career Options for Mental Health Counselors Practicing in Community Settings

Category	Description
Outreach/prevention	This career option typically involves services aimed at promoting mental health and wellness and reducing the risk of mental disorders. Prevention services are often offered at schools, businesses, and community events.
Clinical	Mental health counselors working in this capacity are generally responsible for offering interventions aimed at decreasing symptoms associated with mental disorder and improving functioning at home, school/work, and the community. Clinical services are often offered in community mental health clinics, private offices, or home/school/employment settings of clients.
Administrative	This career option commonly includes the managerial and clinical supervision of staff who are working in outreach/prevention or clinical roles. Nonprofit organizations, state/county mental health agencies, and private practices represent some of the settings in which administrative work is located.

As mentioned, there may be no "typical day" in the life of a mental health counselor. Moreover, any one position may be varied in its typical tasks. Table 9.2 overviews general foci that may be present in community mental health counseling positions.

SPECIAL TOPICS IN MENTAL HEALTH COUNSELING IN COMMUNITY SETTINGS

One of the most exciting aspects of MHC in community settings is the variety of approaches used to address the multilayered needs of individuals and families experiencing struggles associated with mental disorders and related community problems. Many of these approaches, which direct counselors to additionally focus on social change, center on promoting mental health and empowering individuals and communities. This trend toward attending to the person and their environment is unique to the practice of MHC in community settings. The following paragraphs describe major treatment approaches used by mental health counselors in community settings. The CC model previously described is extended to organize categories of service to help the reader make direct links between previously described models and intervention approaches.

Direct Client Services

This category of service directly addresses the immediate mental health needs of clients and related systems (e.g., home, workplace/school, community). Each of these services involves helping individuals improve experiences with the immediate systems they interact with and often informally and formally includes members of those systems (e.g., family members, social support networks) in treatment. The following section provides a brief introduction to services commonly provided by mental health counselors practicing in community settings.

Case Management

Individuals seeking mental health services in community settings often have needs that cross various and oftentimes fragmented systems (e.g., education, justice, social service, family) and, recognizing the negative impact of uncoordinated and redundant services, mental health counselors working in community settings often provide case management. Case management seeks to decrease service fragmentation and redundancy by facilitating, coordinating, and organizing interventions across systems (Summers, 2006). There are generally three levels of case management: administrative, resource, and intensive.

Administrative case management services are typically targeted to individuals with mental health needs who are functioning well at home, work/school, and in the community but need some assistance organizing and facilitating services across multiple providers. For example, a mental health counselor working at a local nonprofit youth organization may provide case management services to a family that has a 15-year-old daughter who is pregnant and believes she may also be HIV positive. In this role, the case manager may help the family navigate the multiple organizations (e.g., public health, education, mental health) that may provide needed services (e.g., prenatal care, child care, counseling).

Resource case management services address the needs of individuals with mental health concerns who have difficulty managing multiple details, but with assistance, are able to function well in community settings. A mental health counselor, for example, may help an individual with bipolar disorder find housing in the community or organize transportation to and from work.

Intensive or clinical case management is generally targeted toward persons who are experiencing chronic crisis and who are not functioning well in the community without frequent intervention. A family that has called the local crisis line three times in one month for problems managing the behavior of their child may be referred to intensive case management services. A mental health counselor working with this family may identify that the mother has an untreated mental health concern, the father is abusing alcohol, and the child has been diagnosed with bipolar disorder but has not yet received any treatment. Intensive case management services may be used to link family members to additional services, teach the family specific parenting and coping skills, and develop a crisis plan to help the family identify solutions for common crises before they begin. While case management involves coordinating services and some clinical interventions, mental health counselors practicing in community settings also offer psycho-education services as a part of case management or as a separate service, depending on the needs of clients and the programming structure of the agency.

Community-Based Counseling Services

Individuals experiencing mental health concerns often seek individual, family, or group counseling services in the community. As counseling practice has evolved over the past two decades, services are increasingly being offered outside of traditional clinic settings (Woodford, Bordeau, & Alderfer, 2006). In addition to office-based interventions, mental health counselors working in the community can be expected to offer counseling services in homes, schools, workplaces, parks, and other settings. The extension of traditional outpatient counseling to community settings was prompted by the realization that progress made and skills developed in clinical settings often did not generalize to other settings (e.g., school, work, home, community). Additionally, counseling services offered in the community are viewed as helpful to improving access to care for individuals who may not have transportation or schedules that allow them to make contact with community mental health centers. The provision of counseling services in the normative environments of individuals can also provide some productive contexts for sessions. A mental health counselor working with a family on establishing achievable expectations for a child diagnosed with Asperger syndrome, for example, has a new set of tools to use when counseling occurs in the home. During an in-home counseling session, the family may report that the mother and son just had an intense argument about whether he cleaned his room. The mental health counselor in this situation can suggest that the session briefly move to the child's room to identify differences in expectations and, if appropriate, negotiate more realistic prospects between the mother and child. This same intervention offered within a traditional office-based setting, however, may not be as effective given the lack of access to directly observe and discuss the issue (e.g., whether the room was clean). The following narrative provides a glimpse into a day in the life of a mental health counselor working in a community setting:

A Day in the Life of a Mental Health Counselor

Wearing Many Hats

Working with children and adolescents in a community mental health setting is an intensely challenging and yet deeply rewarding experience. I've been fortunate in that I've been able to wear many hats in my work. I've had the opportunity to provide intensive in-home counseling, conduct assessments, engage clients in individual and family counseling, and manage a group counseling program and presently. I serve as a mental health counselor in a school-based setting though a federal grant awarded to our local community mental health agency in conjunction with the local school district. My current position involves an innovative approach to intervention that is generally more intensive and ongoing than school counseling. In this position, I work closely with school counselors, social workers, and administrators to address social-emotional issues impacting academic performance, discipline referrals, and attendance. A typical day consists of completing assessments and treatment plans, providing counseling to a caseload of clients and their families, coordinating care with school staff, and attending meetings in the school and the community.

Mental health counseling in community settings offers a rich diversity of presenting clinical concerns. While there are days I leave exhausted, I continually feel very connected to my work. With ongoing feedback from a good supervisor and progressive training in your professional interests, mental health counseling in community settings offers a plethora of experiences to build a strong foundation as a counselor. Mental health counseling in the community is an ideal place to exercise social justice and advocacy skills daily. Those served are often marginalized, silenced, and accustomed to being in a cyclical role of oppression based on socioeconomic and mental health status. These individuals need intelligent, compassionate counselors to empower them to break cycles in their lives.

Kim Hayes, Mental Health Counselor, Cobb County School District, Georgia

Crisis Intervention

This is another service that is often offered in community settings such as homes, schools, and local detention centers. Many individuals experience crises that can precipitate new or exacerbate existing mental health problems. Specific events that ignite crisis states vary among individuals, but common triggers can include losing a job, termination of a romantic relationship, unexpected death of a loved one, incarceration, and diagnosis of a terminal illness. When individuals are in crisis, according to Roberts and Ottens (2005), they experience the event as being significantly distressing, and coping skills normally used to manage upsetting events in their lives fail. The goal of crisis intervention, therefore, is to reestablish emotional balance and reinstate or develop coping skills for managing the crisis in the short term. Many community agencies have mobile 24/7 crisis teams that assess and intervene with individuals in crisis. While the outcome (e.g., going to stay at a friend's house, contracting for safety, referral to additional community resources) of crisis intervention varies by individual and the severity of the psychological stress, some individuals who are in need of multiple crisis interventions are referred to intensive outpatient services such as day treatment.

Day Treatment

This treatment approach is designed for individuals who are experiencing acute mental health concerns or substance use issues that can be managed outside of inpatient settings but need more intensive and regular intervention than those provided by traditional outpatient services. Two types of day treatment are generally available: partial hospitalization programs (PHPs) and intensive outpatient programs (IOPs) (Gladding, 2004). PHPs are typically available six to eight hours a day, five days a week and may be a step down in treatment for someone who has recently been discharged from inpatient care or may serve as a preventative step for keeping an individual from needing psychiatric hospitalization. PHPs generally include a wide variety of services such as psychiatric medication monitoring, individual counseling, case management, group psycho-education, life skills training, and vocational rehabilitation. Comparatively, individuals involved in IOPs generally receive group counseling services two to five days per week for two to three hours at a time and can similarly be used as a step down from more intensive levels of services or as a preventive step for psychiatric hospitalization. IOPs are typically focused on a specific issue (e.g., substance use disorders, eating disorders) and targeted toward individuals who are in need of less supports than those involved in PHPs, but still need more regular and organized services than traditional outpatient treatment approaches (e.g., counseling, psycho-education) that are commonly offered once a week for one hour.

Indirect Client Services

This category of service focuses on approaches for addressing the various ecological systems that influence the client. This category of service may address relationships between the client and specific systems, or relationships among two or more systems that influence the client. Mental health counselors working in community settings often provide indirect services to clients. The following section provides an overview of indirect services offered by mental health counselors.

Advocacy

Through advocacy, many counselors work to improve the quality of life for both individuals and communities (Prilleltensky & Prilleltensky, 2006). As a result of stigma and misunderstanding, many individuals and systems unknowingly penalize or fail to effectively address mental health problems. Persons with mental illness, for example, are significantly overrepresented in the criminal justice system. According to the Criminal Justice/Mental Health Consensus Project (2008), 16 percent of incarcerated individuals have a mental illness, and offenders with mental health issues stay in jail longer than those without disabilities, are more expensive to detain because of necessary increased staffing patterns and psychotropic medications, and are more likely to return to incarceration after release. Individuals are often arrested for behaviors associated with untreated mental illness rather than criminal activity. A person may, for example, be arrested for disorderly conduct for walking around a store with his pants down to his ankles, while a woman might be charged with trespassing after falling asleep in her neighbor's yard. These behaviors may be related to untreated mental health problems that would be more effectively and efficiently addressed by community-based treatment rather than incarceration. A mental health counselor working, for example, with either of these two individuals may petition the court to refer them to treatment rather than incarceration. This is just one of many examples of the type of advocacy work with which mental health counselors are involved.

Consultation

Another indirect service that focuses on the ecological systems of the client is consultation. Mental health counselors providing consultation services often work with systems the client directly interacts with to provide information, address specific problems, and teach them how to better respond to particular events or behaviors. Mental health counselors who work with children and adolescents often consult with school counselors about specific behavioral issues related to mental health concerns (Hall & Gushee, 2000). For example, a child who has been diagnosed with attention deficit disorder may easily get frustrated when too many directives are given at one time. A mental health counselor working with this child may spend time consulting with his schoolteacher and parents about less confusing approaches for asking the child to complete something, such as presenting one step of an activity at a time or writing the directions out. Consultation services can be especially useful for creating consistent expectations for children and adolescents with mental health problems across settings, helping improve relationships among microsystems, and helping the mental health counselor identify additional resource needs.

Direct Community Services

The philosophical orientation of MHC in community settings directs practitioners to address not only individual problems but also larger community concerns that influence mental health. Instead of restricting intervention for substance abuse issues to individuals, mental health counselors practicing in community settings often directly intervene at the community level to prevent the development of additional substance use disorders. The following section provides a brief introduction to the efforts of counselors to affect change.

Prevention Programming

This category of service typically involves universal, selective, and indicated approaches (Mrazek & Haggerty, 1994) for promoting mental health and reducing the risk of mental illness and substance abuse. Universal prevention programming targets risk factors in a specific population. For example, many community mental health organizations offer programs for adolescents focused on preventing substance abuse. Selective prevention programs, comparatively, target specific groups of individuals that share a specific risk factor. Children from neighborhoods with high levels of violence may be targeted for after-school programs that focus on gang prevention. Indicated prevention approaches are designed to address the needs of persons who exhibit some, but not all, symptoms of a mental health disorder or substance use problem. Adolescents who are failing classes, showing early signs of substance abuse, and exhibiting delinquent behaviors may be offered opportunities for alternative education paths, graduation coaching, mentoring programs, and/or family counseling.

Educational Programming

Mental health counselors practicing in community settings also provide information to systems that commonly encounter the unique needs of individuals with mental health concerns or substance use issues. A mental health counselor may be asked to provide a workshop to local police officers about deescalating an individual who is experiencing a psychiatric crisis, while another practitioner may be invited to a professional development day at a local school to discuss how to identify symptoms of mental health problems among children. Educational programs offered by mental health counselors include information about specific diagnoses, recommendations for addressing specific behaviors, and contact information for local resources that may be useful to the particular group being addressed. These programs may be useful in helping decrease stigma and increase mental health awareness among members of the immediate community. Mental health counselors practicing in community settings can also accomplish similar goals at the macrosystem level through indirect community services.

Indirect Community Services

This category of services helps extend change made at the local level to larger cultural and social institutions that influence the community. Often these services address stigma, inequalities, and supports available to individuals with mental health or substance use disorders.

Shaping Public Policy

Based on their knowledge and expertise, counselors and other practitioners are often invited to respond to proposed changes in public policy that relate to mental health (ACA, 2008). For example, realizing the impact of untreated mental health concerns on the ability for young people to succeed at school, many clinicians have been involved in developing promotional materials, letters to key government officials, and educational information to support the creation of additional funding for school mental health programming linked to the reauthorization of No Child Left Behind (Center for Mental Health in Schools, 2008). Similarly, mental health counselors have also been involved in efforts to require private sector health plans to provide equal levels of reimbursement for mental health and substance abuse services as they do for general medical care. Stigma regarding mental health and substance abuse has often resulted in limited coverage for services and, as a result, many individuals have not been able to access the level of care they need. While these are just two examples, mental health counselors are helping to effect change at the local, state, and national levels through influencing public policies.

Promoting Social Change

Counselors also work to promote social change through counseling and acting as change agents within community settings. Activities may involve reducing stigma through hosting events during children's mental health awareness month, maintaining a public blog about the media's representation of mental illness, or starting an action group or task force focused on a specific issue related to mental health (e.g., hate crimes, poverty, gangs). Regardless of the specific approach, mental health counselors seek to address cultural and social factors that influence the mental well-being of the individuals and communities they serve. Mental health counselors seeking to learn more about how to promote social change are encouraged to connect with Counselors for Social Justice, a division of the ACA that focuses on addressing issues of equality and oppression that impact a wide variety of individuals and systems.

Active Learning Exercise **9.3**

Visit home page of Counselors for Social Justice (http://counselorsforsocialjustice.com). Review the position statements, journal, newsletters, and announcements. What type of direct and indirect client and community services are members involved in? What specific activities and issues interest you? What specific skill sets and attitudes do counselors need to participate in social justice–oriented activities? Develop a plan for learning more about how to incorporate social justice activities into your practice as a counselor.

FURTHER CONSIDERATIONS IN MENTAL HEALTH COUNSELING IN COMMUNITY SETTINGS

Parallel to the mental health concerns experienced by individuals and families, the practice of MHC in community settings is dynamic and complex, involving a variety of different systems. At the same time, the mental health system has experienced significant and rapid changes over the past 15 years such as managed care, recovery-oriented services, and evidence-based practice (Hoge, Huey, & O'Connell, 2004). These changes, combined with the multilayered context in which mental health counseling is situated within communities, have expanded potential ethical issues. The following narrative introduces the reader to ethical issues that have begun to emerge from recent trends in mental health counseling in community settings.

Confidentiality

Because mental health counselors practicing in community settings intervene at both the individual and community level, they are often involved with multiple systems that impact the client. While this approach to care has many benefits, one key limitation is often the unintentional disclosure of confidential information to others. For example, Samuel is a counselor who works for a local nonprofit youth center. He is working with a young woman whose parents were killed in a car accident approximately six months earlier. Last week, the young woman also disclosed to Samuel that she was recently diagnosed with a terminal illness. At the start of services, Samuel obtained the appropriate release of information forms from the client and her guardians to talk with the school counselor to coordinate appointments to see the client at school. Earlier this week when Samuel went to the school to visit the client, he stopped in to greet the school counselor. The school counselor asked how the young woman was doing and Samuel mentioned that he was worried about her following the recent diagnosis of a terminal illness. Much to his surprise, the client had not disclosed the diagnosis to the school counselor. On his way home, Samuel wondered if he had violated the client's rights to confidentiality even though he had a signed release of information form for the school counselor.

Even when appropriate release of information forms are signed, client confidentiality is often inadvertently compromised when treatment coordination and services span multiple systems. *ACA Code of Ethics* Standard B.2.d, minimal disclosure, provides some guidance for Samuel in evaluating his response in the current situation and navigating confidentiality in future similar circumstances. This standard directs counselors to reveal only essential information and to consult, if possible, with the client before disclosing confidential information. In this situation, Samuel did not involve the client in making a decision about whether to disclose her diagnosis to the school counselor. When Samuel did disclose the confidential information, it was not essential to the stated purpose of the informed consent, which was coordination of counseling appointments within the school setting. In this particular situation, Samuel should not have disclosed any confidential information to the school counselor. In addition, if there were specific reasons for disclosing the diagnosis, then the appropriate course of action would have been for Samuel to support his client in making that decision, involving the legal guardians, and if the client and her legal guardians decided the information should be disclosed, the informed consent form should be revised to expand the scope of purpose.

The Counseling Relationship

As previously discussed, mental health counselors practicing in the community often provide services in nontraditional treatment settings such as homes, schools, and detention centers. With the trend toward provision of mental health services in nontraditional settings, ethical issues regarding the counseling relationship often emerge. For example, Kristin is a mental health counselor who provides in-home services to children, adolescents, and their families. During one of her recent visits, the family invited Kristin to share a meal with them after the counseling session was over. Kristin, sensing a potential ethical dilemma, politely declined the offer by informing the family that she had another appointment to be at in 30 minutes. One week later when Kristin returned to work with the family, she found that they had prepared a dinner to share with her and included a place setting for her at the table. Kristin recognized that the family was genuinely trying to make her feel welcome in their home and treating her as they would other guests; they did not know that there is an ethical issue associated with offering her a meal.

This situation is not unique and represents one of numerous ethical dilemmas encountered by mental health counselors practicing outside of traditional treatment settings. When counseling services are offered in homes and other normative settings, the boundaries of the counseling can easily become blurred to both counselors and clients. While the ethical standards of the ACA provide some guidelines regarding professional boundaries, directives specific to sexual and romantic relationships with clients (A.5.a and A.5.b) appear more clear than those specific to other nonprofessional interactions (A.5.c. and A.5.d). The *ACA Code of Ethics* (2005, p. 5) directs counselors to avoid nonprofessional interactions with clients, family members, and other supporters except when "the interaction is potentially beneficial to the client." While the standards do provide some examples of potentially beneficial nonprofessional client-counselor interactions (e.g., attending an important ceremony, purchasing a product made by the client), they do not appear to directly address interactions that are more common to in-home counseling, such as offers to share a meal or meet extended family.

In the absence of clear ethical guidelines for psychologists, Knapp and Slattery (2004) provide some recommendations that may be useful to mental health counselors practicing in community settings. First, when practicing in nontraditional settings, at the start of services professionals should discuss with clients and their families how traditional professional relationships can be challenged and establish some set boundaries (e.g., family is welcome to eat dinner during the session, but the counselor will not be able to eat with them). The previously described situation with Kristin may not have occurred had expectations about professional boundaries been discussed with the family at the outset of counseling. Second, Knapp and Slattery suggest providing a handout at the start of services that emphasizes the professional role of the helper within the home. If the family Kristin was working with offered her dinner after that was established as a professional boundary, Kristin could have reminded them of the discussion and referred them back to the original handout. Finally, as challenges to professional boundaries emerge, Knapp and Slattery recommend consideration of the long- and short-term outcomes as they relate to the plan of care. Identifying and addressing strengths and challenges to family interactions may be a key goal on the treatment plan for the family Kristin is working with. While Kristin may decline to share dinner with them, she may take the opportunity to sit at the table to assess and intervene in family interaction patterns.

While this is one of numerous examples of challenges to professional boundaries that occur outside of traditional treatment settings, mental health counselors interested in working in such settings should seek ongoing consultation before deciding on a course of action. Anticipation of potential ethical conflicts specific to in-home practice and related responses may also be helpful for situations that require more immediate action.

Professional Responsibility

The increasing use of psychotropic medications for the treatment of various mental health problems has created new roles and ethical issues for counselors. One of the primary ethical issues to emerge is professional competence given that few counseling training programs offer or require training specific to psychopharmacology. Adam, a counselor in a local community mental health center who has never had any formal coursework or training specific to psychopharmacology, is strongly against the use of psychotropic medications. During a recent session, one of Adam's clients, who recently started to take an antidepressant medication, reported that he has experienced some relief of his symptoms. Adam, however, based on a recent book he read about holistic approaches to treating depression, recommended that the client discontinue use of the psychotropic medication and instead take vitamin supplements to alleviate his symptoms.

The trend toward integrated treatment approaches, according to King and Anderson (2004), to address mental health problems has resulted in potential ethical issues for counselors as exemplified in the previous scenario. As research on the brain continues to produce new knowledge about the etiology of SMI, managed care organizations have increasingly moved toward standards of care that support combined medical and psychological approaches to treatment. Individuals with SMI receiving community-based treatment, therefore, often meet with a psychiatrist or a physician three to four times a year to monitor psychopharmacological care in addition to receiving counseling services. The ethical issue of professional competence, however, is evident in the example of Adam and his client. Is recommending that a client discontinue use of a psychotropic medication within the boundaries of competence for Adam? According to *ACA Code of Ethics* Standard C.2.a (ACA, 2005), it is not. This standard directs counselors to practice only in areas in which they have the requisite training, supervision, and credentials. Because Adam is not a medical professional, he should not be directing a client to use or not use a certain medication. An alternative approach, which would more closely reflect practice within boundaries of competence, would have been for Adam to educate his client about all available treatments for depression and related efficacies, and if the client were interested in complimentary and alternative treatment approaches, encouraged him to talk about it with his prescribing physician.

Active Learning Exercise **9.4**

As noted throughout this chapter, mental health services are increasingly offered in nontraditional treatment settings such as homes, schools, and libraries. Take a few moments to think about potential ethical issues that might be related to offering services in these nontraditional settings. Consult the *ACA Code of Ethics* (ACA, 2005) for guidance about these issues. To prepare for practice in nontraditional settings, based on the advice of Knapp and Slattery, create a handout or brochure for clients that highlights and provides boundaries for potential ethical issues.

CONCLUSION

This chapter has highlighted the challenging and exciting evolution of mental health counseling in community settings. With the recent change in CACREP standards, the professional will likely continue to evolve and improve as community mental health and MHC preparation programs merge. The practice of MHC in community settings is dynamic and provides counselors with a rich context for their work. The philosophical orientations and models give direction for addressing both individual and community concerns and the related categories of services that involve counselors in a wide variety of roles and responsibilities. Throughout their careers, many mental health counselors practicing in community settings are involved in direct and indirect individual and community services in preventative, clinical, or administrative roles. Recent significant and rapid changes in the mental health service system have also contributed to emerging ethical issues, and consultation with supervisors and other colleagues will be key to effective mental health counseling practice in community settings.

CHAPTER REVIEW

1. Mental health counselors working in community settings recognize the reciprocal interactions between persons and their environment and work to empower both individuals and related social systems to engage in activities that promote mental health and wellness.
2. Credentials available to mental health counselors who practice in community settings include the CCMHC, the MAC, and licensure as a professional counselor. Career options for this specialty area of practice also include outreach and prevention, direct clinical service provision, and administrative roles.
3. Services offered by mental health counselors working in the community can generally be categorized as direct client services (counseling, crisis intervention), indirect client services (advocacy, consultation), direct community services (prevention programming, educational programs), and indirect community services (shaping public policy, promoting social change).
4. Recent changes in mental health services—such as managed care, recovery-oriented services, integrated treatment, and evidence-based practice—in addition to the multilayered context in which mental health counseling is situated present some unique ethical concerns. These include confidentiality, boundaries within the professional relationship, and professional responsibility.

REVIEW QUESTIONS

1. Describe the history of specialization in community and mental health counseling and the recent merging of these two areas into clinical mental health counseling.
2. Identify and describe the three major models that provide a framework for understanding the philosophical orientation of mental health counselors who practice in community settings.
3. Describe the role of counselors in affecting social change. How does this relate to the philosophical orientation of mental health counseling in community settings?
4. What are some of the major treatment approaches used by mental health counselors who practice in community settings?
5. Describe some potential ethical considerations that are related to emerging trends in mental health such as managed care, recovery-oriented services, integrated care, and evidence-based practice.

ADDITIONAL RESOURCES

- American Mental Health Counselors Association (http://www.amhca.org/)
- Counselors for Social Justice (http://counselorsforsocialjustice.com/)
- Society for Community Research and Action (http://www.scra27.org/)
- Substance Abuse and Mental Health Services Administration (http://www.samhsa.gov/)
- National Alliance on Mental Illness (http://www.nami.org/)

REFERENCES

American Counseling Association (2005). *ACA code of ethics*. Retrieved July 14, 2008, from http://www.counseling.org/Resources/CodeOfEthics/TP/Home/CT2.aspx.

American Counseling Association. (2007). *Licensure requirements for professional counselors*. Retrieved July 11, 2007, from http://www.counseling.org/PublicPolicy/TP/ResourcesAndReports/CT2.aspx.

American Counseling Association. (2008). *Current issues*. Retrieved August 22, 2008, from http://www.counseling.org/PublicPolicy/PositionPapers.aspx.

Bronfenbrenner, U. (1989). Ecological systems theory. In R. Vasta (Ed.), *Annals of child development* (Vol. 6, pp. 187–249). Boston: JAI Press.

Center for Mental Health in Schools. (2008). An open letter to Congress: Re: reauthorizing the elementary and secondary school education act to better address barriers to learning and teaching. Retrieved August 22, 2008, from http://smhp.psych.ucla.edu/pdfdocs/congress%20letter.pdf.

Council for Accreditation for Counseling and Related Educational Programs. (2008). *2009 standards*. Retrieved August 28, 2008, from http://www.cacrep.org/2009Standards.html.

Criminal Justice/Mental Health Consensus Project. (2008). *About the problem*. Retrieved June 26, 2008, from http://consensusproject.org/the_report/intro/about-problem

Drake, R. E., Green, A. I., Mueser, K. T., & Goldman, H. H. (2003). The history of community mental health treatment and rehabilitation for persons with severe mental illness. *Community Mental Health Journal, 39,* 427–440.

Gerig, M. S. (2007). *Foundations for mental health and community counseling: An introduction to the profession.* Upper Saddle River, NJ: Pearson Merrill Prentice Hall.

Gladding, S. T. (2004). *Community and agency counseling* (2nd ed.). Upper Saddle River, NJ: Pearson.

Hall, A. S. & Gushee, A. G. (2000). Diagnosis and treatment with attention deficit hyperactive youth: Mental health consultation with school counselors. *Journal of Mental Health Counseling, 22,* 295–306.

Hershenson, D. B., & Berger, G. P. (2001). The state of community counseling: A survey of directors of CACREP-accredited programs. *Journal of Counseling & Development, 79,* 188–193.

Hershenson D. B., Power, P. W., & Waldo, M. (1996). *Community counseling: Contemporary theory and practice.* Boston: Allyn & Bacon.

Hoge, M., Huey, L. Y., & O'Connell, M. (2004). Best practices in behavioral workforce education and training. *Administration and Policy in Mental Health, 32,* 91–106.

King, J. H., & Anderson, S. M. (2004). Therapeutic implications of pharmacotherapy: Current trends and ethical issues. *Journal of Counseling & Development, 82,* 329–336.

Knapp, S., & Slattery, J. M. (2004). Professional boundaries in nontraditional settings. *Professional Psychology: Research and Practice, 35,* 553–558.

Knoph, D., Park, M. J., & Mulye, T. P. (2008). *The mental health of adolescents: A national profile, 2008. Research brief.* San Francisco, CA: National Adolescent Health Information Center.

Lewis, J. A., Lewis, M. D., Daniels, J., & D'Andrea, M. J. (1998). *Community counseling: Empowerment strategies for a diverse society.* Pacific Grove, CA: Brooks/Cole.

Mrazek, P. J., & Haggerty, R. J. (Eds.). (1994). *Reducing risks for mental disorders: Frontiers for preventive intervention research.* Washington, DC: National Academy Press.

National Board for Certified Counselors. (2008). *NCC.* Retrieved August 22, 2008, from http://www.nbcc.org/certifications/ncc/Default.aspx.

National Center for Children in Poverty. (2007). *Who are America's poor children?* Retrieved September 2, 2008, from http://www.nccp.org/publications/pub_787.html.

Pistole, M. C., & Roberts, A. (2002). Mental health counseling: Toward resolving identity confusions. *Journal of Mental Health Counseling, 24,* 1–19.

Prilleltensky, I. & Prilleltensky, O. (2006). *Promoting well-being: Linking personal, organizational, and community change.* Hoboken, NJ: John Wiley & Sons.

Roberts, A. R., & Ottens, A. J. (2005). The seven-stage crisis intervention model: A road map to goal attainment, problem solving, and crisis resolution. *Brief Treatment and Crisis Intervention, 5,* 329–339.

Summers, N. (2006). Case management: Definitions and responsibilities. In N. Summers (Ed.), *Fundamentals of case management practice: Skills for the human services* (2nd ed., pp. 37–57). Belmont, CA: Thomson Brooks/Cole.

Orfield, G., Losen, D., Wald, J., & Swanson, C. (2004). *Losing our future: How minority youth are being left behind by the graduation rate crisis.* Retrieved August 22, 2008, from http://www.urban.org/url.cfm?ID=410936.

U.S. Bureau of Labor Statistics. (2009). *Employment situation summary.* Retrieved May 7, 2009, from http://www.bls.gov/news.release/empsit.nr0.htm.

U.S. Department of Health and Human Services. (2008). *National consensus statement on mental health recovery.* Retrieved June 26, 2008, from http://mentalhealth.samhsa.gov/publications/allpubs/sma05-4129/.

Wilcoxon, S. A. (1990). Community Mental Health Counseling: An option for the CACREP dichotomy. *Counselor Education and Supervision, 30,* 26–36.

Woodford, M. S., Bordeau, W. C., & Alderfer, C. (2006). Home-based service delivery: Introducing family counselors in training to the home as a therapeutic milieu. *The Family Journal, 14*(3), 240–244.

CHAPTER **10**

Student Affairs and Counseling in College Settings

LEARNING OBJECTIVES

After reading this chapter, you should be able to

- relate the definitions of student affairs and college counseling;

- outline the history of student affairs and college counseling;

- explain the differences and similarities of student affairs and college counseling;

- discuss the theoretical base for student development; and

- describe the challenges and future trends facing the profession of student affairs and college counseling.

CHAPTER OUTLINE

Introduction

Defining Student Affairs

Student Affairs: A Brief History

Defining College Counseling

College Counseling: A Brief History

Theoretical Bases of Student Affairs and College Counseling
Psychosocial Theories
Cognitive Theories
Typological Theories

Special Topics in Student Affairs and College Counseling

Diversity
Increasing Student Stress and Pathology
Student Suicidal Behavior
Ethical Issues Regarding Parents
Violence on Campus

The Future of Student Affairs and College Counseling

Changing Role and Function
Limited Funding and Resources

Conclusion

CHAPTER REVIEW
REVIEW QUESTIONS
ADDITIONAL RESOURCES
REFERENCES

INTRODUCTION

Professionals who work within student affairs on college and university campuses serve many functions and include deans of students; academic affair officers; academic advisors; directors of housing and residential life; orientation and first year success staff; judicial affairs officers; career, counseling, and psychological services professionals; and more. Historically, those persons who worked in student affairs came from the academic ranks of the university, especially to fill the roles of deans and directors. But as the field developed and the profession began to take form, more and more of these professionals came with education and training from student affairs programs specifically designed to prepare them to support student learning and deal with the everyday administration of an institution of higher education (Hamrick, Evans, & Schuh, 2002). Additionally, within the counseling profession, a specialty emerged in the area of college counseling that focuses primarily on providing developmental and clinical counseling services to the college age population and nontraditional students. All of these professionals can be considered to work within student affairs or student life services (Gladding, 2004).

This chapter will focus on the identity, practice, and profession of student affairs, especially as it relates to the profession of counseling from which it takes it roots (Hamrick et al., 2002). It will seek to define student affairs and review the history of the profession. Additionally, current models of student development will be reviewed, trends and challenges for the professional will be presented, and the ethics that guide the profession will be discussed.

This chapter will also focus particular attention on the specialty of college counseling. College counseling can be seen as an essential service on the university campus, providing support, treatment, and remediation of mental health issues as well as career, assessment, retention, consultation, education, and training services to the students, faculty, and staff (Gladding, 2004; Nugent & Jones, 2005). While part of student services, often under the direct administrative control of a dean of students or vice president of student affairs, the counseling center provides services that are distinct and confidential and whose records are unavailable to the college administration except in extreme or emergency circumstances (Nugent & Jones, 2005).

DEFINING STUDENT AFFAIRS

There have been several efforts over the years to define the role and function of student affairs in higher education. This is a reflection of the changing role and identity of the university in America and in the student's life while on campus. As Rentz (2004) points out,

> The role, mission, and goals of student affairs have never been, and hopefully never will be, static. For it is in the dynamic tension that resides within and between the field and higher education's changing institutions that the seeds of our power and value can be found. (p. 54)

This "dynamic tension" has historical roots that reflect the development of the profession and the understanding of its role as an integral part of the mission of the university. Understood in its broadest fashion, a student affairs professional's role in the university is to enhance student learning by supporting the academic mission of the institution, being proactive in making changes in the institution, and facilitating the development and self-knowledge of the whole person (Neukrug, 2007; Nuss, 1996).

A Day in the Life of a College Counselor

Being the Only Student Affairs/Counseling Staff Member at a Small Open Enrollment College

As the only academic advisor and counselor at a small open enrollment college a "typical day" can be hard to find. It is common place for counselors at smaller institutions to take on many job duties and wear many diverging hats. As I walk into the office and review my schedule for the day, I notice that the day is filled with a small amount of students. I check my messages and respond to letters and emails. The first appointment is a student who wants to know about transferring to a different school. The second student of the day is a continuing client that I have been working with on issues regarding depression due to past trauma and abuse. I quickly write up a case note and the phone rings; the administrative assistant asks if I can see a walk-in student. The walk-in student is frustrated about classes and failing in a few of them. As I talk more to the student I learn that he is unhappy with his selected course of study and yearns to be a professional chef but he feels family pressure to pursue a degree in pre-med to later become a doctor. The appointment is running long and there is only 5 minutes until my next student. I schedule the student to come in next week to talk further about career and personal issues. The next appointment arrives and I quickly pick up that the student is upset as she yells about the perceived unfair rules regarding academic probation. I calmly explain the college's policies and procedures and attempt to not internalize or personalize the student's misdirected anger.

Following lunch a new student comes by to inquire about academic accommodations for a learning disability. We review the paperwork and determine that the student is eligible to receive accommodations. The student receives this news with a smile that quickly fades once he learns that his new accommodations cannot be used retroactively to retake an old exam that he failed. I reassure him that one exam will not make or break his entire academic career. After that appointment I head off to a different building for a meeting with financial aid, it is time to review appeals. As the only counselor on campus my presence is needed at these meetings in order to provide a sense of fairness and compassion. The rest of the day is spent behind closed doors with three other college administrators attempting to review students' written appeals to receive more financial aid money in order to continue their education. The reason that the students' financial aid money is being withheld is due to poor academics or a pattern of non-matriculation or a combination of both. The rest of the day is long, tiring, and intense. We deliberate quickly on several students' appeals because they are straightforward. The next student's appeal is not that easy and we end up having to contact the student to request more documentation that substantiates their probable story as to why they have continuously done poorly with their academics. After the meeting I have just enough time to get back to the office and attempt to answer several voicemails from students and from parents. I make as many phone calls as possible and then create a list of things to complete for the next day when I arrive back to the office.

JB, Michigan

STUDENT AFFAIRS: A BRIEF HISTORY

At the genesis of American colleges and universities was the goal to prepare students to be good citizens of this country. This was accomplished by teaching the student the principles of religion and nurturing the student's ability to govern oneself and the country. As most of the colleges at this time were chartered by religious denominations, they were also charged with educating men for work as clergy in the church. The environment was one that would gather the faculty and students together in a common place that offered a moral environment and was intellectually stimulating. These colleges and universities were empowered to act in loco parentis (in place of the parent) and often had a system of discipline that was harsh, authoritarian, and paternalistic. Those who did work in student services were drawn from the ranks of the board of trustees, presidents, faculty, teaching fellows, and tutors (Neukrug, 2007; Nuss, 1996).

The notion of activities beyond the classroom and official curriculum began to emerge in the mid-19th century. This reflected the desire for the development of the whole student, mind, body, and soul. Additionally, the university began to evolve from a center for classical studies and religious instruction to a growing intellectualism and focus on the hard sciences of mathematics, physics, chemistry, and so forth (Rentz, 2004). From the beginning of the university system to this time, the work of those who cared for and supported the education of students consisted mostly of insuring students led a moral life and encouraging extracurricular religious activities. This began to change as more and more faculty were engaged in research and teaching and had less time to devote to monitoring student life beyond the classroom. Then, in 1870, Harvard University appointed its first college dean. Other universities followed suit and appointed deans to oversee advising, counseling, and discipline, thus relieving the presidents to administer the ever growing institutions. At the same time, the Morrill Act of 1862 and 1890 created land grant colleges and publicly funded segregated Black colleges. Women's colleges were also developing at a quick pace as the student bodies on all colleges and universities grew rapidly (Hamrick et al., 2002; Nuss, 1996; Rentz, 2004). While the profession of student affairs did not exist at this point, these events began to lay the ground work for the emergence of the profession.

The beginning of the 20th century saw tremendous evolution in the field of student affairs. Faculty had moved from being heavily involved in student personnel matters to detachment. Colleges and universities had hired deans to take over the job of regulating student behavior, providing discipline as needed, and fostering student development. Students were taking more responsibility for their own behavior as these institutions were employing some form of an honor code or system (Nuss, 1996).

During this time professionals in the field began to gather together to discuss their work, share common concerns, and find solutions to common issues. Professional associations began to form around the different functions of student services, some based upon gender and race issues (Nuss, 1996; Rentz, 2004). For example:

- The National Association of Deans of Women (NADW) formed at the 1910 meeting of the American Association of University Women.
  The NADW would eventually become (after two more name changes) the National Association for Women in Education, reflecting its change in mission and function only to later be dissolved in 2000 due to a decline in membership (Gangone, 2008).
- The Conference of Deans and Advisors of Men held its organizing meeting in 1919 at the University of Wisconsin. In 1951 the organization adopted a new name that recognized the changing roles and functions of its members on campus and became the National Association of Student Personnel Administrators (NASPA). As the organization broadened its appeal, women began to join the association in equal numbers, eventually taking on positions of leadership.
- The American College Personnel Association (ACPA) began in 1924 as the National Association of Appointment Secretaries, whose job it was to assist teachers and other college graduates with finding employment. The organization changed its name in 1929 to the National Association of Placement and Personnel Officers and again in 1952 to its current moniker as its role within higher education broadened. Also in 1952 the ACPA helped form the American Personnel and Guidance Association, which later became the American Association for Counseling and Development (AACD) (later becoming the American Counseling Association). The ACPA was a division of the AACD until 1992, when it voted to disaffiliate and become independent.
- Formed as a result of ACPA's disaffiliation from AACD was the American College Counseling Association (ACCA) in 1992. It was created to fill the needs for a professional organization for college counselors who did not disaffiliate with ACPA. ACCA's mission statement states, "The mission of the American College Counseling Association is to be the interdisciplinary and inclusive professional home that supports emerging and state of the art knowledge and resources for counseling professionals in higher education" (American College Counseling Association, 2009).

Racial tension and barriers prevented minorities from joining and leading many of these and other student affairs professional associations. The National Association of Student Affairs Professionals (NASAP) began in 1954 when the Association of Deans of Women in Colored Schools and the National Association of the Deans of Men in Negro Education Institutions organized the National Association of Personnel Workers (NAPW). This organization was focused upon the "hopes, aspirations, and goals of 'Negro' education" (Barrett, 1991, p. 2 as cited in Nuss, 1966). In 1994 the NAPW changed its name to NASAP. Membership today consists of a wide variety of administrators and student affairs professionals from an array of colleges and universities (NASAP, 2009).

It was also during this time that the first graduates of professional preparation programs that focused specifically on student affairs began to graduate from colleges and universities. These degrees were focused on advising and education and included masters and doctoral programs (Nuss, 1996). Today those same programs include 20 that are accredited by the Council for the Accreditation of Counseling and Related Educational Programs (2009) and 127 that are listed by ACPA (2009). The minimum degree in this field is a master's with many programs providing doctoral training.

Active Learning Exercise **10.1**

The purpose of this activity is to help you think about joining the student affairs and counseling profession. Professional associations have been a part of student affairs and professional counseling since the early 1900s. These associations have evolved as the professions have evolved. In years past, professionals joined their corresponding association as part of their obligation to the profession and as a sign of professionalism. Additionally they joined to network with other professionals and to participate in continuing education. Today's associations work hard to attract new members and to keep current members. They offer a myriad of services, products, and continuing educational opportunities.

Which professional organization corresponds with your future career choice? What do they have to offer you? What leadership opportunities might they offer to a new professional? Take a moment to explore the different associations that relate to your future career choice. You may find more than one association that relates to your choice. Almost all associations offer student and new professional rates that are must less than the regular/professional rate.

- NASPA—Student Affairs Administrators in Higher Education (http://www.naspa.org/)
- ACPA—American College Personnel Association (http://www.myacpa.org/)
- ACCA—American College Counseling Association (http://www.collegecounseling.org/)
- NACADA—National Academic Advising Association (http://www.nacada.ksu.edu/)
- APA, Div 17—American Psychological Association, Counseling Psychology: Section on College and University Counseling Centers (http://www.div17.org/SCUCC/default.htm)

While there was the creation of many professional organizations, the field of student affairs was going through its own ups and downs on colleges campuses. The Depression of the 1920s and 1930s brought a decline in students at all higher educational institutions. Many student affairs programs were cut back and colleges once again focused solely on the intellectual development of the student. As the country recovered from the Depression and into the 1940s, especially with the return of World War II veterans who enrolled into colleges and universities with the help the G.I. Bill, the field of student services saw a recovery (Neukrug, 2007). This was supported by the Student Personnel Point of View of 1937 and 1949. These two documents focused the work of student affairs programs for decades to come and continue to guide professional work into the future (Carpenter, 2003).

The next several decades present a colorful picture for student affairs and the university system in the United States. The 1950s and 1960s brought about greater federal government monies and involvement in higher education and student affairs. It was also during this period that the concept of in loco parentis changed as students sought increasing freedoms and less oversight from university administrators. Civil rights rallies, anti-war (Vietnam) protest rallies and riots, and strains in race relations spilled onto college campuses. The women's movement and sexual revolution began to impact American culture and college student services as health and counseling centers increased their service offerings to meet student needs with crisis centers, women's centers, and increased substance abuse treatment options. Rentz (2004) notes that this era, especially the 1960s, was "the age of student activism" (p. 46). Caught between students and administration, student affairs personnel often found themselves trying to foster student development by advocating for students, helping students with social causes while trying to navigate the bureaucratic structure of the institution, and providing counseling and advising services (Neukrug, 2007; Nuss, 1996; Rentz, 2004).

It was during this time that student affairs moved from a reactive approach to proactive action with students seeking to foster student development as they struggled with their role in the academic mission of the university (Rentz, 2004). During this time and into the 1980s, student developmental theory began to take on a more preeminent role. Additionally, federal laws governing access to services, the rights of persons with disabilities, sexual harassment, and affirmative action all increased the need for services, while decreases in funding caused student services offices to downsize or offer more focused services to a broader array of people (Neukrug, 2007).

In 1986, NASPA appointed a committee to look at the past and future of student affairs practice on college campuses. Colleges and universities were continuing to feel the affects of budget cuts, and the profession of student affairs was struggling with the shifts to a student development philosophy. They hoped the work of the committee would provide discussion, debate, and understanding about the role and identity of student affairs, contribute to an appreciation of the profession's work in academia, and provide direction for the future. The "Plan for a New Century Committee" core assumptions were developmental in nature and would echo the many core values from decades earlier. The core assumptions follow:

- The academic mission of the institution is preeminent.
- Each student is unique.
- Each person has worth and dignity.
- Bigotry cannot be tolerated.
- Feelings affect thinking and learning.
- Student involvement enhances learning.
- Personal circumstances affect learning.
- Out-of-class environments affect learning.
- A supportive and friendly community life helps students learn.
- The freedom to doubt and question must be guaranteed. Effective citizenship should be taught.
- Students are responsible for their own lives. (Sandeen et al., 1987)

As the 1990s arrived, so too did a challenge to the student developmental model as the only philosophical underpinnings of the profession. In 1993, the ACPA convened a group of leaders to consider how the profession could enhance student learning and development while being seen as a valued part of the academic institution and not an ancillary unit that could be dispensed with (ACPA, 1994). They proposed five characteristics that reflected the transition of student affairs in institutions that were more diverse and demanding greater accountability in the face of public scrutiny:

1. The student affairs division mission complements the institution's mission with the enhancement of student learning and personal development being the primary goal of student affairs programs and services.
2. Resources are allocated to encourage student learning and personal development.
3. Student affairs professionals collaborate with other institutional agents and agencies to promote student learning and personal development.
4. The division of student affairs includes staff who are experts on students, their environments, and teaching and learning processes.
5. Student affairs policies and programs are based on promising practices from the research on student learning and institution-specific assessment data. (ACPA, 1994)

As can be seen in this review, the profession of student affairs is hard to define and in a constant state of transformation. This is a reflection of the environment in which it exists—the university—which is also constantly evolving with the ever-changing student body that comes to learn from the faculty and develop as human beings in the environment of higher education.

DEFINING COLLEGE COUNSELING

A definition of college counseling is more complex than simply stating that it is the delivery of counseling services by trained professionals (counselors, psychologists, clinical social workers, and psychiatrists) to a specific population (college students) in a specified environment (the college campus). That is because college counseling has evolved to include more than providing short- or long-term professional counseling services. It now includes consultation, teaching, training, supervision, assessment, outreach and prevention services, career planning, crisis and emergency services, and much more (Spooner, 2000). The amount and type of services offered by the counseling center on campus is dictated by budgets, staff size and training, mission of the center, configuration of student services on campus, campus culture, and size and type of the educational institution (e.g., community or technical college, small liberal arts college, large research university). Small centers may only be able to provide short-term, primary services that lead to community referrals of the more complex cases. Well-funded counseling centers connected to health centers may provide comprehensive services including psychiatric evaluations for medication and long-term psychotherapy. Therefore the definition of college counseling "as the delivery of counseling services by trained counseling professionals in a postsecondary setting" (Spooner, 2000, p. 4) is as deceptively simple as it is complex.

A Day in the Life of a College Counselor

My Life as the Director of Counseling and Advising at a Community College

I believe that most college counselors in the community college and small-staff college counseling world would agree: there are very few typical days and there are very few dull moments! These factors alone are what keep the spice and energy continuously flowing in this profession. As both a college counselor and student services administrator in the community college counseling and academic advising arenas, I simply never go home at night wondering about the purpose for my work or what I need to add to my to-do list. It truly is an amazing and fulfilling profession.

On a recent day in our counseling services department, things started as most do: checked and returned emails and voice mails and reviewed the schedule to prepare for client appointments and meetings. And as most days evolve, the neat and tidy schedule changed periodically as clients scheduled and rescheduled and last-minute tasks presented themselves. On this particular day, five clients were scheduled, three of whom were coming for career counseling and assessment, one coming for academic advising, and one for on-going personal, mental-health counseling. During the administration of the Strong interest interview with the second client, a faculty member stopped by to consult about disturbing language and content discovered in a student's English Composition I paper. A plan for contacting the student by the counselor was agreed upon by faculty and counselor. The student coming for academic advising brought with her numerous other issues negatively affecting her academic success including depressive symptoms and possible domestic violence; the advising session quickly turned to personal counseling and a follow-up session was scheduled. By lunch, the schedule had changed for the afternoon as a client rescheduled and another quickly filled his spot. At 1:00, the classroom presentation about Stress Management and Resilience was conducted and then a speedy return to the office was met with a call from campus safety and security who had requested assistance with a student reported crying in the Atrium. After finally catching up to the student as she raced across the parking lot to her car, the counselor and security officer assessed the situation and made necessary follow-up plans with her.

The remainder of the afternoon was significantly quieter than the first six hours. Career testing results were reviewed with a client; intakes and progress notes were completed; visits, consults, and laughs were made with fellow colleagues; and follow-up phone calls were made. The day wrapped up with a bit more work being completed toward the development of the campus Behavioral Intervention Team procedures and a check of daily mail. The to-do list for the next day was made to include preparation for an upcoming classroom presentation, GED test administration, and research for an off-campus organization of which the counseling staff are members.

Perhaps there are no "typical" days in the college counseling profession. There is one thing that I can count on, however: never a dull moment!

JRT, Missouri

COLLEGE COUNSELING: A BRIEF HISTORY

The histories of college counseling and student affairs are closely intertwined. Yet there are enough specific milestones for college counseling that warrant separate treatment in the historical record of student affairs. Additionally, the rise of college counseling centers is also inextricably linked to the rise of the profession of counseling psychology and professional counseling (Meadows, 2000).

As institutions grew in size and complexity, so too did the mental health and advising needs of the student body. At the beginning of the 1900s three events took place that would bring about the creation of counseling centers on some college campuses.

1. The development of psychometrics during World War I (Brandel & Yarris, 2004).
2. The publication of *A Mind That Found Itself* (Beers, 1908) by a former Yale student. Beers wrote about his deplorable experience as a patient in a mental institution and the treatment of the mentally ill. His work helped begin the mental health movement in the United States (Gladding, 2004). This lead to the establishment of mental hygiene clinics at Princeton University, the University of Wisconsin, Washburn College, and the U.S. Military Academy (Brandel & Yarris, 2004; Meadows, 2000).
3. The publication of Frank Parsons' book *Choosing a Vocation* (Parsons, 1909), which proposed a model of assessment and counseling that helped people find suitable employment in the world of work (Nugent & Jones, 2005).

These three separate events, when brought together, would create the essential functions of counseling and the early counseling center:

*   To measure and assess intelligence, mental health, adjustment, and so forth

- To support and promote good mental health and care
- To assist in proper choices and decisions (often called guidance and centered on moral choice and vocations) (Brandel & Yarris, 2004; Gladding, 2004)

An example of how these principles were brought together can be seen at the University of Minnesota in 1932 in one of the first counseling centers. This counseling center offered professional educational and vocational guidance at the University Testing Bureau. Their work at the bureau was recognized for a model of student counseling that would later be referred to as the "Minnesota point of view" (Brandel & Yarris, 2004; Meadows, 2000).

This time was followed closely by the devastation of the Great Depression that not only affected college enrollment, but influenced college counseling. Meadows (2000) notes that the National Youth Administration specifically helped young people with testing and career counseling and placement services. This helped counseling emerge as a separate function of higher education within student personnel work. Additionally, Ohio State University opened a remedial counseling center that helped with "how to study" courses that involved college seniors in teacher education programs helping beginning students. This would eventually lead to a graduate program in student personnel work using a student personnel counseling model. Other universities would follow this example with the addition of mental health programs for the treatment of students (e.g., University of Missouri, University of Chicago). By the time World War II (WWII) began, many other colleges would have counseling centers and graduate counseling programs. While the devastation of WWII on the economy of higher education brought about the closing of many counseling centers, the counseling programs and counseling was strongly entrenched in higher education.

During WWII and following, counseling was in a state of transition from a vocational-, assessment-, and guidance-dominated field to a more client-centered field. Carl Rogers' seminal work *Counseling and Psychotherapy* emerged in 1942 along with works by pioneers in counseling college students—*How to Counseling Students* (Williamson, 1939) and *A Student Personnel Program for Higher Education* (Lloyd-Jones & Smith, 1938) that would not only affect the field of student personnel counseling but the profession of counseling itself (Meadows, 2000). It was from the mid-1940s through the 1990s that the focus on personal adjustment and good mental health became a major influence and focus of many counseling centers across the country (Brandel & Yarris, 2004).

The end of WWII brought governmental funding to universities to support the veterans returning to begin or complete their education. That funding also included money for vocational guidance and psychological assessment. As the veterans graduated and moved on, much of the government funding declined and the institutions took over the budgetary and administrative responsibilities for the emerging modern counseling centers.

In 1951, directors of counseling centers from 33 colleges and universities came together at the University of Minnesota to share their common concerns, challenges, and programming. This group became known as the Association of University and College Counseling Center Directors. This association has expanded and now has a professional conference and an electronic listserv, and provides support and information for over 748 institutional members (Association for University and College Counseling Center Directors, 2009).

The 1960s through the 1980s brought many changes and challenges to college counseling just as they did for student affairs practice. Counseling centers were asked to provide more outreach and consultation services as well as crisis interventions. The developmental model that was gaining ground in student affairs work was also affecting counseling, as more emphasis was being placed on prevention and developmental activities while moving away from a medical- or pathology-based model. All this was being asked of the counseling center as administrations were also cutting budgets.

From the beginning of the 1980s and continuing well into the 1990s, counseling centers were providing a greater array of services to a more diverse student body. This in part was created by the needs of the previous decade and also by a need for the counseling center to be seen as an integral part of the university. Campus enrollment of traditional age college students (18–25) was leveling off or declining, and there was an increase in nontraditional students (older, part-time, ethnic minorities) (Meadows, 2000). Institutions had to find ways to control or cut budgets, and counseling centers that did not demonstrate their worth to the institution often found themselves merged with other entities on campus (e.g., health centers or advising offices) (Aiken, 1982). At the same time, much of the career assessment and testing was now being transferred to placement offices or career centers (Brandel & Yarris, 2004). While this was occurring, counseling center directors were reporting a perceived increase of students seeking services with more severe clinic issues (Bishop, Gallagher, & Cohen, 2000; Robbins, May, & Corazzini, 1985).

Coinciding with the rise of these issues was a movement within the insurance industry that would take full bloom in the 1990s and would affect college counseling. Managed health care and the movement to control and contain costs in the medical field led to discussions of outsourcing mental health services on college campuses (Webb, Widseth, & John, 1997). This discussion was preceded by the decline in funding for higher education on the state government level. Administrators were looking for ways to preserve resources as they faced declining funds. Outsourcing health care, including mental health services, to a managed care service was seen as a possible way to limit costs and still provide some level of service (Brandel & Yarris, 2004; Meadows, 2000). What was generally not taken into account was the impact of using mental health professionals who did not understand student development and who underestimated the campus environment. This led, in some cases, to an overly clinical approach that excessively pathologized the student and provided inadequate interventions and services (Phillips, Halstead, & Carpenter, 1996; Widseth, Webb, & John, 1997). This outsourcing movement did not generally succeed, and those that tried outsourcing found it difficult to maintain or brought the services back to the college campus. Counseling centers naturally resisted this movement by increasing their profile on campus as a training center for interns in the mental health professions, attaining accreditation for the center itself and for the internships, and using research (e.g., client data and student retention data) to demonstrate their worth to the educational mission of the institution (Brandel & Yarris, 2004).

The new century brought about new concerns for counseling centers with an increased awareness of suicide and violence on the college campus (L. J. Schwartz & Freeman, 2009). Organizations such as the Jed Foundation (2009) and the American Foundation of Suicide Prevention (2009) have created many resources to help counseling centers create procedures and policies to help prevent suicide. While the rate of suicide for traditional college-aged students is half that of their counterparts who are not attending college (Francis, 2003), the increased attention from well-publicized cases brought about federal grant monies and programs that were being implemented nationwide while highlighting the limits of what counseling centers can do and what their staff can share with administrators (Farrell, 2002).

A Day in the Life of a College Counselor

My Life as the Counseling Center Director at a Mid-Sized University

The thing about a typical day is in a college counseling center is there is no such thing as a typical day. A few students come in to see me for therapy. Together, we create quiet conversations. "Tell me more about how your roommate sets the snooze alarm" or "How much is too much when your mother calls three times a day to check on you?" Therapy at its best is like a talk with a good friend. I am someone who will listen and who will try to understand.

Other times, the conversations are more powerful. A distant-eyed student recalls how her grandfather would try to touch her breasts while her grandmother made dinner in the kitchen. A scared freshman worries he is becoming like his alcoholic father. "Is 10 beers in one night too much? Does that make me an alcoholic?" The question hangs. I listen and care; reflect and help.

The day moves on. No more students with problems. I'm attending a departmental staff meeting. There are 25 department heads, each sharing their reports to attract the attention of the Vice President or avoid the attention of the Vice President to move on to the next meeting. And that's the choice. Be a talking head or stay quiet. Today, I check messages on my Blackberry. Catch up on overdue case notes.

Now back to the office. I'm scheduled to supervise a graduate student learning about therapy. I spend my time focused on the relationship. I've learned that graduate students often become a good therapist in spite of their graduate school training, not because of it. I help them understand that therapy is about listening. It's about understanding problems from another person's perspective. It's an uphill battle. They want to fix things. To help people who aren't ready to change. They get the gist, but will try to help too much with their clients anyway. I'll give this talk again and they will catch on eventually.

I'm behind on my case notes. Like Sisyphus pushing that rock up the hill for all eternity only to watch it roll back down again. I write. They come back. I write some more. I try not to think about 98 percent of the notes will never be read by anyone. It's those 2 percent that will be read by a lawyer or judge. So I write. Push the rock uphill.

The day ends with a parent calling. The mom is worried about their stepson. "He's depressed. I just know things are going well for him. He hasn't been going to class. Can someone check on him? He doesn't like talking, but

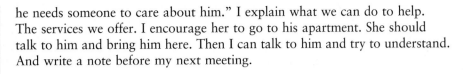

he needs someone to care about him." I explain what we can do to help. The services we offer. I encourage her to go to his apartment. She should talk to him and bring him here. Then I can talk to him and try to understand. And write a note before my next meeting.

BVB, Kentucky

Violence, legal issues, and the mental health of college students also came to the forefront after the tragic shootings at Virginia Tech in April of 2007 and at Northern Illinois University in February of 2008 (Flynn & Heitzmann, 2008). The full report detailing the mistakes and misinterpretations of federal and state privacy laws and mental health law in the aftermath of the Virginia Tech shootings has led counseling centers and university administrations to focus more attention on student mental health, the creation of crisis teams, and regular review of student issues by behavioral intervention teams on many college campuses (Flynn & Heitzmann, 2008; Rasmussen & Johnson, 2008; Virginia Tech Review Panel, 2007).

Counseling centers generally function as an important and integrated part of the university community. They have evolved from providing only moral and academic guidance and vocational assessment and counseling provided by the presidents, deans, and faculty of the institution to offering a full range of services provided by professionally trained mental health experts. Those services include counseling, outreach, training and education, supervision, research, crisis intervention, and more. This has come about due to the evolution of the needs of the student body and the higher education environment (Archer & Cooper, 1998; Stone & Archer, 1990). The type and levels of services are often decided by the size and type of the institution along with the student affairs philosophy of the administration. One issue that continues to plague college counseling centers is the requirement that they continue to provide more services to a greater number of student with increasingly complex issues and to do so with less resources (Guinee & Ness, 2000).

THEORETICAL BASES OF STUDENT AFFAIRS AND COLLEGE COUNSELING

College students of all ages present professionals in student affairs and college counseling with unique developmental and intellectual challenges. Their growth as individuals, learners, and future or current professionals can be understood from many different theoretical points of view. Having an understanding of those developmental theories enhances the professional's ability to design and implement educational programs and psychological interventions that benefit the student and support the mission of the institution. Unfortunately, many student affairs professionals do not have an in-depth knowledge of these theories (Gladding, 2004). While it is beyond the scope of this chapter to present a comprehensive overview of student developmental theories, a brief review of selected theories will be presented. They will include theories from a psychosocial, cognitive perspective, and typology perspective.

Psychosocial Theories

Erikson's (1959) seminal work on psychosocial development presents a comprehensive model that has become the basis of other developmental theories that focus on student development. The most notable of these is the work of Chickering in 1969, later revised with the help of Reisser in 1993 (Chickering & Reiser, 1993; Reisser, 1995). Chickering noted that the central developmental task during a student's college years is the establishment of identity, building upon the Erickson's notion of identity and intimacy.

Chickering theorized that students move through seven developmental stages, which he classified as vectors. Each developmental vector contributes to the student's identity formation along with seven key environmental factors that are found in the educational setting (Chickering & Reisser, 1993). This development takes place at different rates for each student, with vectors building upon and interacting with one another. Issues and conflicts that may have been settled in one developmental vector may be revisited in the proceeding vector with new understanding developing as the student's identity becomes more nuanced and complex (Evans, 1996).

The seven vectors as presented in the revised theory include the following:

1. Developing Competence: This competence is identified as the "three-tined pitchfork" of intellectual, physical and manual skills, and interpersonal competence, the student develops self assurance that "one can cope with and achieve goals successfully" (Chickering & Reisser, 1993, p. 53).

2. Managing Emotions: Student develops their ability to identify, manage, and accept the variety of emotions that they bring to campus and that develop during their tenure at the university.

3. Moving Through Autonomy Towards Interdependence: Traditional students develop emotional independence (which may or may not include physical independence) as well as a sense and acceptance of their interdependence with others. Nontraditional students may continue their clarification of goals, a reordering of priorities, and acceptance of familial help as they seek new direction in their lives.

4. Developing Mature Interpersonal Relationships: The college student learns to manage increasingly complex relationships. These new relationships with a diverse student body help the student develop the ability to have healthy, lasting relationships with increasing intimacy.

5. Establishing Identity: Chickering and Reisser identified several areas that help a student develop a positive identity (Reisser, 1995):

   - Comfort with one's gender and sexual orientation
   - An acceptance and appreciation of one's social, historical, and cultural identity
   - Through experience with others, a clear conception of self-identity and chosen lifestyle
   - A sense of or comfort with self in response to feedback from significant people in one's life
   - Self-acceptance and self-esteem
   - A sense of personal stability and integration

6. Developing Purpose: The student develops a clearer vocational plan based on personal priorities and interests. This is a more conscious choice that is driven by a clearer purpose or goal that is sought despite obstacles that may be in the way.

7. Developing Identity: Moving away from black/white, right/wrong thinking, the student develops more relativistic thinking that takes more contexts into account as well as personal values and beliefs. Additionally, the student has learned that she or he is not the only person in the world and takes into account other's viewpoints when making decisions.

This development does not take place in a vacuum, but in the environment of the college or university. Those key environmental factors include the institutional objectives, size of the institution, faculty-student interaction, curriculum, teaching practices, diversity of the student communities, and the level of student affairs programming and services.

Cognitive Theories

Cognitive views of development encompass theories of intellectual development as well as moral development. William Perry (1970) proposed a system of cognitive development that included both an intellectual and ethical or moral scheme. Made up of nine positions that are grouped into four levels, this system proposes a developmental model from which the student views and interacts with the environment.

- Dualism: We live in a dichotomous world.
    1. The student experiences the world in a dichotomous fashion, with either right or wrong answers. Authorities have the right answers.
    2. As the student experiences more of the world, uncertainty begins to develop. This can be viewed as a challenge to find the "correct" answer.

- Multiplicity: Not all answers are known, but soon will be.
    3. The student sees uncertainty as a temporary state where authorities have yet to determine the correct answer.
    4. As uncertainty becomes more extensive, the student begins to see all opinions as equally valid. The student relies less on authorities.

- Relativism: There is not always a right answer.
    5. The student begins to understand that knowledge is contextual and relative to that context.
    6. Analytical thinking becomes more prominent as the student evaluates his or her own ideas and those ideas of others.

- Commitment in Relativism: The student is learning to make personal commitments in a relativistic context.
    7. The student commits to certain ideals and values within a relative context.
    8. The student experiences and explores the responsibilities that come with his or her commitment to chosen values and ideals.

9. The student realizes that commitment is a continuous activity that impacts his or her ongoing identity development and investment in personal ideals and values.

Typological Theories

Theories in this area focus on individual differences in characteristics such as temperament, personality type, or how one views and/or relates to the world (Evans, 1996; Gladding, 2004). Not truly developmental in nature, typological theories are helpful in understanding how people with different traits, interests, or ideals relate to one another. These traits are varied between people and within individuals and persist over time. They influence motivation, achievement, and interpersonal relationships among other things. The information derived for the many different psychological inventories and assessments is often used in career services and consulting.

One of the most common and widely used measures of personality type is the Myers-Briggs Type Indicator (MBTI) (Myers, McCaulley, Quenk, & Hammer, 2003). Based on Jung's theory of psychological types (Jung, 1971), the MBTI seeks to measure how individuals perceive their environment, how they make judgments and conclusions, how they relate to people and their external environment, and their orientation to the world.

Using Jung's work, the MBTI determines a person's type based on answers to items related to four type dichotomies.

1. Perception: The way of becoming aware of things, people, events, or ideas
   - (S) Sensing—This refers to observations made by way of the senses in the here and now.
   - (N) Intuition—This refers perception made through possibilities, meanings, and relationships through insight.

2. Judgment: The way of coming to conclusions from what has been perceived
   - (T) Thinking—This refers to the linking of ideas and thoughts through logical associations.
   - (F) Feeling—Decisions are weighed and made through the understanding of personal and group values and the merit of the issues at hand.

3. Approach or Orientation Toward Life: How a person interacts with their world
   - (I) Introverted Attitude—The energy a person has toward life is drawn from the environment and brought to an inner experience and reflection.
   - (E) Extroverted Attitude—A person's energy is drawn out to the objects and persons in the environment.

4. Attitude or Orientation to the Outer World: Not part of Jung's work, this area is described by the authors of the MBTI as a dichotomy of how one interacts with the outer, extraverted world (Myers et al., 2003).

- (J) Judging—The person is concerned with planning, organizing, deciding, or seeking closure (purposeful behavior) based upon analysis (Thinking) or consideration of values (Feeling).
- (P) Perceiving—The person is accustomed to a myriad of incoming information to help make decision (spontaneous and curious) based upon what is happening in the environment currently (Sensing) or consideration for new ideas, patterns, and possibilities (Intuitive).

The MBTI results in a four-letter label that can help people understand their interaction with other individuals, the world around them, and how they best acquire and integrate knowledge. It has been used on college campuses to help students with major and career choice, living arrangements, programming, and counseling.

No one theory explains all the development that goes on during a student's time on campus, but they do supply pieces to the larger puzzle. Taken together they can provide a clearer picture of the student and help to customize education, programming, and interventions. This is especially true in the counseling arena where these theories serve as support to the counseling theories that mental health professional use to guide their work. No one counseling theory is used predominately in the college counseling profession, and therefore a review of all counseling theories is beyond the scope of this chapter.

SPECIAL TOPICS IN STUDENT AFFAIRS AND COLLEGE COUNSELING

The challenges in higher education are as different and plentiful as the students who populate the colleges and universities in our country. There are challenges that are faced in a large research university that are never thought about at the small private college. But the reverse of that is also true; the small private college faces hurdles that are not dealt with at the larger university. Each college administration and counseling center will deal with issues that are unique to their setting. Yet there are common issues that each faces in different ways.

Diversity

The American university has been a crucible of social change for decades. It is also one of the major pathways to social, professional, and economic success in our country and the world (Sandeen & Barr, 2006). So it was natural that the university was one of the first places where racial, sexual, religious, and disability barriers would be challenged so that all people could gain access to the opportunities that education provided. Enrollment continues to increase for minority students and other underrepresented populations on most college campuses today (Cook & Cordova, 2007) (See Table 10.1).

Colleges and universities have a long way to go before they are barrier free. In order to accomplish this, student affairs and college counseling professionals need to become cognizant of the needs of a diverse student body. This includes helping students learn about their classmates and roommates who come from increasingly different parts of the country and world, as well as different social and economic classes; it also includes helping the faculty devise

TABLE **10.1**

Total Fall Enrollment in Higher Education, 1994 and 2004

Race/Ethnicity	1994	2004
White	10,042,776	10,641,522
African American	1,407,705	2,030,542
Hispanic	1,005,965	1,679,924
Asian American	737,784	1,013,011
American Indian	123,797	166,228
Foreign Student	455,653	599,607
Race/Ethnicity Unknown	471,922	1,151,210

Source: (Knapp, Kelly-Reid, & Whitmore, 2006)

new modalities of instruction to reach students with different ways of learning. Additionally, the minority student (e.g., students of color, gay, lesbian, bisexual, transgender, international students) faces several issues when stepping onto a college campus for the first time. Lack of role models, difficulty with the academic transition, navigating the campus milieu, overt and covert discrimination, communication barriers, and role overload make the transition from home or country more difficult for the minority student. For student affairs professionals this means working to make the institution more accessible, open, and inclusive. There are several ways to accomplish this task, which include insuring the existence of

- a diversity of staff;
- policies and procedures practiced by the institution that are sensitive to the diversity of students on campus;
- equal access to funding for student organizations;
- support services for underrepresented or underprepared students;
- first-year experiences or capstone courses that promote understanding of diverse cultures, orientations, and ideas; and
- programming that promotes learning and understanding of a diversity of cultures, orientations, and values.

This is not a comprehensive list, but rather suggestions that provide a direction for student affairs professionals to use as a starting point to create a learning environment that is supportive of the development and success of all students (Brent, Cornish, Leslie-Toogood, Nadkarni, & Schreier, 2006; Sandeen & Barr, 2006).

The college counselor is also challenged to provide support to a diverse body of students (Archer & Cooper, 1998; Brent et al., 2006; Wright, 2000). Wright (2000) identifies challenges in the five critical areas of the counseling process where the counselor will need to make changes to increase their effectiveness with a multicultural client. In each area (intake, goal setting, working phase, solidifying growth and gains, closure and termination) the question must be asked how the student's cultural, racial, or ethnic background influences his or her perception of the issues, what direction to take the session and goals, how one chooses to work on the problem, how one measures and generalizes change and growth, and what factors need to be considered when bringing the relationship to a close. As diversity means more than race, culture, and ethnic background, I would also incorporate other variables, including sexual orientation, social economic status, differing abilities, and age (Archer & Cooper, 1998).

Additionally, the counseling center faces the challenge of how to reach out to underrepresented populations on campus while continuing to provide services to the rest of the institution with limited resources. This is the challenge faced by all programs at an institution that has no easy answer. Yet, if the campus community is to be welcoming to all learners, it is a challenge that must be wrestled with by the administration and staff of the university.

Active Learning Exercise **10.2**

While there is no single profile for today's college student, there are several historical characteristics that help define the environment that has impacted the college student's worldview. For 12 years researchers at Beloit College have complied the Mindset List (http://www.beloit.edu/mindset/index.php) to help identify the events and experiences that have impacted the worldview of the students entering higher education. As a learning experience, go the Beloit Mindset Web site. Once there, you can explore the different events and issues that have impacted the worldview of the entering freshman for the past 12 years. Ask yourself the following questions:

- How does my understanding or experience of these events impact my worldview?
- How does my worldview differ from the students who I am hoping to help in the future as a college counselor or student affairs administrator?
- What adjustments might I have to make in order to connect with these students?
- How does the students' experience (or lack thereof) impact their understanding of what being successful in college means?

If you have the opportunity, meet with a current traditional undergraduate student to discuss the Beloit list and see how your view of the list differs from his or hers.

Increasing Student Stress and Pathology

There is a perception among college counseling center directors and staff, as well as student affairs professionals, that incoming students are facing greater levels of stress, working more part-time jobs to pay for school, coming to college with more psychotropic medications and complex psychiatric diagnoses, and dealing with other major issues that are distracting them from the task at hand—obtaining an education to move forward in a career or profession (Archer & Cooper, 1998; Cooper, 2006; Gallagher, 2006; Kadison & DiGeronimo, 2005; VonSteen, 2000). While research in this area continues to produce mixed results (Males, 2007), it is clear that more students are showing up on campus with a higher level of stress then ever before. Added to this mix is the fact that college students with mental illnesses and/or developmental concerns and problems are taking increasing advantage of the services at the counseling center or are more aware that the services are offered (Megivern, 2001). Centers that are already doing more with less financial support are being stretched thin (Benton & Benton, 2006).

A Day in the Life of a College Counselor	**My Life as the Only Counselor on a Small College Campus**

My Life as the Only Counselor on a Small College Campus

Care team, disability services, crisis situations, faculty and/or staff consultation, family/parent concerns, and administrative commitments are but a few of the responsibilities that I face during any "typical" day. My primary function as the sole counselor on a small campus (~500 fulltime traditional students and ~300 residential traditional students) is to provide individual counseling sessions to students. In a typical week, I meet with anywhere between 15 and 25 students.

When I'm not in individual session, in an emergency situation or unscheduled meeting of any type, I'm working to set a schedule for campus-wide programming to include depression screening, eating disorders screenings, freshman seminar programming, parent orientation presentations, etc. I'm also preparing and planning for the presentations themselves.

GV, Michigan

It is important to make a distinction between students who are struggling with serious mental illnesses and those whose behavior is "disturbing" or disruptive (Ragle & Justice, 1989). Those students who are struggling with mental illnesses are eligible for disability services, have diagnosable mental health issues, and often fall through the cracks by not seeking and obtaining help (Megivern, Pellerito, & Mowbray, 2003). Disturbing students are those whose actions and behaviors can be described as impulsive, immature, and manipulative. These are students who live on the edge of their community and may be testing the boundaries of behavior as they seek to individuate. Clear expectations and policies and procedures that are consistently applied will assist the student affairs professionals in working with this population of students as they travel through the educational system.

At times both types of students (those with clear and serious mental illnesses and those with behavioral problems) create problems on campus. It is important that the student affairs professionals work closely with the counseling center staff to be able to understand the differences so that appropriate counseling services can be offered, when necessary, and disruptive student behavior is addressed, insuring that all students are safe. It is also important for counseling services and student affairs to have clear lines of communication and appropriate boundaries so that it is clear who provides what services and how those services impact student success (Sandeen & Barr, 2006).

Student Suicidal Behavior

The rate of suicide among college students is about half that of the same aged population that is not attending college. Additionally, the rate of suicide for both populations is declining, while the public's attention is increasingly focused on this issue due to well-publicized cases (Pavela, 2006; A. J. Schwartz, 2006). Yet these facts do not lessen the powerful impact the death of a student by suicide has on a college campus and the helplessness felt by students, faculty, and staff (Levine, 2008). The impact is magnified if it takes place within the close confines of a residence hall where students live in high-density housing (Farrell, 2002). Not only is the student's roommate affected, but all the other students on the floor where he or she lived are affected. Added to this are any close friends, classmates, residence hall staff, faculty, administrators, and family (Haas et al., 2003).

While the rate of suicide for college students is lower than the comparable population who are not attending college, the rates of suicidal thinking is high. Research suggests that 1 in 10 students seriously considers attempting suicide in an academic year (L. J. Schwartz & Freeman, 2009; Stanley & Manthorpe, 2002), and 1 in 4 students who has sought out mental health care at a college counseling center has seriously considered ending his or her life (Locke et al., 2009). Other students report high levels of depression and anxiety. This potent mix, along with higher levels of stress and needs to excel, make suicide a growing concern on college campuses.

Student affairs professionals and college counseling centers are creating procedures and programs to deal with students who demonstrate suicidal ideation or behavior that protect not only the student, but the community of learners and educators who surround that student (Francis, 2003). To not do so invites confusion and disaster that can result in the unnecessary interruption of a student's education or mental health treatment (Rawe & Kingsbury, 2006) or, in extreme cases, the death of a student, the loss of a child to a family, and the disruption of the lives of all persons who have contact with that student (Sontag, 2002). One such program that has shown positive results in reducing the number of completed suicides on a college campus can be found at the University of Illinois at Urbana-Champaign (Joffe, 2007). Beginning in the fall of 1984, it has been the policy of the university to mandate any student who has demonstrated suicidal ideation or threat to four sessions of assessment at the university counseling center. Failure to comply with the mandate could result in range of sanctions, including an involuntary psychiatric withdrawal. The program differentiates between mandated counseling, which has been shown to have limited effectiveness, and mandated assessment, which has four functions: (1) assess current ideation, intent, and access to means; (2) reconstruct with the student the circumstances, feelings, and thoughts leading to the suicidal threat or attempt; (3) completion of a lifetime history of the student's suicidal intent and its meaning and beginnings; and (4) explaining the university's standard of self-welfare to the student (Joffe, 2007). Students are free to explore the meaning of their behavior with the mental health staff member, who also points out the requirements of a standard code of conduct that all students are expected to follow. This report is submitted to and reviewed by a team of mental health professionals who accept, modify, or deactivate the report. While this description is simplistic, the process and results are much more complicated and have produced a reduction in completed suicides.

This is not always an easy task as there are varying levels of law and ethics that govern the use and dissemination of information gathered by mental health professionals and university administrators and educators. One challenge here is not how this information can be kept confidential, but instead who is going to share what specific information with whom so that the student is safe and the institution can continue to carry out its mission of providing a safe and secure environment for students to learn and faculty members to teach (Farrell, 2002; Francis, 2003; Pavela, 2006). Pavela emphasizes this point when he quotes Paul R. McHugh, former chairman of the department of psychiatry at John Hopkins School of Medicine (cited in the article "Parents Were the Last to Know" by Eileen McNamara in the January 30, 2002 *Boston Globe*): "Privacy isn't everything; life is everything. We lock people up, we take their civil liberties away if they are a danger to themselves. But we can't call the parents? What kind of nonsense is that?"(p. 15).

Ethical Issues Regarding Parents

Generally traditional aged college students are over the age of 18. The consequence of this is that they are considered adults in the eyes of the law concerning their mental health records, which must remain confidential unless written permission is given to release the record to a specific person or agency or the event of an emergency. The codes of ethics of all mental health professions clearly define the limits of confidentiality and when a counselor may breach that confidentiality in the best interest of the client or identified others (See *ACA Code of Ethics*, Section B; American Counseling Association, 2005). Parents do not have unfettered access to their students' counseling files. Yet, when a student presents as a danger (suicide) to himself or herself, should you call the parents so that they might be able to offer their care and support? Do you call the parents if the student has shared with you that his or her family of origin is one of the major factors contributing to his or her self-destructive behavior? One more question that arises for college counselors and student affairs professionals is, Who makes the call, the counselor, the dean of students, or the student with the help of one of the college professionals? As a future college counselor or student affairs professional, you will be asked to wrestle with these questions and many others like them in dealing with students' right to privacy and confidentiality.

College counselors and legal scholars have struggled making that decision for the past decades (Pavela, 2006). Added to this discussion is the fact that many college students are still developing their decision-making skills and may not be the best ones to decide if their parents should be notified when they are in psychological distress. What will you do—call the parents, help the student call their parents, or keep all information confidential?

A place to begin is by bringing together all the representatives of the different offices that could come into contact with the student who demonstrates suicidal ideation or behavior (e.g., campus safety, residence life, dean of students, counseling center, judicial services). This group can create a step-by-step protocol that focuses on insuring that each office (staff members) knows who to contact and under what circumstances so that the student is safe; provided an evaluation by a trained professional; offered appropriate options (e.g., treatment, hospitalization, medical withdrawal), if necessary; and given follow-up care (Francis, 2003; Meilman, Pattis, & Kraus-Zeilmann, 1994; Pavela, 2006; Stanley & Manthorpe, 2002).

Violence on Campus

On April 16, 2007, 49 students were shot and 32 were killed at Virginia Tech before the gunman, Seung-Hui Cho, turned the gun on himself and committed suicide (Flynn & Heitzmann, 2008). On February 14, 2008, Steven Kazmierczak entered a large auditorium-style lecture hall in Cole Hall on the campus of Northern Illinois University with a shotgun and three handguns and open fired. He killed 6 students and wounded 18 others. In both cases the shooters were mentally ill and current or former university students. The repercussions of these and others similar events include a heightened awareness of the mental health issues of college students, violence on campus, and, in the case of the state of Virginia, the mandating of crisis teams being established at every state university. Generically called College or University Behavior Intervention Teams (CUBITs), they are staffed by student affairs professionals (dean of students, public safety, judicial services, etc.) who meet periodically to review students whose behavior are a concern to the institution (National Center for Higher Education Risk Management, 2009). Additionally these events and teams have given rise to a small industry of consultants and companies that specialize in training faculty, staff, and administrators in identifying and managing crisis, violence, or aggression (e.g., the National Center for Higher Education Risk Management, the Center for Aggression Management).

CUBITs are in their infancy and are still trying to define their purpose and boundaries within the institution. The college counseling staff is also defining their role within these teams, often acting as consultant providing mental health information and interventions. In some cases they find themselves having to protect the confidentiality of a client who is also being discussed by the CUBIT for behavior that is being dealt with in therapy. This balance between confidentiality of the client and the safety of the campus is one that student affairs professionals and college counselors are negotiating as they seek to work together for the benefit of all.

It is noteworthy to point out that violence on campus is one of the most significant issues of the decade on campuses and will define many students' educational experience (Virginia Tech Review Panel, 2007). At the same time the vast majority of students are not at risk of being harmed or harming others, and those with mental illnesses, whether they be students on a college campus or in the general population, are more likely to be victims of violence rather then perpetrators of violence (Locke et al., 2009).

THE FUTURE OF STUDENT AFFAIRS AND COLLEGE COUNSELING

Student affairs and college counseling have been part of the American university system for over 100 years. In that time each has seen its place in the educational environment change for several reasons, most often due to changes in its role and function as a result of reorganization and changes in funding.

Changing Role and Function

If student affairs offices and college counseling centers are to succeed on the college campus of the future, they need to be able to define their role and function as it relates to the mission of the institution (Mattox, 2000; Sandeen & Barr, 2006). The broad mission of any college or university is to provide a safe and secure environment that is supportive of student learning (and at research institutions, to promote the expansion of knowledge) (Archer & Cooper, 1998; Francis, 2000).

Where the office of student affairs or college counseling center is located in the organizational structure of the institution is not as important as is how effective the leadership is on the campus and how well they communicate their successes in helping students achieve whatever their goal may be as it relates to their education. Mattox (2000) points out,

> Successful college counselors recognize that positive campus relationships are essential in promoting the mission of the counseling centers and solidifying the presence of college counseling on campuses. If college counseling is to thrive in the new millennium, counselors and counseling centers must initiate, cultivate, and maintain meaningful ties with academic affairs and the academic mission of the institutions. Likewise, they must educate the campus community about the integral contributions that college counselors make on a daily basis. (pp. 221–222)

While Mattox is speaking specifically about counseling centers, the same point can be made about student affairs in general. Linking the role and function of the offices of student affairs to the mission of the institution and demonstrating its effectiveness in supporting this mission is essential.

A Day in the Life of a College Counselor

My Day as a Counseling Center Director of a Small College

Each day begins with the same basic routine; I walk into my office around 7:30 A.M. and open my Titanium schedule to review my day. Next I read email, responding first to those from the dean of students or directly from a client, relegating the remaining mail to review between clients/meetings.

The next step is perhaps the most important of the day. I walk down the hall at 8 A.M., grab a cup of coffee and sit down with our director of health services for about 10–15 minutes. We review the day past (in the case of Monday we discuss our weekends) and the day ahead. This may seem trivial or a "time waster" but it is truly one of the most productive moments of the day. Walking back up the hall from her office I stick my head into each of the counseling offices, say good morning and if we have a pressing case coming in that day maybe take a moment to touch base about that specific case. Typically this is just a "good morning" drop in.

I move from there to the chart room to pull my charts for review and prep. If am lucky I haven't been interrupted with three phone calls before I sit down at my desk to review charts. I will see anywhere from three to five clients a day, typically one out of office meeting that takes about one hour, and no less than one either staff supervision, staff meeting, or case consultation each day. During the day, between meetings and clients, I may answer 50+ emails and 8–10 phone calls. Assuming no emergencies and no administrative projects (budget

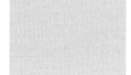

review, staff evaluations, programming planning, report writing, etc.), I can complete my therapy notes and be out the door by 6 P.M. to start the entire process over again at 7:30 A.M. the next morning.

MJR, Maryland

Limited Funding and Resources

State universities and colleges continue to receive a smaller and smaller portion of state budgets (Humphrey, Kitchens, & Patrick, 2000). In order to make up for the loss in state support, institutions have been raising tuition at rates that far exceed inflation. This has raised concern across the country as to the cost of higher education and who can afford a college education (Sandeen & Barr, 2006).

Student affairs and college counseling centers have not been insulated to these cuts in resources or cost analysis reviews. For example, institutions have contracted out student housing to private companies to reduce the costs of running residence halls. Student affairs programming to these residences may have been affected. The number of counseling sessions has been limited on some campuses with more serious and long-term clients being referred out to community resources (Webb et al., 1997; Widseth et al., 1997). In this way counseling center staff can see more students with less staff if they are not tied up with long-term clients. If this trend is to be stopped, student affairs and college counseling centers must concretely demonstrate their value to the institution.

Funding for student affairs and college counseling centers comes from a variety of sources, yet their stakeholders (the students) remain the same. Often these professionals have been reluctant to gather information on the effectiveness of their services. For example, counseling centers have often cited their need to maintain the confidentiality of client information. Yet there are a myriad of different ways that both student affairs and counseling centers can survey their clients/students and ask if or how their services have helped retain the student on campus, enhanced their ability to learn, increased their understanding of the world (i.e., diversity workshops), prevented catastrophic events that can interfere with or end a student's career on a campus (i.e., date rape, violence to others, substance abuse education), or provided support for the faculty to provide a quality education. Additionally, the senior professionals in both areas need to educate themselves about the budgeting process of their institutions so that they can become strong advocates for their services to the different funding sources (Sandeen & Barr, 2006).

CONCLUSION

Student affairs professionals are faced with a myriad of different responsibilities and tasks. Their work is as diverse as the student body of their institutions and as complex as the different types of colleges and universities that provide higher education across our country. The field is dynamic and constantly growing and changing as the population of students grows and changes. At the same time, it is built upon a solid foundation of theoretical constructs and a philosophical grounding that provides stability to the profession and informs its practice. The application of this knowledge to the tasks and responsibilities at hand aids in the overall goal of the institution to provide support for student learning and comprehensive development in both formal and informal ways (Sandeen & Barr, 2006).

The college counselor impacts student development and mental health in a way unlike any other on the college campus. This professional uses the art and science of counseling and psychology at a critical time in the development of a human being. Providing services that include career development and education, crisis counseling, psychotherapy, developmental counseling, and referral services to appropriate providers of other mental health services, this professional also seeks to support the goal of the university while supporting the education and development of the whole person (Archer & Cooper, 1998; Davis & Humphrey, 2000).

CHAPTER REVIEW

1. The professionals who work in student affairs and college counseling have historically worked together to help students develop into successful contributors to society. This work began tangentially as a way to develop men for the clergy and has evolved into numerous services that encompass everything from academic advising, residence life, disabilities services, fraternity and sorority affairs, international education, judicial affairs, counseling services, and more. The profession has also developed theoretical understandings of how students develop while in college and applied those to the different programs that have been created over the years to help students learn and education to proceed.

2. The profession of student affairs has faced many challenges during its development. It is constantly working to remain relevant as the incoming student body evolves. This means that the professionals are always creating new programs and revising current programs to meet the goal of helping a diverse body of students develop into successful learners and future participants in the global community.

3. College counseling has evolved from student affairs to be a related, but separate profession. The work of college counselors is diverse, as are the types of institutions in which they are employed. They provide services that span academic advising to short- and long-term psychotherapy in an effort to help students overcome academic, career, developmental, and psychological problems so that they can focus on the task of learning and growing.

4. The student body is growing more diverse year by year. Each student brings to the college or university not only their eagerness to learn, but their own unique stresses and coping skills. Many of these students are bringing higher levels of stress and, in some cases, increased levels of mental distress in the forms of mild to serious mental illnesses that may be managed by psychotropic drugs. College counselors are seeking to help by increasing prevention services, outreach programs, and educational programs, and by adding staff in a time of limited or decreased funding for all services.

5. Student affairs and college counseling continues to be a dynamic profession due to the evolving needs of the students coming to college. Because of this, it will continue to be an exciting field to work in that requires creative, compassionate, and energetic professionals to help students develop into productive members of our global community.

REVIEW QUESTIONS

1. How do the definitions of *student affairs* and *college counseling* differ? How are they the same?
2. How did the concept of in loco parentis evolve from the late 1880s to the 1980s? What impact did that have on student affairs work?
3. What are the two major developmental models for traditional students (18–25)?
4. What ways can a college counseling and/or student affairs office address the task of making the institution more accessible to a more diverse student body?
5. What are some of the legal and ethical challenges in working with students who present with suicidal or violent behavior?
6. How has decreased levels funding impacted student affairs and counseling services?

ADDITIONAL RESOURCES

- American College Counseling Association (http://www.collegecounseling.org)
- American College Personnel Association (http://www.myacpa.org)
- American Psychological Association, Div 17: Counseling Psychology: Section on College and University Counseling Centers (http://www.div17.org/SCUCC/default.htm)
- National Academic Advising Association (http://www.nacada.ksu.edu)
- Student Affairs Administrators in Higher Education (http://www.naspa.org)

REFERENCES

Aiken, J. (1982). Shifting priorities: College counseling centers in the eighties. *NASPA Journal, 19*(1), 15–22.

American College Counseling Association. (2009). *ACCA mission statement*. Retrieved May 27, 2009, from http://www.collegecounseling.org/ms.html.

American College Personnel Association. (1994). *The student learning imperative: Implications for student affairs*. Washington, DC: Author.

American College Personnel Association. (2009). *Directory of graduate programs*. Retrieved May 26, 2009, from http://www.myacpa.org/c12/directory.htm.

American Counseling Association. (2005). *ACA code of ethics*. Alexandria, VA: Author.

American Foundation for Suicide Prevention. (2009). Home page. Retrieved May 27, 2009, from http://www.afsp.org/.

Archer, J., Jr., & Cooper, S. (1998). *Counseling and mental health services on campus: A handbook of contemporary practices and challenges*. San Francisco, CA: Jossey-Bass.

Association for University and College Counseling Center Directors. (2009). *Mission statement*. Retrieved May 26, 2009, from http://www.aucccd.org/.

Beers, C. (1908). *A mind that found itself*. New York: Longman Green.

Benton, S. A., & Benton, S. L. (2006). Responding to the college student mental health problem. In S. A. Benton & S. L. Benton (Eds.), *College student mental health: Effective services and strategies across campus* (pp. 233–244). Washington, DC: National Association of Student Personnel Administrators.

Bishop, J. B., Gallagher, R. P., & Cohen, D. (2000). College students' problems: Status, trends, and research. In D. C. Davis & K. M. Humphrey (Eds.), *College counseling: Issues and strategies for a new millennium* (pp. 89–110). Alexandria, VA: American Counseling Association.

Brandel, I. W., & Yarris, E. (2004). Counseling centers. In F. J. D. MacKinnon & Associates (Eds.), *Rentz's Student Affairs Practice in Higher Education*. Springfield, IL: Charles C Thomas.

Brent, M. E., Cornish, J. A. E., Leslie-Toogood, A., Nadkarni, L. I., & Schreier, B. A. (2006). College student mental health and special populations: Diversity on campus. In S. A. Benton & S. L. Benton (Eds.), *College student mental health*. Washington, D.C.: NASPA.

Carpenter, D. S. (2003). The philosophical heritage of student affairs. In F. J. D. MacKinnon & Associates (Eds.), *Rentz's Student Affairs Practice in Higher Education* (3rd ed., pp. 3–26). Springfield, IL: Charles C Thomas.

Chickering, A. W., & Reisser, L. (1993). *Education and identity* (2nd ed.). San Francisco, CA: Jossey-Bass.

Cook, B. J., & Cordova, D. I. (2007). *Minorities in higher education twenty-second annual status report: 2007 supplement.* Washington, DC: American Council on Education.

Cooper, S. E. (2006). Counseling and mental health services. In S. A. Benton & S. L. Benton (Eds.), *College student mental health: Effective services and strategies across campus* (pp. 151–167). Washington, DC: NASPA.

Council for the Accreditation of Counseling and Related Educational Programs. (2009). Council for the accreditation of counseling and related educational programs. Retrieved May 26, 2009, from http://www.cacrep.org

Davis, D. C., & Humphrey, K. M. (2000). *College counseling: issues and strategies for a new millennium.* Alexandria, VA: American Counseling Association.

Erikson, E. H. (1959). *Identity and the life cycle.* New York: International Universities Press.

Evans, N. J. (1996). Theories of student development. In S. R. Komives, J. Dudley B. Woodard & Associates (Eds.), *Student services: A handbook for the professional* (3rd ed., pp. 164–187). San Francisco, CA: Jossey-Bass.

Farrell, E. F. (2002, May 24). A suicide and its aftermath: An MIT sophomore's death underscores the balancing act between students' privacy and administrators' obligations. *The Chronicle of Higher Education, 48,* A-37–39.

Flynn, C., & Heitzmann, D. (2008). Tragedy at Virginia Tech: Trauma and its aftermath. *The Counseling Psychologist, 36*(3), 479–489.

Francis, P. C. (2000). Practicing ethically as a college counselor. In D. C. Davis & K. M. Humphrey (Eds.), *College counseling: Issues and strategies for a new millennium* (pp. 71–86). Alexandria, VA: American Counseling Association.

Francis, P. C. (2003). Developing ethical institutional policies and procedures for working with suicidal students on a college campus. *Journal of College Counseling, 6*(2), 114–123.

Gallagher, R. P. (2006). *National survey of counseling center directors.* Alexandria, VA: International Association of Counseling Services.

Gangone, L. M. (2008). National association for women in education: An enduring legacy. *NASPA Journal About Women in Higher Education, 1,* 1–22.

Gladding, S. T. (2004). *Counseling: A comprehensive profession* (5th ed.). Upper Saddle River, NJ: Prentice Hall.

Guinee, J. P., & Ness, M. E. (2000). Counseling centers of the 1990s: Challenges and changes. *Counseling Psychologist, 28*(2), 267–280.

Haas, A. P., Hendin, H., Mann, J. J., Duane, E. A., Stewart, C. S., & Bridgeland, W. M. (2003). Suicide in college students: College student suicidality and family issues. *American Behavioral Scientist Special Issue: Suicide in Youth, 46*(9), 1224–1240.

Hamrick, F. A., Evans, N. J., & Schuh, J. H. (2002). *Foundations of student affairs practice: How philosophy, theory, and research strengthen educational outcomes.* San Francisco, CA: Jossey-Bass.

Humphrey, K. M., Kitchens, H., & Patrick, J. (2000). Trends in college counseling for the 21st century. In D. C. Davis & K. M. Humphrey (Eds.), *College counseling: Issues and strategies for a new millennium* (pp. 289–305). Alexandria, VA: American Counseling Association.

Jed Foundation. (2009). Home page. Retrieved May 27, 2009, from http://www.jedfoundation.org/index.php.

Joffe, P. (2007). An empirically supported program to prevent suicide in a college student population. *Suicide and Life-Threatening Behavior, 38*(1), 87–103.

Jung, C. G. (1971). *Psychological types* (H. G. Baynes, Trans.). Princeton, NJ: Princeton University Press.

Kadison, R., & DiGeronimo, T. F. (2005). *College of the overwhelmed: The campus mental health crisis and what to do about it.* San Francisco, CA: Jossey-Bass.

Knapp, L. G., Kelly-Reid, J. E., & Whitmore, R. W. (2006). *Enrollment in postsecondary institutions, Fall 2004; graduation rates, 1998 & 2001 cohorts; and financial statistics, fiscal year 2004* (No. NCES 2006–155). Washington, DC: National Center for Education Statistics.

Levine, H. (2008). Suicide and its impact on campus. *New Directions for Student Services, 121,* 63–76.

Lloyd-Jones, E. M. & Smith, M. R. (1938). A student personel program for higher education. New York: McGraw-Hill.

Locke, B., Crane, A., Schendel, C., Castonguay, L., Boswell, J., McAleavey, A., et al. (2009). *2009 pilot study: Executive summary.* Center for the Study of Collegiate Mental Health, Penn State University.

Males, M. (2007, May 27). The kids are (mostly) all right: Statistics and surveys don't support fears of a mental health crisis at our colleges. *Los Angeles Times, Section M, 6.*

Mattox, R. (2000). Building effective campus relationships. In D. C. Davis & K. M. Humphrey (Eds.), *College counseling: Issues and strategies for a new millennium* (pp. 221–237). Alexandria, VA: American Counseling Association.

Meadows, M. E. (2000). The evolution of college counseling. In D. C. Davis & K. M. Humphrey (Eds.), *College counseling: Issues and strategies for a new millennium* (pp. 15–40). Alexandria, VA: American Counseling Association.

Megivern, D. M. (2001). *Educational functioning and college integration of students with mental illness: Examining the roles of psychiatric symptomatology and mental health service use.* Unpublished dissertation, The University of Michigan, Ann Arbor.

Megivern, D. M., Pellerito, S., & Mowbray, C. (2003). Barriers to higher education for individuals with psychiatric disabilties. *Psychiatric Rehabilitation Journal, 26*(3), 217–231.

Meilman, P. W., Pattis, J. A., & Kraus-Zeilmann, D. (1994). Suicide attempts and threats on one college campus: Policy and practice. *Journal of American College Health, 42,* 147–154.

Myers, I. B., McCaulley, M. H., Quenk, N. L., & Hammer, A. L. (2003). *MBTI manual* (3rd ed.). Mountain View, CA: CPP.

National Association of Student Affairs Professionals. (2009). Home page. Retrieved May 26, 2009, from http://www.nasap.net/.

National Center for Higher Education Risk Management. (2009). *The CUBIT model.* Retrieved June 9, 2009, from www.ncherm.org/cubit.html.

Neukrug, E. S. (2007). *The World of the Counselor* (3rd ed.). Pacific Grove, CA: Brooks/Cole.

Nugent, F. A., & Jones, K. D. (2005). *Introduction to the profession of counseling* (4th ed.). Upper Saddle River, NJ: Prentice Hall.

Nuss, E. M. (1996). The development of student affairs. In S. R. Komives, D. B. Woodard Jr., & Associates (Eds.), *Student services: A handbook for the profession* (3rd ed., pp. 22–42). San Francisco, CA: Jossey-Bass.

Parsons, F. (1909). *Choosing a vocation.* Boston: Houghton Mifflin.

Pavela, G. (2006). *Questions and answers on college student suicide: A law and policy perspective.* Asheville, NC: College Administration Publications.

Perry, W. G., Jr. (1970). *Forms of intellectual and ethical development in the college years: A scheme.* New York: Holt, Rinehart, and Winston.

Phillips, L., Halstead, R., & Carpenter, W. (1996). The privatization of college counseling services: A preliminary investigation. *Journal of College Student Development, 37*(1), 52–59.

Ragle, J., & Justice, S. (1989). The disturbing student and the judicial process. In U. Delworth (Ed.), *Dealing with the behavioral and psychological problems of students.* San Francisco, CA: Jossey-Bass.

Rasmussen, C., & Johnson, G. (2008). *The ripple effect of Virginia Tech: Assessing the nationwide impact on campus safety and security policy and practice.* Minneapolis, MN: Midwestern Higher Education Compact.

Rawe, J., & Kingsbury, K. (2006, May 14). When colleges go on suicide watch. *Time.* p. 62.

Reisser, L. (1995). Revisiting the seven vectors. *Journal of College Student Development, 36*(6), 505–511.

Rentz, A. L. (2004). Student affairs: An historical perspective. In F. J. D. MacKinnon & Associates (Eds.), *Rentz's student affairs practice in higher education* (3rd ed., pp. 27–57). Springfield, IL: Charles C Thomas.

Robbins, S. B., May, T. M., & Corazzini, J. G. (1985). Perceptions of client needs and counseling center staff roles and functions. *Journal of Counseling Psychology, 32*(4), 641–644.

Rogers, C. R. (1942). *Counseling and psychotherapy: Newer concepts in practice.* New York: Houghton Mifflin Co.

Sandeen, A., Albright, R. L., Barr, M. J., Golseth, A. E., Kuh, G. D., Lyons, J. W., et al. (1987). A perspective on student affairs: A statement issued on the 50th anniversary of *The Student Personnel Point of View.* Retrieved May 28, 2009, from www.naspa.org/pubs/files/StudAff_1987.pdf.

Sandeen, A., & Barr, M. (2006). *Critical issues for student affairs: Challenges and opportunities.* San Francisco, CA: Jossey-Bass.

Schwartz, A. J. (2006). College student suicide in the United States: 1990–1991 through 2003–2004. *Journal of American College Health, 54*(6), 341–352.

Schwartz, L. J., & Freeman, H. A. (2009). College student suicide. *Journal of College Student Psychotherapy, 23,* 78–102.

Sontag, D. (2002, April 28). Who was responsible for Elizabeth Shin? *The New York Times Magazine,* p. 57, Section 56.

Spooner, S. E. (2000). The college counseling environment. In D. C. Davis & K. M. Humphrey (Eds.), *College counseling: issues and strategies for a new millennium* (pp. 3–14). Alexandria, VA: American Counseling Association.

Stanley, N., & Manthorpe, J. (2002). Responding to student suicide. In N. Stanley & J. Manthorpe (Eds.), *Students' mental health needs: Problems and responses* (pp. 243–260). Philadelphia, PA: Jessica Kinglsey Publishers.

Stone, G. L., & Archer, J. (1990). College and university counseling centers in the 1990s: Challenges and limits. *Counseling Psychologist, 18*(4), 539–607.

Virginia Tech Review Panel. (2007). *Mass shootings at Virginia Tech: Report of the review panel.* Virginia Polytechnic Institute and State University.

VonSteen, P. G. (2000). Traditional-age college students. In D. C. Davis & K. M. Humphrey (Eds.), *College counseling: Issues and strategies for a new millennium* (pp. 111–131). Alexandria, VA: American Counseling Association.

Webb, R. E., Widseth, J. C., & John, K. B. (1997). Outsourcing and the role of psychological services on the college campus. *NASPA Journal, 34,* 186–198.

Widseth, J. C., Webb, R. E., & John, K. B. (1997). The question of outsourcing: The roles and functions of college counseling services. *Journal of College Student Psychotherapy, 11*(1), 3–22.

Williamson, E. G. (1939). *How to counsel students: A manual of techniques for clinical counselors.* New York: McGraw-Hill.

Wright, D. J. (2000). College counseling and the needs of multicultural students. In D. C. Davis & K. M. Humphrey (Eds.), *College counseling: Issues and strategies for a new millennium* (pp. 153–168). Alexandria, VA: American Counseling Association.

PART 3

Professional Counseling Specialties

CHAPTER **11**

Career Counseling in the 21st Century

LEARNING OBJECTIVES

After reading this chapter you should be able to

- understand the importance of career counseling in all settings in which professional counselors work;

- describe a career counselor's roles and activities;

- identify the definitions of key career counseling terms;

- understand the historical context of career counseling;

- discuss the role of social justice in career counseling; and

- discuss ways to make career counseling relevant to the current work context.

CHAPTER OUTLINE

Introduction

Defining Terms in Career Counseling
Career
Career Development
Career Development Interventions
Career Counseling
Career Development Programs

Career Counselors' Roles and Functions
Career Counseling Competencies
Career Counseling Across the Life Span

The Parsonian Model
The Early Context for Career Interventions
The Trait-and-Factor Approach
Recent Approaches

INTRODUCTION

Today, one would be hard-pressed to identify a counseling setting in which knowledge and skills related to career counseling would not be relevant. Children, adolescents, and adults experience career development challenges on an almost daily basis. Children must learn about themselves and the world-of-work in ways that are not influenced by bias and discrimination related to gender, race/ethnicity, heterosexism, and so on. Adolescents must develop clear and accurate pictures of who they are and what educational and career options exist for them. They must also learn how to access the options they choose to pursue. Adults must cope with unstable employment situations while they also live their lives as partners and parents. They must learn skills and acquire knowledge that will allow them to remain viable to current and prospective employers. The world-of-work is not what it used to be, and therefore, the work performed by career counselors must evolve in ways that result in effective responses to the current career context.

We also know that when experiences such as unemployment increase, incidents of partner abuse, substance abuse, depression, and suicide increase. The ripple effects of employment situations going awry are dramatic, substantial, and, unfortunately, negative. Thus, virtually every professional counselor will encounter either directly or indirectly clients/students attempting to cope with career concerns.

Despite the prevalence of career issues confronting people in contemporary society, many students in counseling and related educational programs react less than enthusiastically to enrolling in the required "career development" course (Heppner, O'Brien, Hinkelman, & Flores, 1996). Perhaps some students imagine course requirements forcing them to memorize sections of occupational information books or spending hours learning how to administer and interpret tests to tell clients what occupations they should choose. Perhaps they view career development interventions as separate from more general counseling interventions, with the skill requirements of the former involving information dissemination, advising, and test administration and the skills of the latter involving more "sophisticated" therapeutic techniques. Maybe they envision career development interventions that resemble mechanistic processes in which the counselor acts in directive ways and takes complete responsibility for career intervention outcomes. Or, perhaps, they simply view career development interventions as irrelevant to their future work as a professional counselor. Whatever the reasons for the lack of enthusiasm many students feel toward courses related to career development, I take this opportunity to challenge such views and assumptions. To understand the roles and functions of career counselors, it is first necessary to understand the key terms that describe the activities and foci of career counseling.

DEFINING TERMS IN CAREER COUNSELING

Career development interventions are shaped, in part, by how we define our terms. A major issue within the area of career development interventions is the misuse of terminology among career practitioners as well as clients. For example, it is not uncommon for professional counselors to use the terms *career* and *work* interchangeably. It is also not unusual to hear professionals talk about "doing career development" as if career development were an intervention rather than the object of an intervention. Similarly, counselors often confuse the terms *career guidance* and *career counseling*. This lack of precision confuses practitioners, students, clients, and policy makers, and therefore is a barrier to advancing the efficacy of, and legislative support for, career development interventions. When language lacks precision, the implication is that terminology does not matter. Words have power, however, in that career counselors are "engaged in a verbal profession in which words and symbols frequently become the content of the interactions they have with clients" (Herr, 1997, p. 241). Thus, the need exists for greater clarity and specificity with regard to the key terms related to career development interventions. Such specificity enhances the credibility of our profession and provides a common ground for devising, implementing, and evaluating career development interventions. In this chapter, I define key terms as follows.

Career

Rather than limiting the definition of career to work, Niles and Harris-Bowlsbey (2009) advocate viewing *career* as a lifestyle concept. Super's (1976) view of career as the course of events constituting a life, and Herr, Cramer, and Niles' (2004) notion of career as the total constellation of roles played over the course of a lifetime, provide more wholistic definitions of *career*. Broader definitions highlight the multiple life roles people play and acknowledge differences across people regarding life-role salience generally and provide flexibility regarding the areas in one's life where work is located. For example, broad definitions of career apply to those locating work in the life role of homemaker or in volunteer activities.

Career Development

Career development refers to the lifelong psychological and behavioral processes as well as contextual influences shaping one's career over the life span. As such, career development involves the person's creation of a career pattern, decision making style, integration of life roles, values expression, and life-role self-concepts (Niles & Harris-Bowlsbey, 2009).

Career Development Interventions

Career development interventions, defined broadly, involve any activities that empower people to cope effectively with career development tasks (Spokane, 1991). For example, activities that help people develop self-awareness, develop occupational awareness, learn decision-making skills, acquire job-search skills, adjust to occupational choices after they have been implemented, and cope with job stress can all be labeled as career development interventions. Specifically, these activities include individual and group career counseling, career development programs, career education, computer-assisted career development programs, and computer information delivery systems, as well as other forms of delivering career information to clients.

Career Counseling

Career counseling involves a formal relationship in which a professional counselor assists a client, or group of clients, to cope more effectively with career concerns (e.g., making a career choice, coping with career transitions, coping with job-related stress, or job searching). Typically, career counselors seek to establish rapport with their clients, assess their clients' career concerns, establish goals for the career counseling relationship, intervene in ways that help clients cope more effectively with career concerns, evaluate clients' progress, and, depending on clients' progress, either offer additional interventions or terminate career counseling (Niles & Harris-Bowlsbey, 2009).

Career Development Programs

Career development programs can be defined as "a systematic program of counselor-coordinated information and experiences designed to facilitate individual career development" (Herr & Cramer, 1996, p. 33). These programs typically contain goals, objectives, activities, and methods for evaluating the effectiveness of the activities in achieving the goals.

CAREER COUNSELORS' ROLES AND FUNCTIONS

Career counselors seek to empower people to make positive life choices leading to increased career and life satisfaction. Career counselors help others decide how to structure the basic roles of living into a life. These are exciting activities that focus on maximizing human potential.

Active Learning Exercise **11.1**

Consider the counseling specialty for which you are preparing and identify ways in which career issues could confront the students or clients with whom you will work. Try to identify both direct and indirect career issues. Regarding the latter, think about how career issues could confront a loved one of your student or client and what the "ripple effects" might be. Make a list of the potential issues you identify. Then, brainstorm how you might be able to help your student or client deal with the issues you identify.

Career Counseling Competencies

To help others maximize their potential, competent career practitioners must possess expertise in a broad and challenging array of counseling-related competencies. The knowledge and skills required for providing career counseling effectively encompass and go beyond those required in more general counseling. For example, the career counseling competencies identified by the National Career Development Association (NCDA, 2003) indicate that career counselors need knowledge and skills in career development theory; individual and group counseling; individual/group assessment; career information/resources; program promotion, management, and implementation; career coaching/consultation; multicultural counseling; supervision; ethical/legal issues; and using technology effectively in the career intervention process. These skills are in addition to the requisite skills for effective counseling practice.

Moreover, the topics related to career development interventions are exciting and challenging. Essentially, career practitioners seek to help their clients increase their life satisfaction. Career counselors help people consider how they will develop and use their talents as they live their lives. Career counselors in the 21st century seek to empower people to construct meaning out of their unique life experiences and then translate that derived meaning into appropriate occupational and other life-role choices. Translating life experiences into career choices requires people to possess a relatively high level of self-awareness (Niles & Harris-Bowlsbey, 2009). Accordingly, career counselors strive to provide interventions that help their clients clarify and articulate their self-concepts. These interventions can include formal, standardized assessments as well as informal, nonstandardized assessment activities that actively and creatively engage clients in the career intervention process (Amundson, 1998). Because sorting through career concerns and engaging in career planning are complex processes, competent career counseling practice requires counselors to be skilled at developing effective working alliances with their clients (Anderson & Niles, 2000). Career counselors meet their clients at the intersection of what has been and what might be in their clients' lives. When career counselors work collaboratively and innovatively with their clients to construct a clear career direction, both the client and the counselor experience the intervention process as exciting and positive.

| A Day in the Life of a Career Counselor | **Loving My Work as a University-Based Career Counselor** |

It's exciting to me to know that my students are really in the process of constructing their lives in ways that allow them the opportunity to experience success and life satisfaction. Working with my students to help them identify what is important to them, what they enjoy doing, and what they hope to experience in their future is truly my dream job. Of course, there are occasional frustrations and there are some students who I wish would take the process more seriously. I realize, however, that there is a readiness factor. Some students are simply more ready to engage in career planning then others. Finding ways to motivate my students is also one of the challenges that I love most about my work.

Sharon J., Pennsylvania

Career decision-making is rarely a simple task, and therefore, good career counseling is never mechanistic and routine. When we consider the fact that decisions about work are made within a life context that intertwines with other life roles and responsibilities, the complex, and often stressful, nature of career decision making becomes clear. What might seem on the surface to be a relatively straightforward process of making a decision about work can quickly become overwhelming, frustrating, and complicated when important factors such as family expectations, limited occupational opportunities, financial limitations, and multiple life-role commitments are considered (Vondracek, Lerner, & Schulenberg, 1986).

Given the complexity of career decision-making, there should be little surprise that many clients seeking career counseling experience substantial levels of psychological distress (Niles & Anderson, 1993). Obviously, career counselors must address their clients' distress as they also help their clients clarify their values, skills, life-role salience, interests, and motivation. When clients also experience low self-esteem, weak self-efficacy, and little hope that the future can be more satisfying than the past, the career counselor's task becomes even more challenging. Clients coping with such issues require more assistance in resolving their career dilemmas than a test battery can provide. Given this fact, it is not surprising that career counseling clients describe the support and the experience of an effective therapeutic alliance with their career counselors as one of the most helpful aspects of their career counseling experience (Anderson & Niles, 2000). Obviously, skills found to be essential counseling skills (e.g., establishing rapport, reflective listening, expressing empathic understanding) are also essential career counseling skills.

Working collaboratively and effectively with clients also requires career counseling practitioners to possess multicultural competencies at an advanced level (Leong, 1995). For instance, clients operating from a collectivistic orientation engage in the career planning process in important ways that differ from clients operating from an individualistic orientation. Working with the client's cultural context is essential to providing effective career assistance. For example, Kim, Li, and Liang (2002) found that career counselors focusing on the expression of emotion were perceived as having greater cross-cultural competence than counselors focusing on the expression of cognition when working with Asian American college students with high adherence to Asian values. Leong (2002) found acculturation to be positively related to job satisfaction and negatively related to occupational stress and strain. Gomez and colleagues (2001) found that Latina career development is strongly influenced by sociopolitical, cultural, contextual, and personal variables. Specifically, factors such as socioeconomic status, family, cultural identity, and the existence of a support network all helped to shape the course of career development for the Latinas participating in the Gomez et al. study. The client's constellation of cultural/contextual variables clearly matters in the career intervention process. Thus, similar to general counseling interventions, the career development intervention process is a dynamic, complex, and challenging one that requires career counselors to draw upon multicultural counseling skills to effectively help their clients move forward in their career development (and, like general counseling, all career counseling is also multicultural counseling).

Active Learning Exercise **11.2**

Consider the values you that express in your work. You might do this by answering the following questions: To me, being a good worker means _____. What are the values embedded in your answer to this question? In what ways do these values reflect your cultural background? How do they influence your career goals?

Indications are that the career development process will become more, rather than less, complex in the near future. The current work context requires workers to demonstrate an extensive set of skills, behaviors, and attitudes to manage their careers effectively. Among other things, effective career self-management today requires workers to engage in lifelong learning, interact effectively with diverse coworkers, develop the ability to adjust quickly to changing work demands, and use technology effectively (Niles & Harris-Bowlsbey, 2009). To help people acquire these competencies, career development interventions must be holistic, comprehensive, and systematic. Moreover, because career development is an essential aspect of human development, career practitioners must be skilled at helping their clients cope with their career concerns within a developmental context. Because children, adolescents, and adults are presented with career development tasks, professional counselors must be skilled at providing career interventions and understanding the career development process, regardless of their work setting (Niles & Pate, 1989).

Career Counseling Across the Life Span

It is clear that the need for providing systematic assistance to individuals attempting to deal more effectively with the influence of work in their lives is tremendous. The young, the elderly, the unemployed, the underemployed, the displaced homemaker, the displaced worker, and members of diverse racial, ethnic, and socioeconomic groups are each confronted with work-related issues that have significant implications for their lives. How well they are able to cope with these issues may well be the difference between living a life that is meaningful and productive and one that is largely void of meaning and satisfaction.

Professional counselors provide career assistance to their clients in a number of ways. For example, counselors in high school, postsecondary, and community settings can teach clients the types of skills (e.g., self-assessment, job search, and career information acquisition) that are necessary for effective career planning and career decision making. Professional counselors in all settings can also help their students/clients to realize that decisions about work influence one's total life. Correspondingly, counselors can help clients develop realistic expectations for what work can provide in terms of personal satisfaction. When work is lacking in personal satisfaction, meaningful participation in other life roles helps offset this lack of satisfaction. Given the extreme emphasis we place on intra-individual variables in career development, a major task confronting counselors involves helping people to realize that self-worth is not defined by one's work situation. Self-worth relates more to how one lives rather than where one works. These are important lessons, especially in traditional Western cultures, that professional counselors in school, postsecondary, and community settings can teach and reinforce in their students/clients.

A Day in the Life of a Career Counselor	**My Day as a High School Counselor**
	Providing my students with career assistance is the part of my job I love the most. I challenge students to consider the possibilities for their futures. I work a lot with students considering career and technical education options. Their eyes light up when I talk to them about the potential earnings for many of these occupations. Many students are also relieved to know that they don't necessarily have to leave the area to pursue on occupation that they can prepare for in the career and technical program. Plus, when I tell them about the job security related to many of the occupations they can prepare for in the career and technical program, that is just "icing on the cake." One of the challenges related to this is addressing some parents' attitudes towards these jobs. Many parents think that a four-year degree is the only viable option. I try to help them learn about other options. Sometimes, they will share with me that they wished someone had told them about these jobs when they were in high school!
	Jennifer N.

THE PARSONIAN MODEL

The definitions of the terms described earlier have evolved over the decades. Early approaches to career development interventions reflected an emphasis on helping students or clients develop self-knowledge, acquire occupational information, and implement "true reasoning" in deciding which occupational choices seemed to offer a reasonable chance for experiencing occupational success. This was the approach articulated by Frank Parsons in the early 1900s.

An engineer by training and a social reformer by personal commitment, Parsons merged his training and commitment to outline a systematic process of occupational decision making, which he referred to as "true reasoning." Zytowski (2001) notes that Parsons delivered a lecture in 1906, entitled "The Ideal City," to the Economic Club of Boston. In this lecture, Parsons discussed the need for young people to receive assistance in the choice of a vocation. The lecture generated interest and requests by recent high school graduates for personal meetings with Parsons. From these activities, Parsons generated his systematic approach to vocational guidance. This approach was described in detail in Parsons' book *Choosing a Vocation* (1909). In his book, published one year after his death, Parsons discusses various principles and techniques that he found useful in helping the adolescents with whom he worked, first at the Breadwinners' College at the Civic Service House, a settlement house in Boston, and then at the Boston Vocation Bureau.

Parsons helped young people achieve the goal of "choosing a vocation." Parsons advocated activities such as reading biographies, observing workers in their settings, and reading existing occupational descriptions. These techniques were incorporated into the "Parsonian model," which consisted of three steps or requirements for helping someone make an occupational choice. These steps involved first developing clear self-understanding, then developing occupational knowledge, and, finally, using "true reasoning" to identify appropriate occupational options.

The Early Context for Career Interventions

Parsons developed his model against a background of social (e.g., rapid urbanization, child labor, immigration), economic (e.g., the rise of industrialism and the growing division of labor), and scientific (e.g., the emergence of human and behavioral sciences) changes occurring in the United States. These changes resulted in the need to place workers in jobs requiring specific skills and aptitudes, to help young people develop career plans, and to protect young people from child abuse in the labor force. Parsons' approach also fit nicely with the dominant scientific thinking of the 20th century, which emphasized positivism and objective methodology. That is, the Parsonian model encouraged practitioners to objectify interests, values, and abilities through the use of standardized assessment to guide people in identifying where they fit within the occupational structure.

The Trait-and-Factor Approach

The three requirements of the Parsonian approach formed the basic elements of what is now labeled as the *actuarial* or *trait-and-factor* approach to career counseling. The trait-and-factor approach emphasizes the identification of a person's relevant traits or characteristics, usually through the use of standardized tests or inventories. The same approach is used in describing occupational factors or requirements (i.e., occupations are profiled according to the degree to which they require certain traits such as aptitudes). Then the individual's profile of traits is matched with the factors or requirements of specific occupations. The goal of this type of matching is to identify the degree of fit between the person and an occupation. It is also the goal that Frank Parsons had in mind when he noted that he sought to help others find a vocation and not merely hunt for a job (Parsons, 1909). Emerging theories such as cognitive information processing (Reardon, Lenz, Sampson, & Peterson, 2000) advance the traditional Parsonian model by incorporating a cognitive dimension to the career decision-making process. Such theories contend that decisional processes include metacognitions that can either foster or inhibit effective career decision making.

Recent Approaches

It is important to note that career counseling theories have evolved significantly beyond traditional trait-factor approaches. The work of John Holland, Donald Super, John Krumboltz, Linda Gottfredson, and others represents important advances in the evolution of career development theory and practice. These theories embrace developmental perspectives, cognitive approaches, and person-environment interactions in addressing career development. Although this chapter focuses on the role and activities of the career counselor and not the theories they might use, I recommend that readers become familiar with the work of the theorists mentioned above. The theories represent a rich tapestry of important statements that guide the work of career counselors.

SPECIAL TOPICS IN CAREER COUNSELING

There are many special topics worthy of discussing relative to career counseling. We will consider three of them: using the Internet, professional credentialing, and advocating for social justice.

Utilizing the Internet

The increased use of the Internet, for example, certainly provides both promises and pitfalls regarding the provision of career services. Career counselors can use vehicles such as Skype to provide access to career assistance to anyone with a computer and Internet connection. This is a significant step forward for students/clients residing in more rural locations. Of course, challenges arise as one considers such issues as how to intervene in crisis situations and how confidentiality could be compromised related to Web access. For counselors using Internet-based career assessments, there is also concern regarding whether the assessments used have psychometric evidence supporting their use (many Web-based career assessments do not).

Credentialing

Career counselor credentialing is also a major issue currently. Career counseling practice is often embedded within more general counseling licensure. There is no license that applies solely to career counseling practice. Unfortunately, many licensed professional counselors have very little expertise in providing career counseling services. Thus, a license to practice counseling may not indicate that the practitioner is qualified to provide career counseling. There are also many who claim the title of "career coach" with no training at all in the counseling field, let alone in career counseling. Certificate designations are available through the National Career Development Association (NCDA), but many potential consumers of career services are not aware of the relevance of these designations. Thus, there is the need for career counseling credentialing that is widely adopted and rigorous to provide some assurance to the public that a potential career counselor is, in fact, trained to provide career counseling.

Social Justice

A third area for special topics relates to the need to integrate social justice initiatives into the work that career practitioners perform. Interestingly, acknowledging the multiple ways in which the societal context artificially limits career development for many people has led commentators to remind career theorists and practitioners of the importance of addressing social justice in career development interventions in the 21st century (Blustein, 1994; Herr & Niles, 1998). Indeed, striving for social justice through career interventions commenced with the work of Frank Parsons and, therefore, is an important theme throughout the history of the career development field. In this regard, Herr and Niles note,

> For most of the last 100 years, whether or not it has been explicit, counseling and, in particular, career counseling have become sociopolitical instruments, identified by legislation at the federal level, to deal with emerging social concerns such as equity and excellence in educational and occupational opportunities, unemployment, human capital development, persons with disabilities, child abuse, AIDS, teenage pregnancy, substance abuse, career decision making relative to the preparation for entrance into emerging skilled occupations, and the identification and encouragement of students with high academic potential to enter higher education in science and mathematics. (p. 121)

Recapturing the spirit of social justice by acting as agents of social change to maximize the career development opportunities available to all members of our society is emerging as an essential aspect of career interventions for many career practitioners today. Theoretically, Blustein, McWhirter, and Perry (2005) emphasize the need for reclaiming the historical tradition of socially just career intervention. Drawing upon the work of Prilleltensky (1997), they call for an emancipatory communitarian (EC) approach to career development. The EC approach describes five mutually dependent values that are central to creating a good life and a good society. These values are caring and compassion, self-determination, human diversity, collaboration and democratic participoation, and distributive justice (Prilleltensky, p. 319). Constructing career interventions that manifest these values requires providing assistance that moves beyond the traditional career counselor-client relationship to include efforts aimed toward creating systemic change. Blustein and his associates (2005) note the need for incorporating social advocacy and activism in theory and practice in order to achieve these goals.

Other more recent career development theories also integrate the impact of the social context into the career decision-making process. For example, social cognitive career theory, developed by Lent, Brown, and Hackett (2002), seeks to address ways in which contextual factors serve as either facilitators or restrictors in the career development process. Likewise, the systems theory framework developed by Patton and McMahon (1999) offers a contextual framework that integrates systems theory into conceptualizations of career development.

Conducting career interventions for social action requires counselors to provide multifaceted career interventions and to expand their roles beyond traditional individual career counseling practice. Career counseling for social action begins with career counselors possessing the multicultural competencies (i.e., knowledge, skills, and attitudes) necessary for understanding how the environments their clients occupy interact to influence the interpretations and meanings clients attach to work and occupational opportunities. Multicultural competencies serve as the foundation for identifying social action strategies aimed at facilitating career development.

Career counselors engaged in social action also use community resources to provide clients access to information and opportunities (e.g., employment offices, "one-stop career shops," support groups). Learning about career resources available in the community facilitates appropriate referrals and increases the probability that clients will receive the services they need. Therefore, career counselors engaging in social action play the role of facilitator by providing information, referrals, and encouragement to clients (Enright, Conyers, & Szymanski, 1996). Playing this role effectively requires career counselors to maintain files of useful resources, including names of potential mentors representing a diversity of backgrounds (e.g., African American, Asian American, individuals with disabilities, gay men and lesbian women), information on accommodations for disabled individuals with different functional limitations, names of employers willing to provide opportunities for job shadowing and internship experiences, and names of individuals willing to participate in informational interviewing experiences (Enright et al., p. 111). Having a thorough knowledge of career resources available in the community also allows counselors to identify areas in which services are lacking. In these instances, counselors once again take on a strong advocacy role and seek to rectify service deficiencies in their communities.

Advocacy is also important when clients' career concerns are the result of external factors such as large-scale downsizing, wage stagnation, and salary inequities experienced by women, persons of color, and persons with disabilities. More often than many care to acknowledge, workers struggle to earn a living. On average, women must work 66 weeks to earn what men earn in 52 weeks (Armendariz, 1997). The inequities experienced by persons with disabilities are even greater. According to Uchitelle and Kleinfeld (1996), in the past 20 years, nearly 75 percent of all households in the United States have experienced a job loss either directly or indirectly (i.e., they have a friend or relative who has lost a job). Those in the dwindling minority of persons not experiencing an encounter with job loss are also acutely aware of the tenuous nature of job security and experience high levels of guilt, fear, and anxiety.

In each of these instances, career counselors concerned with social action address not only the career concerns of individual clients, but also the career concerns of the community at large. This is accomplished by integrating individual career counseling skills with community counseling and advocacy skills. Integrating career counseling and community counseling strategies is especially critical in rural communities in which economic restructuring can threaten the very existence of the community. Community career counseling builds on the strength of individual career counseling and offers assistance to people in their struggle to maintain their communities as they create opportunities for career development. Thus, in addition to individual career counseling skills, career practitioners need skills in facilitating group problem solving and consensus building, and an understanding of social and economic factors that affect careers in contemporary society.

Essentially, career counselors who instill hope in their clients and empower them to manage their careers are multiculturally competent, act as facilitators of information and referrals, advocate for their clients when employment practices and community traditions stand in the way of equity in the workplace, and integrate individual career counseling skills with community counseling skills to assist people in their struggle to maintain their communities and create opportunities for career development. Only time will tell if the recent attention related to addressing social justice issues in career development interventions will blossom into a more common and prominent role for career counselors.

FURTHER CONSIDERATIONS IN CAREER COUNSELING

Bingham and Ward (1994) note that "if vocational counseling was born from the changing demographics and economic needs of this century, then clearly career counseling will need to change in response to the changing needs of the coming century" (p. 168). Indeed, the rapid changes occurring in the world-of-work influenced by technological developments, the emergence of an interdependent global economy, and an increasingly diverse workforce bring into question whether career development interventions need to be revised to meet the career development tasks confronting people in the 21st century. The evidence seems clear that people, both young and old, are struggling to cope more effectively with these tasks. Research results also indicate clearly that when an individual's career situations go awry, the effects are far-reaching and often negative, for both the person and society (Herr, 1989).

We are confronted daily with news reports citing statistics about high levels of global unemployment, corporate downsizing, and a jobless economic recovery. These statistics provide examples of the fact that the social contract between employer and employee is gone. Other evidence that the nature of work is changing is found in the number of companies now offering day care and parental leave; increases in the number of families requiring dual earners; and increases in the number of people working at home. These themes reflect the strong intertwining of work and family roles. Thus, career theories, career interventions, and career development professionals must respond to these evolutionary shifts occurring in the nature of work. Moreover, career interventions must be embedded in assumptions that reflect the shifts we are experiencing in work (e.g., that adults change occupations many times over the course of their lives, that lifelong learning is essential to maintaining one's marketability, that life roles interact, that rapid changes in the world-of-work are a constant, and that everyone must become skilled at interacting with diverse coworkers). Herr (2003) contends that the demand for career assistance will expand due to rising unemployment rates and an increase in part-time work.

How we intervene in the lives of the people we serve is guided by our understanding of how these shifts influence what is required for people to move forward in their careers. The emerging career concerns people experience in contemporary society point to the need for career counselors to continue their historical tradition of responding to current concerns with current interventions. Precious little appears in the professional literature proposing future directions for career counseling. Because the discourse barely exists, the direction remains unclear. Thus, career counseling's identity status resembles that of a client who lacks vocational identity and clearly articulated goals (Niles, 2003).

Savickas (1993) discusses his interpretation of what is required to move the profession forward. Specifically, he notes that in the 21st century, career development professionals will shift from supporting the 20th-century notion of careerism to fostering self-affirmation in their clients. Career counselors, Savickas contends, will teach people to be more critical of authority. People will need to be encouraged to make a commitment to their culture and community as well as learn how to develop and express their values in the real world. Rather than providing clients with predefined services in a sort of "one size fits all" approach, career counselors will collaborate with their clients to help them interpret and shape their career development. Rather than emphasizing a singular truth and objectivity, career counselors will move toward appreciating multiple realities, perspectivity, and relationships in their work with clients (Savickas, 1993). In the emerging scenario, it seems clear that a primary task of career practitioners involves clarifying (rather than assuming) how they can be *useful* to their clients. Achieving this basic and essential understanding requires career practitioners to be skilled at providing culturally appropriate career interventions.

In addition to the Savickas (1993) article, a special issue of *The Career Development Quarterly* (September 2003) stands as one of the few examples in the literature in which future directions for career counseling are identified. Building upon these contributions, I identify several ways in which career development professionals can construct career interventions that respond to clients' career concerns in the 21st century.

Viewing Career Decisions as Values-Based Decisions

Brown (2002) has presented an emerging career theory that highlights the importance of addressing clients' values in career development interventions. Brown reminds us that career decisions are essentially values-based decisions. Some values will figure prominently in a future scenario and others will be left behind, subordinated, or perhaps even distorted in a career transition. Indeed, career decisions entail determining what is to prevail and what is to be sacrificed (Cochran, 1997). Without the promise of gain and the threat of loss, there is no decision to make. One could just follow a "perfect" possibility that was presumably all positive. Yet, in an ordinary decision, one must evaluate to decide. It can be argued that these evaluations are primarily values based and that the way one evaluates defines the person one is to become and the life one is to live. Our identity is defined by these fundamental evaluations. Thus, helping clients clarify and articulate their values will become even more important in providing career development interventions in the 21st century. Career practitioners can empower clients to make choices that implement their declared values through serving as a counselor, coach, and advocate for their clients.

Moving Beyond Objective Assessment

An increased emphasis on values clarification reflects the fact that today, perhaps more than ever, it should be clear that providing clients with information about themselves and the world-of-work (through objective assessment) is necessary, but not sufficient, for empowering people to manage their careers effectively. To be sure, having information about how one's interests compare with others and where one stands on the normal curve is helpful in the process of identifying viable career options. However, most people do not think of themselves as locations on a normal curve. Rather, they focus on the process of trying to make meaning out of their life experiences. Certain life experiences capture more attention in this regard than others do. Most likely, the experiences that capture the most attention are those that have been the most painful. A painful or negative experience creates a yearning for its opposite, which becomes an ideal toward which to strive (Watkins & Savickas, 1990). In this sense, one's early life preoccupations provide the direction for what later in life can become one's occupation. Our life experiences provide the crucial backdrop against which we sort through our values, interests, and skills and then try to connect them to career options. Career development interventions in the 21st century must be directed toward helping people clarify and articulate the meaning they seek to express in their career activities.

Moving to Counseling-Based Career Assistance

Implicit in what has been discussed thus far is that "personal" and "career" concerns are inextricably intertwined. Research by Niles and Anderson (1995) indicates that many adults in career counseling are coping with concerns related to uncertainty, ambiguity, self-efficacy, and personal, as well as occupational, information deficits. Career counseling clients also report valuing the relationship dimension of the career counseling experience, and they often take advantage of the opportunity to discuss general concerns in the career counseling process (Anderson & Niles, 2000). Accordingly, many researchers now conclude that there are few things more personal than a career choice and that the overlap between career and general concerns is substantial (Anderson & Niles, 1995; Krumboltz, 1993; Multon, Heppner, Gysbers, Zook, & Ellis-Katton, 2001; Subich, 1993). Career development practitioners can respond to this overlap by offering counseling-based career assistance.

Career practitioners offering counseling-based career assistance do not view their clients as the problem and the counselor as the solution (Savickas, 1993). Rather, they seek to empower clients to articulate their experiences and construct their own lives. Savickas notes that career counselors operating from this perspective function as collaborators in the career counseling process and pay special attention to the relationship within career counseling (Anderson & Niles, 2000). Functioning in this way also requires career development practitioners to possess multicultural counseling skills.

Moving to a Stronger Emphasis on Advocacy and Multicultural Career Development Theories and Interventions

Concern about meeting the career development needs of culturally diverse clients has been a significant issue in the literature since the early 1980s (Sue et al., 1982). This issue becomes even more critical given the increasing diversity within the workforce. Career development interventions must address the "effects of social and economic barriers such as economic hardship, immigration disruption, and racial discrimination on the career behavior of ethnic minority individuals" (Leong, 1995, p. 550). Certainly, Leong's list can be expanded to include persons with disabilities and persons who are gay, lesbian, or transgendered. Moreover, career practitioners must be aware of the worldview embedded in their interventions and offer assistance that is congruent with the client's worldview. Thus, providing multicultural career development interventions requires counselors to be culturally aware, sensitive to their own values, and sensitive to how their cultural assumptions may affect their clients.

These statements are in contrast to many career theories and practices that have limited relevance for clients not adhering to Eurocentric worldviews emphasizing individualistic and self-actualizing perspectives regarding career behavior (Leong, 1995). Such statements also reinforce the importance of context in career development. Blustein (1994) defines context as "that group of settings that influence developmental progress, encompassing contemporary and distal familial, social, and economic circumstances" (p. 143). Diversity in clients and client concerns makes it clear that context must be considered in the construction and implementation of career development interventions. To act otherwise is to risk providing "culturally encapsulated" (Wrenn, 1962) career assistance.

A Day in the Life of a Career Counselor	**My Day as a Career Counselor in Private Practice**

Many of my clients start their work with me with very clear assumptions about what happens in career counseling. They expect to be tested and then told what occupations they should pursue. It is a little unsettling for them when I explain what does and what doesn't happen in the career counseling work that I do. One of the latter is that I don't EVER tell my clients what occupation they should pursue. I let them know right away that there is no such test. I explain that any assessments we use together will be used as a springboard for us to explore their self-understanding and how that may relate to occupational options. I also am clear with them that they are free to discuss whatever they wish in their career counseling with me. Many times on the surface a concern may not seem career related in the traditional sense but once we begin to explore those concerns, clients make the connections to work. They also seem to appreciate a holistic approach to career counseling in which they can address the primary life roles that they play. After all, that's how they live their lives! One of the challenges I experience is that many of my clients are not in a financial position that allows them to pay for career counseling. Then, we discuss reduced fees and/or referrals to other agencies. Despite the challenges, I find my work to be rewarding and very satisfying.

Rick B.

CONCLUSION

Careers are person specific and created by the choices we make throughout our lives. Careers emerge from the constant interplay between the person and the environment. They include activities engaged in prior to entering the workforce and after formal activity as a worker has been completed. Careers are personal and encompass the total constellation of life roles that we play. Thus, managing our careers effectively also involves integrating the roles of life effectively. In a very real sense, careers are the manifestations of our attempts at making sense out of our life experiences. The career development process is, in essence, a spiritual journey reflecting our choices concerning how we will spend our time on Earth. Professional counselors must be mindful of these facts as they attempt to intervene in the lives of their clients and assist them in their journeys.

CHAPTER REVIEW

1. All professional counselors will encounter students/clients experiencing career concerns, either directly or indirectly.
2. Career concerns arise across the life span.
3. How we define key terms related to career development is important as it creates the language that both professional counselors and their students/clients use to understand and construct appropriate interventions.
4. Career counseling has a long history that addresses both the individual career decision maker as well as systemic structures that often restrict career opportunities.
5. Emerging career counseling theories incorporate the context into describing how

careers develop, attend to social justice issues, and draw upon multicultural competencies to construct effective career interventions.
6. To address career concerns arising from the current context, career counselors may want to consider viewing career decisions as values-based decisions; moving beyond objective assessment in their career counseling; moving to providing counseling based career assistance; and moving to a stronger emphasis on advocacy and multicultural career development theories and interventions.

REVIEW QUESTIONS

1. In what ways might counselors in the schools, higher education, and community settings encounter students/clients with career concerns?
2. Define key career-related terms.
3. Why is it important for career practitioners to address social justice issues?
4. What are some recent trends in career development theory and practice?
5. How has your particular social and political context helped or impeded your career development?

ADDITIONAL RESOURCES

- National Career Development Association (http://www.ncda.org)
- Relevant journals:
  - *The Career Development Quarterly*
  - *Journal of Vocational Behavior*

- *International Journal for Educational and Vocational Guidance*
- *Journal of Employment Counseling*
- *Journal of Career Development*

REFERENCES

Amundson, N. E. (1998). *Active engagement.* Richmond, Canada: Ergon Communications.

Anderson, W. P., & Niles, S. G. (1995). Career and personal concerns expressed by career counseling clients. *The Career Development Quarterly, 43,* 240–245.

Anderson, W. P., Jr., & Niles, S. G. (2000). Important events in career counseling: Client and counselor descriptions. *Career Development Quarterly, 48,* 251–263.

Armendariz, Y. (1997, April 11). Today women's pay catches up to men's. *El Paso Times,* p. C1.

Bingham, R. P., & Ward, C. M. (1994). Career counseling with ethnic minority women. In W. B. Walsh & S. H. Osipow (Eds.), *Career counseling for women* (pp. 165–196). Hillsdale, NJ: Lawrence Erlbaum Associates.

Blustein, D. L. (1994). "Who am I?" The question of self and identity in career development. In M. L. Savickas & R. W. Lent (Eds.), *Convergence in career development theories: Implications for science and practice* (pp. 139–154). Palo Alto, CA: Consulting Psychologists Press.

Blustein, D. L., McWhirter, E. H., & Perry, J. (2005). An emancipatory communitarian approach to vocational development theory, research, and practice. *The Counseling Psychologist, 33,* 141–179.

Brown, D. (2002). The role of work values and cultural values in occupational choice, satisfaction, and success: A theoretical statement. In D. Brown & Associates (Eds.), *Career choice and development* (4th ed., pp. 465–509). San Francisco, CA: Jossey-Bass.

Cochran, L. (1997). *Career counseling: A narrative approach.* Thousand Oaks: Sage.

Enright, M., Conyers, L., & Szymanski, E. M. (1996). Career and career-related educational concerns of college students with disabilities. *Journal of Counseling & Development, 74,* 103–114.

Gomez, M. J., Fassinger, R. E., Prosser, J., Cooke, K., Mejia, B., & Luna, J. (2001). Voces abriendo caminos (Voices forging paths): A qualitative study of the career development of notable Latinas. *Journal of Counseling Psychology, 48,* 286–300.

Heppner, M. J., O'Brien, K. M., Hinkelman, J. M., & Flores, L. Y. (1996). Training counseling psychologists in career development: Are we our own worst enemies? *The Counseling Psychlogist, 24,* 105–125.

Herr, E. L. (1989). Career development and mental health. *Journal of Career Development, 16,* 5–18.

Herr, E. L. (1997). Super's life-span, life-space approach and its outlook for refinement. *The Career Development Quarterly, 45,* 238–246.

Herr, E. L. (2003). The future of career counseling as an instrument of public policy. *The Career Development Quarterly, 52,* 8–17.

Herr, E. L., & Cramer, S. H. (1996). *Career guidance and counseling through the lifespan: Systemic approaches* (5th ed.). New York: HarperCollins.

Herr, E. L., Cramer, S. H., & Niles, S. G. (2004). *Career guidance and counseling through the lifespan: Systemic approaches* (6th ed.). Boston: Allyn & Bacon.

Herr, E. L., & Niles, S. G. (1998). Career: Social action in behalf of purpose, productivity, and hope. In C. Lee & G. R. Walz (Eds.), *Social action: A mandate for counselors* (pp. 117–156). Alexandria, VA: American Counseling Association.

Kim, B. S. K., Li, L. C., & Liang, C. T. H. (2002). Effects of Asian American client adherence to Asian cultural values, session goal, and counselor emphasis of client expression on career counseling process. *Journal of Counseling Psychology, 49,* 3–13.

Krumboltz, J. D. (1993). Integrating career and personal counseling. *The Career Development Quarterly, 42,* 143–148.

Lent, R. W., Brown, S. D., & Hackett, G. (2002). Social cognitive career theory. In D. Brown & Associates (Eds.), *Career choice and development* (4th ed., pp. 255–311). San Francisco, CA: Jossey-Bass.

Leong, F. T. L. (1995). *Career development and vocational behavior of racial and ethnic minorities.* Mahwah, NJ: Lawrence Erlbaum Associates.

Leong, F. T. L. (2002). Challenges for career counseling in Asia: Variations in cultural accommodation. *The Career Development Quarterly, 50,* 277–284.

Multon, K. D., Heppner, M. J., Gysbers, N. C., Zook, C., & Ellis-Katton, C. A. (2001). Client psychological distress: An important factor in career counseling. *The Career Development Quarterly, 49,* 324–335.

National Career Development Association. (2003). *Career counseling competencies.* Tulsa, OK: Author.

Niles, S. G. (2003). Career counselors confront critical crossroads: A vision of the future. *The Career Development Quarterly, 52,* 70–77.

Niles, S. G., & Anderson, W. P. (1993). Career development and adjustment: The relation between concerns and stress. *Journal of Employment Counseling, 30,* 79–87.

Niles, S. G., & Anderson, W. P. (1995). A content analysis of career and personal concerns expressed by career counseling clients. *Educational and Vocational Guidance Bulletin, 57,* 59–62.

Niles, S. G., & Harris-Bowlsbey, J. (2009) *Career development interventions in the 21st century* (3rd ed.). Columbus, OH: Merrill Prentice Hall.

Niles, S. G., & Pate, P. H., Jr. (1989). Competency and training issues related to the integration of career counseling and mental health counseling. *Journal of Career Development, 16,* 63–71.

Parsons, F. (1909). *Choosing a vocation.* Boston: Houghton Mifflin.

Patton, W., & McMahon, M. (1999). *Career development and systems theory: A new relationship.* Pacific Grove. CA: Brooks/Cole.

Prilleltensky, I. (1997). Values, assumptions, and practices: Assessing the moral implications of psychological discourse and action. *American Psychologist, 52,* 517–535.

Reardon, R. C., Lenz, J. G., Sampson, J. P., Jr., & Peterson, G. W. (2000). *Career development and planning: A comprehensive approach.* Belmont, CA: Wadsworth/Thompson Learning.

Savickas, M. L. (1993). Predictive validity criteria for career development measures. *Journal of Career Assessment, 1,* 93–104.

Spokane, A. R. (1991). *Career interventions.* Upper Saddle River, NJ: Prentice Hall.

Subich, L. M. (1993). How personal is career counseling? *The Career Development Quarterly, 42,* 129–131.

Sue, D. W., Bernier, Y., Durran, A., Feinberg, L., Pedersen, P., Smith, E. J., & Nuttall, E. V. (1982). Position paper: Cross-cultural counseling competencies. *The Counseling Psychologist, 10*(2), 45–52.

Super, D. E. (1976). *Career education and the meaning of work.* Washington, DC: Office of Education.

Uchitelle, L., & Kleinfield, N. R. (1996, March 3). On the battlefield of business, millions of casualties. *The New York Times,* Section 1, p. 1ff.

Vondracek, F. W., Lerner, R. M., & Schulenberg, J. E. (1986). *Career development: A life-span developmental approach.* Hillsdale, NJ: Lawrence Erlbaum Associates.

Watkins, C. E., Jr., & Savickas, M. L. (1990). Psychodynamic career counseling. In W. B. Walsh, & S. H. Osipow (Eds.), *Career counseling: Contemporary topics in vocational psychology* (pp. 79–116). Hillsdale, NJ: Lawrence Erlbaum Associates.

Wrenn, C. G. (1962). The culturally encapsulated counselor. *Harvard Educational Review, 32,* 444–449.

Zytowski, D. G. (2001). Frank Parsons and the progressive movement. *The Career Development Quarterly, 50,* 57–65.

CHAPTER 12

Substance Abuse Counseling

LEARNING OBJECTIVES

After reading this chapter, you should be able to

- understand the impact of substance abuse on our society;

- understand the impact of substance abuse on individuals and families;

- identify definitions and models of substance abuse and addiction;

- describe substance abuse treatment models and counseling approaches; and

- discuss the role of the substance abuse counselor, substance abuse counseling training, and ethical issues when dealing with substance abuse problems.

CHAPTER OUTLINE

INTRODUCTION

Addiction to alcohol and other drugs has probably existed well before recorded history. The disastrous effects on the addicted individual, the family, and society have made addiction one of our most serious medical, psychological, sociological, and economic problems. The impact of our use of addictive chemicals cannot be overestimated. It is no wonder that this problem has evolved into an area of concern for all counselors. This chapter will provide an overview of the challenges that addiction poses to our society, concepts and models of addiction, the history of addiction counseling, methods used to confront addiction, and ethical issues in addiction counseling.

Counselors in all settings will encounter the issue of substance abuse and addiction in their practice. This chapter contains basic information on these topics that are therefore important for school, clinical mental health, marriage and family, career, and college counselors. Although there is some information about career paths for addictions counselors, it is important for counselors in other settings to understand the specialty area of addictions. This is perhaps even more important since the implementation of the 2009 CACREP (Council for Accreditation of Counseling and Related Educational Programs) standards, which contain stronger emphasis on addiction knowledge and skills than any previous standards.

THE IMPACT OF ADDICTION AND SUBSTANCE ABUSE ON SOCIETY

There are many estimates of the impact of addiction and substance abuse on our lives and our society. In term of pure numbers, the National Survey on Drug Use and Health conducted by the Substance Abuse and Mental Health Services Administration (2006) estimated that of U.S. citizens 12 years and older, about 9.1 percent, or 22.2 million people, were either dependent on or abusers of alcohol and illicit drugs. Of these 22.2 million, 18.7 million, or 7.7 percent of the 12 and older population, were dependent on or abusers of alcohol. About 4.1 million people experienced problems with marijuana, 1.5 million with cocaine, and 1.5 million with pain relievers, .49 million with tranquilizers, and .41 million with stimulants. Overall, these statistics indicate a problem of epidemic proportions.

To put these numbers in perspective, you have to simply look around you and realize the roughly 1 of every 10 people you see have had or will have a serious problem with alcohol or other drugs. A 1-in-10 incidence rate also means that every reader of this chapter is probably acquainted with someone who has a serious problem with addiction or abuse. Many of us have seen or experienced the impact of addition. Even in our nonprofessional lives, we can be affected almost daily by this problem.

The cost of addiction is yet another dimension of this problem. A Brandeis University study (Horgan, Skwara, & Strickland, 2001) indicated that alcohol and drug use costs our economy approximately $276 billion per year in lost productivity, crime, health care, accidents, and other consequences. The same study also estimated that untreated addiction costs are greater than costs associated with diabetes, cancer and heart disease combined. In addition, the emotional devastation of substance abuse and dependence to families, friends, and others close to the problematic user cannot be estimated and can probably not be completely comprehended.

Active Learning Exercise 12.1

Take a few minutes to jot down the people you know who have been affected by the abuse of alcohol and other drugs. There are many ways that individuals can be affected: They may be addicted or abusing drugs themselves and have suffered the legal, medical, social, family, or vocational/educational effects of alcohol and other drugs. Chances are you know several people who have been arrested for alcohol-related offenses or who have suffered injuries when using alcohol. You may have also known people who have been arrested for possession offenses. Even greater might be the number of people who have family members or close friends who are addicted and may have been personally affected by that addiction. There is even a high probability that you may have a member of your extended family who has been addicted. If so, note the impact on your family and the number of people in your family who have been affected. You may also know people who have been injured by drunk drivers. After generating the list, reflect on the depth of the impact of the use of alcohol and other drugs on every person in our culture.

Encountering Addiction and Substance Abuse Issues in Counseling

Counselors in all settings will encounter clients with addiction or substance abuse issues. To put the problem in perspective, depression is one of the most commonly occurring mental health problems, yet the National Survey on Drug Use and Health (Substance Abuse and Mental Health Services Administration [SAMHSA], 2006) indicated that of the population 12 and older, 7.3 percent were depressed during the last year, which is 1.8 million less than those affected by alcohol and other drugs. In addition, 26.3 percent of those who were depressed had substance abuse or dependence issues. The Household Survey also indicated that 21.3 percent of the surveyed population who experienced serious psychological stress had substance dependence or abuse problems.

Despite the devastation, the numbers receiving treatment for substance abuse problems are surprisingly low. The National Survey on Drug Use and Health (SAMHSA, 2006) found that of the 23.2 million individuals who needed treatment, only 20.9 percent actually received it. A 2007 survey by SAMHSA found that only 12.6 percent of those who needed treatment perceived a need for it and only 8.1 percent of those who needed treatment actually received it (see Figure 12.1). These statistics make it clear that we as a society must strengthen our effort to not only provide sufficient treatment

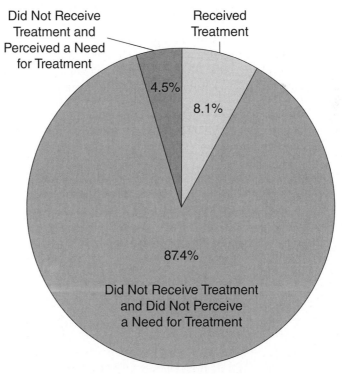

FIGURE **12.1** Receipt of and Perceived Need for Alcohol Treatment in the Past Year among Persons Aged 12 or Older Who Needed Treatment: 2007

options, but also find more effective methods of encouraging addicted individuals to begin the treatment process.

The implications of the results of the National Survey on Drug Use and Health are twofold. The first is that counselors who work with any type of population will have, at minimum, a one in five chance that their client with have a substance dependence or abuse problem. The probability that their client will have a family member with one of these problems is significantly higher. The second implication is that there is a significant proportion of our population experiencing problems in this area, creating a strong need for counselors who have knowledge and skills to work with these individuals.

At this point it should also be clear that every counselor, regardless of setting, will regularly be faced with this problem. Given the severity and impact of addiction and abuse, it should also be no surprise that addiction counseling is a growing specialty within the counseling profession.

The Impact on Adolescents

Adolescents are perhaps the group for which the negative impact of substance abuse is most the most dramatic. The Monitoring the Future survey out of the University of Michigan (Johnston, O'Malley, Bachman, & Shulenberg, 2006) has been surveying students in public schools for decades. Their survey has become a standard indicator of drug use by youth in our society. Their results are often surprising. Taking a look at 12th graders, the 2006 survey indicated that 36.5 percent used an illicit drug in the last year. An examination of specific drugs reveals that 31.5 percent used marijuana, 6.8 percent used tranquilizers, and 5.7 percent used cocaine in the previous year. Alcohol use among 12th graders is equally worrisome. Sixty-six percent have used alcohol in the last year, and 47.9 percent drank to the point where they were drunk. Perhaps surprisingly, 13.9 percent of the eighth graders reported being drunk in the last year. Five percent of the 12th graders reported drinking on a daily basis.

These findings have obvious implication for school counselors and mental health counselors who work with adolescents. They are assured of working with students and clients who are using a variety of drugs. In addition to student use, a survey conducted by Brown University (Lewis, 2000) estimated that over 9 million children live with a parent addicted to alcohol or other drugs. Of all the problems adolescent counselors encounter in their work, alcohol and other drug use will be one of the most common. Thus, it is essential that any counselor who works with adolescents have the knowledge and skills to work with this issue.

A Day in the Life of a Substance Abuse Counselor	**My Rewarding Work with Adolescents**

My Rewarding Work with Adolescents

I work as a counselor in an adolescent outpatient treatment program. Today, most of my work will focus on completing assessments on four new clients who have been referred by the local juvenile court judge, discussing a recent positive urine screen with one of my clients, and running a family group in the evening. Most of my agency's clients are between thirteen and eighteen and are court referred. Others are referred by the local community mental health agency and some are from families who self-refer. The primary focus of my

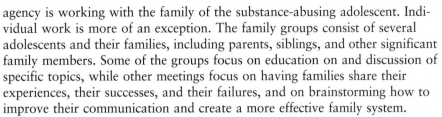

agency is working with the family of the substance-abusing adolescent. Individual work is more of an exception. The family groups consist of several adolescents and their families, including parents, siblings, and other significant family members. Some of the groups focus on education on and discussion of specific topics, while other meetings focus on having families share their experiences, their successes, and their failures, and on brainstorming how to improve their communication and create a more effective family system.

I'm particularly effective in communicating with adolescents. I'm often assigned the tasks of doing assessments because I establish a non-threatening, non-authoritarian relationship that creates a more cooperative relationship with my clients. I also work with the clients involved with the urine screening process, which can be difficult at times.

I find working with adolescents rewarding: "Although they are often resistant at first, if you take the time to listen to them, they can really open up to you. Working with the adolescents and their families also allows you to make changes in the whole system, which is usually what it takes to allow the adolescents to change."

RG, Virginia

DEFINING TERMS

The first issue that must be addressed in understanding substance, abuse, dependence, and addiction is clarification of terminology. The *Diagnostic and Statistical Manual* of the American Psychiatric Association, the *DSM–IV–TR* (American Psychiatric Association [APA], 2000) outlines two general definitions that are relevant in this regard. Each of these definitions can be applied to specific drugs, including alcohol, to create a specific diagnosis. The terms *substance abuse* and *substance dependence* are clarified in Tables 12.1 and 12.2.

The substance abuse definition emphasizes use with potentially dangerous consequences, whereas the substance dependence definition emphasizes physical dependence and withdrawal symptoms, use despite negative consequences, and compulsive use that involves time and effort put into procurement and use of the drug as well as giving up other activities due to the use of the drug. The use must also impair general social and occupational functioning.

The *DSM* therefore provides us with two definitions, with one, substance abuse, outlining harmful use, and the other, substance dependence, outlining harmful and compulsive use. Substance dependence is consistent with what we often label as addiction. The *DSM–IV–TR* nomenclature provides the advantage of clear operationally defined terms. There are, however, two disadvantages that should be noted. The first disadvantage is that the term *substance dependence* can be confused with the concept of physical dependence, which consists of tolerance to a drug and withdrawal symptoms resulting from its use. The problem with this definition is that someone can be physically dependent on a drug, for example, when prescribed opiates or other

TABLE **12.1**

Criteria for Substance Abuse

A. A maladaptive pattern of substance use leading to clinically significant impairment or distress, as manifested by one (or more) of the following, occurring within a 12-month period:

1. Recurrent substance use resulting in a failure to fulfill major role obligations at work, school, or home (e.g., repeated absences or poor work performance related to substance use; substance-related absences, suspensions, or expulsions from school; neglect of children or household).
2. Recurrent substance use in situations in which it is physically hazardous (e.g., driving an automobile or operating a machine when impaired by substance use).
3. Recurrent substance-related legal problems (e.g., arrests for substance-related disorderly conduct).
4. Continued substance use despite having persistent or recurrent social or interpersonal problems caused or exacerbated by the effects of the substance (e.g., arguments with spouse about consequences of intoxication, physical fights).

B. The symptoms have never met the criteria for Substance Dependence for this class of substance. (APA, 2000, p. 199)

TABLE **12.2**

Criteria for Substance Dependence

A maladaptive pattern of substance use, leading to clinically significant impairment or distress, as manifested by three (or more) of the following, occurring at any time in the same 12-month period:

1. Tolerance, as defined by either of the following:
   (a) a need for markedly increased amounts of the substance to achieve intoxication or desired effect
   (b) markedly diminished effect with continued use of the same amount of the substance.

2. Withdrawal, as manifested by either of the following:
   (a) the characteristic withdrawal syndrome for the substance (refer to Criteria A and B of the criteria sets for withdrawal from the specific substances)
   (b) the same (or a closely related) substance is taken to relieve or avoid withdrawal symptoms.

3. The substance is often taken in larger amounts or over a longer period than was intended.
4. There is a persistent desire or unsuccessful efforts to cut down or control substance use.
5. A great deal of time is spent in activities necessary to obtain the substance (e.g., visiting multiple doctors or driving long distances), use the substance (e.g., chain-smoking), or recover from its effects.

6. Important social, occupational, or recreational activities are given up or reduced because of substance use.
7. The substance use is continued despite knowledge of having a persistent or recurrent physical or psychological problem that is likely to have been caused or exacerbated by the substance (e.g., current cocaine use despite recognition of cocaine-induced depression, or continued drinking despite recognition that an ulcer was made worse by alcohol consumption). (APA, 2000, pp. 197–198)

pain killers, but they may not develop the compulsive or harmful use after they stop using the drug. The person would have been dependent, but would not have met the criteria for substance dependence as defined in the *DSM–IV–TR*.

The other disadvantage is that the *DSM* nomenclature omits using the term *addiction*, which is commonly used among all professionals who work with this disorder, thus sometimes creating confusion among both professionals and the public. It might be argued that omitting *addiction* helps clarify the concept and reduce stigma, but it's not clear that the advantages outweigh the disadvantages.

In this chapter, the terms *substance dependence* and *addiction* are used interchangeably, with the term *substance abuse* being used to label the disorder as defined in the *DSM–IV–TR*.

MODELS OF ADDICTION

Addiction and substance abuse have been problems since before recorded history. For centuries, addicted persons, families, communities, law enforcement officers, health professionals, and mental health professionals have strived to understand the nature of addiction. A brief review of the perspectives on addiction will be helpful in giving us insight on how addiction is currently viewed by addiction counselors.

The Moral Model

According to Fisher and Harrison (2005) the first view of addiction was the *moral model*. The moral model, which probably predates history and has been a strong influence on the treatment of addicts in most societies, views addiction as a personal choice. The implication of this view is that the consumption of alcohol or use of drugs is within the control of the addict and that they should be held accountable and probably punished for their use. Within this view, drug and alcohol use is often viewed as a sin. This model also contributes to the development of a high level of stigma surrounding addiction that is not conducive to the addict being provided opportunities for treatment. The implied solution for addiction is for the addict to make a conscious choice to stop his or her use and to use will power to do so. The moral model is still a strong influence on how addiction is viewed by many components of our society.

The Medical Model

Although often viewed the same as the disease model mentioned later, the *medical model* developed in the 19th century as an alternative to the moral model. Proponents of this model viewed addiction as a disease that should be treated through traditional medical methods. The use of hospitalization, medical staff, and medications were consistent with this model that still has a strong influence (White, 1998). In 1956, the American Medical Association (White, 1998) declared addiction to be a disease and, as we have already seen, substance abuse and dependency are classifications in the APA's *DSM–IV–TR*. This model, in particular, influences much of the federally funded research on addiction treatment, which focuses on the development of medications that may be part of a treatment approach for addiction.

The Psychological Model

This model is based on the idea that addiction is a reflection of an underlying psychological problem. This has been another influential model and has been affecting the perception and treatment of addiction for much of the 20th and 21st centuries (White, 1998). The implication of this model is that addiction can be treated not by dealing with the symptoms but by resolving the issues that have been causing the addiction. Although there is little data to support this concept, its intuitive appeal makes it an approach that is attractive to most professionals not trained in addiction counseling approaches.

The Sociocultural Model

For decades researchers have observed that different cultures have differing rates of addiction to alcohol (Fisher & Harrison, 2005). The *sociocultural model* implies that there are cultural variables, such as attitudes toward drunkenness (Fisher & Harrison) and non-moralistic mind-sets (Stevens & Smith, 2005), that appear to affect the level of problematic drinking in a culture. Although the observations have been consistent, there have been few consistent explanations for this phenomenon. There have been no particular components of the culture that seem to explain the difference, and it is not clear whether the difference may be better accounted for by genetics. Despite not knowing the mechanisms of these differences, this model continues to contribute to our understanding of addiction.

The Biological Model

Genetics is one area of addiction about which we seem to know the most. As with the sociological studies there have been clear and consistent findings, particularly for males, that indicate a genetic tendency to become addicted to alcohol and other drugs (Fisher & Harrison, 2005). For females, however, the evidence is not as strong. Both twin and adoption studies have contributed to the observation that there is strong correlation between genetics and addiction. We still do not, however, know the exact genetic mechanism. An "addiction gene" has not been identified. It is also important to note that the genetic connection only indicates a stronger probability of a particular person becoming addicted. There are no indications that anyone is destined to become addicted because of family addiction patterns.

The Disease Model

The model that has perhaps had the strongest impact on counseling and treatment for addiction is the *disease model*. Although the name might imply that it is the same as the medical model, there are significant differences. Although there is not an authoritative definition of the disease model, there is general agreement that it is a biopsychosocial (and, according to some, spiritual) model that posits addiction has, as the label implies, multiple causes (Fisher & Harrison, 2005). In this model, addiction is the result of an interaction of all these variables, which can lead to a point where the symptoms of addiction begin to progress. This model compares addiction to a disease in that the addicted individual is not responsible for getting the disease, and like some diseases, it has a predictable, progressive course. It is also similar in that the disease is primary, meaning that it cannot be treated by resolving underlying psychological problems any more than a cold or flu could be. From this perspective addiction is also viewed as permanent in that, like diabetes, it can be controlled, but not cured.

The disease model is controversial in that it conflicts with both the moral model and the psychological model, which are more intuitively appealing to many. Some also object to the implication inherent in the disease model that addicted individuals are not responsible for the disease, and thus they are absolved of responsibility for their actions, many of which are harmful to others, family, and society. The response to this concern from those who espouse the disease model is that although the addicted individual is not responsible for the disease, they are responsible for getting treatment for the disease and that they are not absolved of responsibility for their actions. This debate has been going on for a long time and it continues. Despite the debate, however, most treatment and counseling programs base their approaches on the disease model (Fisher & Harrison, 2005).

The various models continue to affect the way we view addiction. Substance abuse counselors need to be aware of these models, particularly the disease model. Whether they agree with it or not, it has a strong impact on the way we treat addiction and the vocabulary used in the addiction counseling field.

Active Learning Exercise **12.2**

Now that you have read some of the different ways to view addiction, reflect on how you view addiction. Which of the models above are most similar to your view? As you think about this question, also ask yourself what has affected the development of your view. Was it affected by people you have known who have become addicted? By depictions of addiction in the media? By your religious views or cultural views? By the views of your parents or family members? Chances are that you will find there are many factors affecting the development your attitudes toward addiction and, in many cases, these attitudes lead to stigmatization of individuals who are addicted. Finally, reflect on your reaction to the disease model. Does it make sense to you or is it difficult to think of addiction as a permanent disease for which there is not cure? Your attitudes toward addiction will have a significant impact on how you work with addicted clients. As you encounter addiction in your professional role, you will find these questions coming up on a regular basis.

THE IMPACT OF ADDICTION ON INDIVIDUALS AND FAMILIES

Earlier we looked at the impact of addiction on society. In order to understand addiction it is also important to take a look at the impact on the addicted individuals themselves and on their families.

The *DSM–IV–TR* definition of *substance dependency* (addiction) contains categories of symptoms of addiction to alcohol and other drugs. The first category is tolerance and withdrawal. Although many addicts have these symptoms, which are an indication of heavy alcohol or other drug use over a long period of time, this category of symptoms, while physically uncomfortable, is perhaps the least troubling for the addict. With medication or other medical supervision, these symptoms can be relatively easily resolved in a short period of time. There may be some long-term implications (e.g., cravings and healing from physical damage caused by drugs), but these are, again, usually not the most damaging long-term implications of addiction.

The next category of symptoms is the problems caused by the addiction. Addiction is well documented as causing problems in every aspect of the addicted individual's life. The most devastating impact is usually on family and other relationships. Unless the family or others in some way support the addiction, these relationships are most often irreparably harmed, creating loneliness and isolation for the addicted client. The addiction also usually causes medical problems, legal problems, financial problems, and educational or occupational problems, leaving many addicted individuals unemployed, alone, broke, and with little or no hope of resolving these issues as long as they continue to use. Perhaps the most devastating damage, however, is to the addicted individuals' self-esteem and sense of control of their lives. Because the addiction is often permanent and progressive, they begin to lose any sense of self-efficacy after repeated failures to stop or cut back their substance abuse. Their lives are in a devastating downward spiral from which there seems no hope of escape. This downward spiral, combined with the isolation and the myriad of other problems, leads to a life of despair for which the only apparent solution, self-control, has ultimately proven to be ineffective. The addicts' lives are often ruined, and they perceive that they have nowhere to turn. Although there is a continuum of severity for all these problems, in most cases, if the addiction continues, the impact will progressively lead to the worst-case scenario of physical and psychological deterioration or death.

The last category of symptoms is the compulsive use or loss of control. As implied in the problem category, addicted individuals usually try every means to control their use. These attempts, once addiction has begun, are almost never successful. To many it is the hallmark of addiction that the use of the drug is beyond the individual's power, no matter how hard he or she tries.

The disease is equally devastating to families. From a family systems perspective, it is not difficult to appreciate what would happen to a family system in which there is a member with a progressive disease that leads to occupational, financial, social, legal, and medical problems. It also leads to damaging, unpredictable interactions between the addicted individual and the other family members. As the problems get progressively worse, family members become increasingly desperate for the addicted family member to stop using. Since the dominant model of nonprofessionals in our society is the moral model, the family members usually assume the addicted member could stop if he or she wanted to. This assumption leads to typical first-order change approaches such as coercion, threats, manipulation, and hostility. Because the addicted family member has no control over the alcohol or other drug use, these attempts not only do not work, they usually make the situation worse. Thus, the family begins its own downward spiral that leads to the same level of desperation as with the addicted individual. An old adage in the addiction field is that the rest of the family becomes "sick or sicker" than the addicted member.

The terms *codependency* and *COA* (children of alcoholics) (Brooks & McHenry, 2009) have emphasized the destructive patterns in which family members can find themselves as they attempt to cope with the deterioration and chaos of being in an family with an addicted member. Although these terms do not have research-based definitions, they emphasize the impact of the family system on the addictive process and the importance of counselors' understanding the response of family systems to addiction before they work with addicted clients and their families.

Overall the negative impact on everyone involved with an addicted individual cannot be overestimated. Unfortunately, these consequences ultimately affect us all. There are relatively few people in our society who have not been affected by someone they know or love who is addicted. We only need to reflect on our experiences with addiction to know the devastation it creates.

COUNSELING SUBSTANCE ABUSERS

Substance abuse counseling probably began well before recorded history. Since humans first discovered drugs, it is likely that we have been looking for ways to help those who suffer the consequences of their use. Through most of history, though, the approaches to dealing with this problem have been primarily based on the moral model. In other words, most of the attempts through time have involved trying to convince the addicted individual to stop using. These attempts almost invariably have failed.

The roots of the modern view of addiction treatment began during the latter part of the 19th century. It was during that time that the medical model began to take hold, resulting in the development of both pharmaceutical and hospital-based approaches. By the beginning of the 20th century, there was a wide selection of medications that were touted as cures for alcohol and morphine addiction. Ironically, heroin was sold as a cure for morphine addiction. Despite the popularity of these medications, there is no indication that any of them were effective in any way other than creating an addiction to the medication itself (White, 1998). The hospital-based treatments may have had some very limited success. They at least provided a supportive atmosphere, allowed the addicted individuals to survive withdrawal symptoms (sometimes), and gave them time to recover from some of the consequences of the addiction.

Although interest in the medications dwindled over time due to eventual evidence of ineffectiveness (White, 1998), not much changed in treatment approaches until the 1930s. In the 1930s, substance abuse counseling changed forever with the founding of Alcoholics Anonymous (AA). AA, which will be explored a little later in this chapter, brought about the concept that there was hope for alcoholics, and that recovering alcoholics could play a role in the recovery of others. Although AA, which began in 1935, had its growing pains, it gained strength and greatly influenced the development of substance abuse treatment in the 1940s.

AA contributed to one of the most influential developments in substance abuse treatment and counseling: the Minnesota Model (White, 1998). Developed in three substance abuse hospitals in Minnesota, the Minnesota Model of treatment was based on the implication of the disease model—that addiction is a primary, permanent, and progressive disease. The Minnesota Model integrated the concepts and Twelve Steps of AA, the utilization of recovering addicts as counselors, and abstinence as a goal. The influence of the Minnesota Model grew through the 1950s and 1960s to the point where almost every treatment program for alcoholism was based on the model (White, 1998). The use of recovering counselors became a standard for these programs, but they also emphasized an interdisciplinary team as well. Into the 1970s the proliferation of both in-patient and outpatient treatment and counseling continued, as did the use of recovering counselors. No particular mental health discipline, however, had "claimed" substance abuse counseling as a part of their profession. In the 1970s the federal government recognized that the numbers of trained substance abuse counselors was insufficient and began investing in training and workshops that would increase the skill level of mental health professionals from different disciplines (White, 1998).

Several steps were taken in the 1970s that contributed to the development of substance abuse counseling as a specialty area of counseling. The International Association for Addiction and Offender Counselors was created in 1972 as a division of the American Personnel and Guidance Association (later to become the American Counseling Association) and the National Association for Drug and Alcohol Abuse Counselors (NADAAC) was established in 1975. The professionalization continued with the development of certifications in the field. NADAAC established certifications and in 1981 the precursors of the International Certification Reciprocity Consortium (ICRC) were developed. ICRC also became a strong proponent for certification of substance abuse counselors. In 1995 the National Board of Certified Counselors (NBCC) established the Master Addiction Counselor (MAC) specialty certification in conjunction with NADAAC, which also developed a similar MAC. NBCC's development of the MAC exam was also a landmark in the development of a job analysis for substance abuse counselors, who were also now being referred to as addiction counselors. At the time of this writing, CACREP has proposed a specialty accreditation for addiction counselors that, if approved, would take effect in 2009.

Today, all states have certifications and some states have licensure for addiction counselors. The federal government has established a set of knowledge, skills, and attitudes for addiction counselors (Center for Substance Abuse Treatment [CSAT], 1998). Many counselor education programs have specialty courses and specialty programs in addiction counseling. If the CACREP standards for an Addiction Counseling specialty are approved, the number will likely increase. After several decades of development, the specialty appears to be getting close to a clear professional definition. There are still issues, however, that need resolution. Some addiction counselors still consider themselves a separate profession, not a specialty of counseling and other mental health professions. It is becoming clear, though, that the profession of counseling has embraced addiction counseling as a specialty, and it is likely that the role of addiction counseling within our profession will continue to grow.

| A Day in the Life of a Substance Abuse Counselor | **The Diversity and Intensity of Working in a Residential Facility**

I work as a substance abuse counselor in a private residential treatment facility. My facility's clients are not in-patients because the live in apartments on the grounds that do not require full-time medical care. During the day and some of the evenings, though, they are involved in various aspects of their treatment program seven days a week. Their time in the treatment program may last anywhere from three weeks to several months, depending on the severity of their addiction problem.

On this day I will be leading two family groups in which the clients and their families meet with four or five other families to learn about the effect of addiction on the family and the importance and the process of their participation in the recovery process and relapse prevention. The group will meet for an hour and a half and will be one of three groups that the patients participate in during the day. At other times they may attend individual counseling, attend yoga, meditation, or other self-care programs, attend an education seminar on the impact of addiction, work on their recovery plan and, quite often, attend an AA or other type of twelve-step meeting. There are relatively few times during the day when they do not focus on their addiction, the impact of their addiction, or their recovery.

When not working with clients in the group setting, I may have individual meetings with clients who have been assigned to me, work on paperwork, focus on my administrative tasks as director of the women's transitional

(continued)

A Day in the Life of a Substance Abuse Counselor *(continued)*

housing program, meet with my supervisor, attend a treatment planning meeting, or meet with a client's family.

I enjoy the diversity of my work and the intensity of working in a residential facility: "I feel like the time I have with the patients allows me to develop a genuine connection with the clients and that I can make a significant difference in their lives. It is intense work, but I thrive on that. Not every client who completes the program succeeds but that is usually part of learning what it takes to be in recovery. Sometimes it takes a long time, but when it works, the clients turn their lives around. It's like a miracle."

RG, Virginia

The Recovery Process

In order to understand the work of addiction counselors, it is important to understand the concept of recovery from addiction. Stephanie Brown's book *Treating the Alcoholic: A Developmental Model of Recovery* (1985) provides a good framework for examining this process. Although Brown's model was developed for addiction to alcohol, most of the concepts apply to addiction to other drugs as well. Brown divides the recovery process into four stages: the Drinking stage, the Transition stage, the Early Recovery stage, and the Ongoing Recovery stage. In the Drinking stage, the addict experiences the downward spiral of addiction, denying the existence of the problem and encountering increasingly severe consequences to family, career, finances, and health. Eventually, after many failed attempts to control their drinking, addicts may reach a point when their system of denial collapses. If their denial system continues, they often experience significant deterioration of their life and their health and may die as a final consequence of the addiction. In this stage, counselors need to focus on helping their clients develop the motivation to consider treatment. Because of the strength of denial and resistance at this stage, this can be a difficult task. In the past counselors have relied on more confrontational interventions. More recently, Motivational Interviewing (MI) (W. R. Miller & Rollnick, 2002) has provided counselors with a more effective mode to work with clients in the drinking stage. MI emphasizes rolling with the resistance and helping clients move through stages of change by developing discrepancy in their thinking and by developing within themselves the commitment and confidence to develop a change plan.

The second stage of recovery, the Transition stage, if attained, is usually experienced as a change in how the addicts view themselves, others, and their environment. From Brown's perspective, the addicts must now honestly admit to themselves that they cannot drink and that they have to restructure their lives around this admission. It is a time of emotional and often physical pain, humility, and confusion. In this stage, the addict begins the process, often with the help of AA or other support networks, of learning to live without the use of chemicals. This can be a challenging stage for counselors who are working with addicted clients. Clients in this stage will typically need some type of treatment program, whether it be outpatient or residential. A counselor who may have played a critical role in the patient getting to this stage will probably have to step back and allow the treatment program staff to take over for awhile. It is critical that the client receive a consistent message and support from the treatment staff as well as other clients in the treatment program since most of the treatment will take place in group counseling sessions.

In the next stage, Early Recovery, addicted individuals begin the learning process of being in recovery. Here, they must learn how to use support groups, make significant changes in all parts of their lives, and begin the process of changing their cognitions about using drugs, their sense of control in their lives, their spiritual approach to life, and how they perceive their priorities and their relationships. At this stage they must be open to learning and change, or a relapse is likely. Much of the focus of their lives at this stage has to be on their recovery. They cannot afford many distractions. The role of counselors at this stage is to support the recovery process by encouraging the client to follow the plan developed in the treatment program; a plan that typically entails the development of a positive support system, attendance in Twelve-Step meetings (including working with a sponsor), family counseling, paying attention to signs of a relapse process, and developing the skills to adjust to a life without the use of substances. In this stage, it is important for counselors to remember that recovering addicts will need a lot of support during this time because they are confronted with the task of beginning a new life and letting go of an old one. It is also important that counselors help the client avoid taking on too much during this time. The client's recovery needs to take center stage. Other life concerns need to be addressed as well, but the client needs to balance these with the energy and focus that needs to be directed to the recovery process. Counselors also need to be aware that depressive episodes are common during this stage and that they need to be addressed if they occur.

In Ongoing Recovery, the addicted individuals continue the process begun in Early Recovery, but they also need to begin focusing on other aspects of their lives and integrating these aspects with their recovery. Many need to begin a more mature exploration of their spirituality and begin the process of repairing old, and developing new, relationships. They also need to start focusing more on educational or career issues. The counselor's focus during Ongoing Recovery should be a gradual return to normal functioning and the continual development of life skills. Career, family, and relationship concerns need to be addressed as the client is now able to direct more time and energy toward these areas now that he or she has achieved a stable recovery. Relapse is still a concern in this stage and the counselor will need to be attentive to early signs that the relapse process may be starting. Overconfidence can be particularly problematic during this time. Counselors may also spend time with clients discussing spiritual issues and how spirituality can enhance recovery and most other areas of the client's life. Ongoing Recovery is a process of continual growth in which the counselor often plays a critical role.

This process can take years and obviously takes up a great deal of time and energy. Addiction counselors work with clients in all stages but have varying roles and responsibilities at the different stages. It must be noted that relapse can happen in all the stages of recovery and therefore relapse prevention— which includes activities such as relapse education, client self-assessment, involvement of family and friends, identification of warning signs, and ways to deal with the warning signs—becomes an important role of the addiction counselor (Gorski, 1993). Because addiction can affect every facet of an individual's life and because many different types of counseling services may be needed to support an individual's recovery, it is also important that counselors integrate their role with other health and mental health professionals as well as support groups such as AA. They must also be involved with the family at all stages. This process is extremely difficult and stressful for the family, often leading to separation of the addicted individual from the family. The road to recovery is long and difficult. The recovering person needs to access all the help they can get. We have found that addiction, which was once thought to be a hopeless situation, can lead to recovery, but it takes time, dedication, and expertise on the part of the addiction counseling professionals.

The Contribution of Alcoholics Anonymous

Before discussing treatment approaches, it is important to take a look at AA, its contribution to our understanding of treatment for addiction, and its importance for the work of the addiction counselor. For a complete description of AA's history, its impact, and how it works, see Kurtz's *Not-God: A history of Alcoholics Anonymous* (1979), an authoritative, well-documented volume.

AA began in 1935 with a meeting between Bill Wilson and Dr. Bob Smith in Akron, Ohio. The drama of this meeting and its aftermath are well documented and have been the subject of a made-for-television movie and an off-Broadway play. The early history of AA is full of trial and error, with almost as many errors as trials, which led to an organization that has helped millions. Much of the process of AA is described in the book *Alcoholics Anonymous*, or as it is known among AA members and addiction professionals, "The Big Book" (AA, 2001). The organization took its name from the title of the book (White, 1998). The heart of the AA process is the well-known Twelve Steps, which are shown in Table 12.3.

The first three steps are often used as the foundation of treatment programs: to acknowledge that alcohol is creating unmanageable problems in one's life and to acknowledge the need for help. The other steps encourage self-examination, resolving the problems caused by the addiction, reflection, and helping others. Mutual help was an important dynamic in the first AA encounter between Bill Wilson and Dr. Bob Smith and remains an important part of the process today.

AA, however, is a multifaceted program. Other factors that contribute to its effectiveness are the use of slogans as a method of cognitive change (e.g., "keep it simple," "one day at a time," "easy does it," "nothing is so bad, a drink won't make it worse"), mutual support, unconditional positive regard, the use of sponsors (i.e., asking another AA member to serve as a mentor for the recovery process), asking for help from others, combating isolation, providing structure at a time of disorientation and chaos, 24/7 help when needed, instilling hope, role-modeling, and, of course, encouraging spiritual development (White, 1998).

TABLE **12.3**
The Twelve Steps of AA

1. We admitted that we were powerless over alcohol—that our lives had become unmanageable.
2. Came to believe that a Power greater than ourselves could restore us to sanity.
3. Made a decision to turn our will and our lives over to the care of God as we understood Him.
4. Made a searching and fearless moral inventory of ourselves.
5. Admitted to God, to ourselves, and to another human being the exact nature of our wrongs.
6. Were entirely ready to have God remove all these defects of character.
7. Humbly asked Him to remove our shortcomings.
8. Made a list of all persons we had harmed, and became willing to make amends to them all.
9. Made direct amends to such people wherever possible, except when to do so would injure them or others.
10. Continued to take personal inventory and when we were wrong promptly admitted it.
11. Sought through prayer and meditation to improve our conscious contact with God, as we understood Him, praying only for knowledge of His will for us and the power to carry that out.
12. Having had a spiritual awakening as the result of these steps, we tried to carry this message to alcoholics, and to practice these principles in all our affairs. (AA, 2001)

It is the spiritual piece that has caused much of the controversy about AA. The wording of the Twelve Steps and the Lord's Prayer that is said at the end of many meetings feels to some like an imposed Christianity. It is important for counselors to understand that the spiritual part of AA is purely optional and, despite the references to God in the Twelve Steps and many of the traditions, the emphasis in AA is on spirituality as each member defines it. There is no requirement that anyone be involved in any particular organized religion. In fact, the only requirement for membership in AA is the desire to stop drinking (AA, 2001).

There are other criticisms of AA. Some believe that is it most effective for white males, having been slow to adapt to the needs of women and cultural minorities. Others express concern that there has been little documented effectiveness. Still others feel it has a cultish feel to it and that it has a negative attitude toward addiction professionals. These points continue to be debated and should be. For counselors, however, it is important to remember that the organization has played an important part in the recovery of millions of addicted individuals, many of whom are or will be clients with whom counselors will work. A respectful sense of cooperation, if not a strong understanding of the organization, is important for addiction counselors.

There have been many other offshoots of AA, such as Al-Anon for family members and Narcotics Anonymous (NA) for users of drugs. The Twelve Step programs and their role in recovery have been around for over 70 years now, and it would appear that they will be around for a long time.

Major Treatment Approaches

Addiction is a multifaceted problem and requires a wide range of treatment approaches. Although the 28-day in-patient treatment program based on the Minnesota Model was a dominant model in the 1970s and 1980s, the reluctance of insurance companies to pay for the comprehensive in-patient programs has led to a range of treatment options that are usually tailored to meet the particular needs of the clients (White, 1998). We will take a look at the major types of treatment for substance abuse disorders and then take a look at some of the important issues related to treatment.

Detoxification

In some cases, addiction clients have consumed enough of the drug or drugs over a sufficiently long period of time that they have developed a tolerance for the drug(s). Once they stop using they experience a withdrawal reaction to the cessation of the drug use. Withdrawal effects can range from mild discomfort to a fatal reaction. The fatal reactions most commonly occur in response to alcohol, benzodiazepines (antianxiety medications), and barbiturates. In these cases the client may require either medical assistance in order to avoid a fatal reaction or severe discomfort. Detoxification may be accomplished in in-patient settings or in supervised outpatient situations. When individuals receive detoxification services, they are often required to see or are introduced to a counselor who can help them choose appropriate services after they complete the detoxification process. Sometimes the detoxification occurs as a component of an in-patient treatment program.

In-Patient Treatment

When the addiction is more severe and when finances allow, in-patient treatment is often the recommended modality. An in-patient treatment program is located in a hospital setting in which the addicted individual is admitted as a patient. This type of treatment is intensive, allows for medical care when there are physical consequences to the addiction, and is usually based on the 28-day Minnesota Model. These days the time varies depending on the level of services needed. The program is usually highly structured, includes psycho-educational and group work, as well as some individual counseling, and is typically based on the AA Twelve Steps. The programs are almost invariably abstinence oriented. This was the primary mode of treatment during the 1970s and 1980s, but it less common now due to the expense of a long hospital stay.

Residential Treatment

Residential treatment has supplanted in-patient treatment in many places. The treatment program is usually based on the Minnesota Model as well, but clients stay in non-medically supervised residential units rather than in a hospital. This arrangement makes the whole program less expensive. The treatment program itself usually takes place in a setting where medical personnel are available to assist with the medical consequences of the addiction.

Outpatient Treatment

Outpatient treatment takes place in a variety of settings, including private practices, community mental health centers, and other outpatient community settings. Again, the treatment program is often based on the AA-oriented Minnesota Model, but it is tailored to allow the clients to live at home and sometimes work, depending on the intensity of the program and the severity of the problem. The intensity of the program can range from all day, five days a week, to several evenings a week. The programs typically require AA involvement and are abstinence oriented. Almost all the counseling and education is based in groups. These programs often require outpatient individual counseling and follow-up groups after the program has been completed.

Early Intervention Programs

These programs are usually intended for individuals who have been arrested for either alcohol- or drug-related driving or possession offenses. Their purpose is to prevent substance abuse from becoming addiction or to intervene with addiction at an early stage. Commonly oriented to either adults or adolescents, these programs are conducted in groups and have a strong psychoeducational component. Individual and/or family counseling is often required as a part of participation. These programs are sometimes conducted in conjunction with the criminal justice system.

A Day in the Life of a Substance Abuse Counselor

Providing Counseling as an Alternative to Incarceration

I work for the correctional system as an outpatient counselor in a program that provides alternatives to incarceration. Working in collaboration with the probation officers, the program provides both individual and group counseling for individuals who have received alcohol and other drug violations. Today I will be conducting two group sessions and I will be meeting with three of the clients to provide counseling and to discuss what options they have for an incarceration alternative. The program has several substance abuse groups and programs within the agency and they often refer clients with more serious problems to programs outside the agency. I'm particularly good at my job because I have an in-depth understanding of the connection between substance abuse and offenders, I have a straightforward counseling style that, when combined with my natural empathy, resonates with my client population, I am skilled in Motivational Interviewing techniques that allow me to deal effectively with resistance, and I am patient with the process since I'm familiar with the Stages of Change.

There are many challenges with this type of substance abuse counseling work. I have to coordinate my work with the probation officers and the judges. I also have to deal with non-compliance issue and deciding when my clients need to be referred back to the judge due to the non-compliance.

(continued)

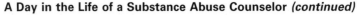

A Day in the Life of a Substance Abuse Counselor *(continued)*

Making these stressful decisions underlines the need for counselors in these settings to engage in self-care and to be able to leave the work behind at the end of the day. It also requires working the evenings when many of the groups are scheduled.

I have an optimism and perspective that seems well suited to meet these challenges: "Despite the recidivism and the frequent non-compliance, I feel that I have the opportunity to help each of my clients make changes that could alter the course of their life. Substance abuse and addition can be devastating, but when my clients start making positive changes, there seem to be no limits as to what they can accomplish."

RG, Virginia

Outpatient Counseling

Sometimes clients are seen on an individual basis in conjunction with support group involvement such as AA or NA. Although group-oriented treatment is almost always the treatment of choice for addiction, individual counseling can be effective if there is some other type of group involvement. Individual counseling is also effective for individuals who have completed treatment and are working on after-care or relapse issues. Individual counseling can also be effective on a pretreatment basis as a transition to treatment for high-functioning clients.

Family Counseling

Family counseling is often conducted for families when a family member is in a treatment program or is dealing with posttreatment adjustment issues. The impact of the family system in all stages of recovery cannot be underestimated. Most treatment programs consider it essential that the family be involved with the treatment process. Family education on the process of recovery, the impact of addiction on the family, and the impact of the family system on recovery and the recovering client are all essential to insure that the family system does not fall back into its previous and sometimes destructive family patterns. Family counseling is also particularly effective in working with substance abusing and substance dependent adolescents. Many adolescent treatment programs base their approach on work working the family system. In fact, working with individual families or families in groups is often necessary if treatment of adolescents is to be effective.

Al-Anon and other Twelve Step–inspired programs play important roles in helping the family deal with an addicted member. These organizations provide support and education both while a family member may be involved with alcohol and other drugs as well as during the recovery process. These programs emphasize self-care and the avoidance of destructive patterns and have been an invaluable resource for families who often have nowhere else to turn.

Pharmacologic Interventions

Over the past 40 years there have been a wider variety of pharmacologic approaches that have added to counselors' arsenal for dealing with addiction.

The oldest is Antabuse, which is taken daily and induces a severe physical reaction when the Antabuse user consumes alcohol. It is best used for motivated clients because the Antabuse reaction can be potentially dangerous and at least extremely unpleasant. There are also several narcotic antagonists and agonists that either block or supplant the user's reaction to narcotic drugs. Methadone is well-known as a drug that supplants opiates. Drugs such as Naltrexone block the effects of opiates. As long as the addicted individual continues to take the drug, they will not be able to experience the effects of the recreational opiates. Buprenorphine is one of the most recent of these drugs that supplant the narcotic reaction, but is not as addictive as methadone. It has also been used to reduce drug cravings for addiction to alcohol and other drugs. At this point, these drugs have rarely been used by themselves as a treatment for addiction, but are more typically used to supplement other approaches.

Other Approaches

These are the primary treatment approaches that are used for dealing with addiction. There are others, though, that are not as commonly used as many of the approaches based on the disease model. "Controlled drinking" and other behavioral approaches have been implemented with success in some settings. There are other support groups such as Women for Sobriety, Secular Organizations for Sobriety, and Moderation Management that have provided alternative approaches to AA. Rational Recovery (RR), a movement based on Rational Emotive Behavior Therapy principles, was another option for some time, but RR groups are no longer in operation (Brooks & McHenry, 2009).

A Day in the Life of a Substance Abuse Counselor

Working in Private Practice

I work in a private practice that specializes in substance abuse problems. Most days I see four or five clients, assesses substance abuse issues in two clients, and conduct one or two group counseling sessions. My schedule varies depending on the day. Some days I may focus mostly on assessments and other days I focus more on either individual or group counseling. The practice I work for serves a mixture of clients who are self-referred, those referred by the criminal justice system, referrals from college judicial officers, referrals from Employee Assistance Programs, and referrals from many other sources. The practice also has a contract with the local Alcohol Safety Action Program that refers clients who have been convicted for drinking and driving. All their counseling is conducted on an outpatient basis. Almost all the clients are seen in outpatient groups. These groups are best described as psycho-educational; combining elements of education about substance abuse and addiction as well as opportunities for each member to work with the other group members in exploring the impact of alcohol and other drugs on their lives.

Working with clients in this setting can be challenging because of their denial and their resistance to taking an honest look at the problems that their use creates in their lives. They can be argumentative, avoidant, and insist on blaming the legal system and anyone or anything else for the legal, medical, and financial problems that their use creates for them. On the other hand,

(continued)

A Day in the Life of a Substance Abuse Counselor *(continued)*

because they are often forced by legal or other reasons to participate in the program, they will face serious consequences if they do not cooperate to some extent. If the counselors in the practice can be effective in helping the clients find the motivation in themselves to make changes, the outcome can be rewarding for both the counselor and the client.

I love the opportunity to make a difference in her client's lives: "Our clients are often in the early stages of abuse or addiction. If we can help them recognize their problems, we can save them and their families years of emotional pain. I have seen the changes people can make when they truly face their problems and the reward of being part of that process goes way beyond anything I get paid."

RG, Virginia

OTHER ISSUES RELATED TO SUBSTANCE ABUSE COUNSELING

In addition to learning some of the basic dynamics of substance abuse recovery and treatment approaches, a number of other treatment issues are important to explore briefly. These include assessment and screening of substance abuse, treatment outcomes, and special considerations in treating adolescents.

Assessment and Screening

One of the most important aspects of treatment for addiction problems is accurate diagnosis and early screening. One of the roles of the addiction counselor is to be familiar with the most accurate and efficient approaches to both. Instruments such the Alcohol Use Inventory (Horn, Wanburg, & Foster, 1986), the Addiction Severity Index (Fureman, Parikh, Bragg, & McLellan, 1990), and the Substance Use Subtle Screening Inventory (G. Miller, 1985) are instruments commonly used for for assessment. The Michigan Alcohol Screening Test (Selzer, 1971), the CAGE Questionnaire (Ewing, 1984), and the AUDIT (Babor, De La Fuente, Saunders, & Grant, 1992) are commonly used screening instruments that can be administered in a matter of minutes. Before using any of these instruments, however, counselors should receive, at the very least, some training in addiction counseling and supervised use of these tools.

Treatment Outcome

Studies over the past 15 years have consistently shown that treatment for substance abuse reduces the impact of addiction on those who go to treatment (CSAT, 1999; SAMHSA, 1998). In fact, a federally funded study in 2001 found that for every dollar spent on alcohol and drug treatment resulted in a savings of $6.40 per patient (Harwood, Koenig, Siegel, Gilani, & Chen, 2001). Project Match (Babor & Del Boca, 2002), the largest clinical outcome study ever conducted, also found that treatment programs were effective; however, those doing the study were not able to determine whether a match of treatment with client characteristics would result in greater effectiveness. Overall, treatment is clearly effective and can a result in a significant financial and emotional savings to society.

Treating Adolescents

The range of treatment for adolescents is similar to that of adults. There have been some interesting trends, however, in treatment for this age group. Some research has indicated that outpatient family therapy and family therapy groups are effective modes for adolescent substance abuse (Fisher & Harrison, 2009). There has also been and increase in the treatment provided through the juvenile justice system and drug courts.

SPECIAL TOPICS IN SUBSTANCE ABUSE COUNSELING

In recent years, much has been learned about substance abuse. This new information has provided new perspectives in the way substance abuse counselors view stages of change, Motivational Interviewing, co-occurring disorders, prevention, and ethical issues surrounding substance abuse.

Stages of Change

One of the more significant concepts in the addiction treatment field over the past 10 years has been Prochaska and DiClemente's Stages of Change (1986). Based on their research on smoking cessation, Prochaska and DiClemente developed a model of change that broke the process into five stages: Precontemplation, Contemplation, Preparation, Action, and Maintenance. The Stages of Change concept has allowed addiction counselors to think of progress not just in terms of success or failure, but in progress through the stages. This has led to a more precise assessment and to a more realistic differential treatment planning that meets the client where they are at, not where we would like them to be. It should be emphasized, however, that progress through the stages is not always linear. In fact, Prochaska and DiClemente emphasized that a regression or relapse could happen at any time, requiring the client to work through the stages again.

Motivational Interviewing

Based on the Stages of Change and developed by W. R. Miller and Rollnik (2002) in the 1990s, the Motivational Interviewing (MI) model for counseling has had a dramatic impact on the process of addiction counseling. Prior to the popularization of MI, addiction counselors commonly used a confrontational approach to counseling that was designed to help clients acknowledge that they were not in control of alcohol or other drugs and their lives. Although successful in some cases, this approach also engendered anger and resistance, which were viewed as an inevitable by-product of the process. Miller and Rollnik envisioned an approach based on client-centered counseling that would assist the client in developing a more internal sense of motivation and hope. The approach relies heavily on having clients explore their own decisional balance, on having the counselor encourage the development of change-talk in the clients, and on rolling with, rather than confronting, the resistance that addicted clients typically display. The research on MI since its development has provided strong evidence of its effectiveness (W. R. Miller & Rollnik, 2002). MI was the basis for one of the treatment protocols for Project Match.

Project Match helped confirm the approach that Miller and Rollnik developed. MI has now become a standard framework for counseling addicted clients.

Co-occurring Disorders

The forces that led to the development of addiction counseling and addiction treatment also led to a separation of addiction counseling and other mental health issues. Those who specialized in addiction tended to view it as a separate process from working with other types of disorders. Over the past 20 years it has become increasingly evident that addiction and other mental disorders tend to go hand in hand. This realization has lead to the term *dual-diagnosis* and, more recently, to *co-occuring disorders*. This recognition has led to approaches that integrate substance abuse treatment with treatment for other disorders, creating a situation where both are treated at the same time instead of separately. It has also led to an increased emphasis on training addiction counselors to work with all types of disorders and for community and mental health counselors to receive increased training in addiction counseling approaches.

Prevention

Since the 1970s addiction professionals have increasingly acknowledged the importance of preventing addiction before it begins to extract a financial and emotional cost from the addicted individual and the family. Since that time, addiction prevention has become its own discipline, and prevention approaches have become far more sophisticated. Most school systems across the country have instituted prevention programs, often using some of the evidence-based practices that have been endorsed by federal agencies (SAMHSA, 2008b). An example of one of the evidence-based prevention program would be the All Stars program; a weekly program in the schools in which teachers or prevention specialists implement small-group activities that are designed to reduce a variety of high-risk behaviors (SAMHSA, 2008a). Prevention programs at the K–12 and higher education levels are based on extensive research, but we still have much to learn. It is clear, however, that prevention will continue to be an important part of our attempt to minimize the negative impact of addiction.

Ethical Issues

Confidentiality related to alcohol or other drug use is perhaps the most significant ethical problem that is specific to addiction counseling. One area of concern is the use of chemicals by minors. If a counselor becomes aware that a minor is using alcohol or other drugs, are they required to report it to parents? This is a complicated question that depends on the counseling setting, state and federal laws, and, in some cases, the age of the minor. If a school counselor is told of drug use, state law or school policy may require the counselor to report the use to the student's parents. Some might also interpret drug use as reportable harm to self, which would also necessitate a break of confidentiality. If the drug use was noted in official school records, the parents would have access to this information due to Family Educational Rights and Privacy Act (FERPA) requirements.

A complicating element involves a law specific to substance abuse and confidentiality. Known to addiction counselors as 42 CFR, this confidentiality regulation is actually the Code of Federal Regulations, Chapter I, Part 2

(SAMHSA, 2004). This section of the federal code outlines a level of confidentiality for substance abuse and dependent clients that is at a higher level of confidentiality than for most other counseling issues. The regulation is meant to encourage addicts to go to treatment by protecting their disclosures about their substance use from law enforcement officials who might try to extract information about drug-related activities from counselors or treatment programs. 42 CFR requires more specific release forms as well as restrictions on the content that courts can access.

Active Learning Exercise **12.3**

Now that you have had a chance to read about and reflect on addictions and the addictions counseling specialty, ask yourself how working with addictions may play into your work as a counselor. Because counselors in all settings will work with clients who are either addicted or affected by addictions, you may decide that you will want to get more training in this area, or perhaps become a specialist yourself. If not, you may just want to know enough about addictions to refer to if you see the problem in your clients, or you may desire to develop some more skills in screening and assessment. Regardless of which option you take, it will be important to remember to not overlook the problem when you see it. Ignoring the problem is what allows it to continue.

TRAINING AND CAREER OPTIONS FOR ADDICTION COUNSELORS

Because recovering addicts have played an important role in the addiction treatment process, there are a number of certification levels with as many different training options for addiction counselors. Some certification levels only require a high school diploma or a GED (General Equivalency Diploma) in addition to several hundred hours of specialized training and supervised counseling experience in addiction counseling. Others require a bachelor's degree along with the specialized training and supervised experience. Although the names for these certifications vary from state to state, typical labels are Certified Substance Abuse Counselor or Certified Addiction Counselor. The NBCC Master Addiction Counselor certification requires that an applicant obtain the National Certified Counselor certification and, in addition, have completed 12 hours of coursework in the area of addictions, which may include up to 6 hours of coursework in group or marriage and family counseling. An applicant may substitute the coursework in addictions counseling with 500 hours of continuing education hours. An applicant must also have three years of supervised experience in addictions and pass the Examination for Master Addictions Counselor.

In its 2009 standards, CACREP (CACREP, 2009) addressed the need for increased training in addition to counseling in several ways: it added an understanding about addictions into its Core Standards; it infused a wide range of addiction counseling learning outcomes into its Clinical Mental

Health Counseling Standards; and it added an Addiction Counseling Specialty. It is likely that these Addiction Counseling Specialty Standards will become the recognized criteria for master's level training in this field.

There are many career options for addiction counselors. All of the programs described earlier in this chapter employ counselors who have specialty training in addictions. In addition, most community counseling and mental health agencies are recognizing that many of their clients have addiction issues and need counselors who have expertise in this area. The Occupational Outlook Handbook (Bureau of Labor Statistics, 2006), states that there are about 76,000 addiction counselors employed in the United States and that the demand for addiction counselors is expected to be strong.

FURTHER CONSIDERATIONS

Perhaps due to an increase in the knowledge base around substance abuse, as mentioned earlier, substance abuse counseling has gained recognition as a special area of counseling. This recognition may well lead to more career opportunities in substance abuse counseling. In any case, "generic" counselors need to and do receive more training in substance abuse counseling than they have in future years.

CACREP and Substance Abuse Counseling

As was noted previously, the 2009 CACREP standards (CACREP, 2009) include a new specialty in Addictions Counseling. This inclusion is an indication that the profession in increasingly recognizing the importance of working with substance abuse clients and of developing a specific body of knowledge in this work. Whether or not counseling programs embrace this new specialty cannot be known at this point. A close examination of the other 2009 CACREP standards would reveal additional trends in the recognition of working with this population. The CACREP Core Standards now include substance abuse content and other specialty standards, most notably the new Clinical Mental Health Standards, include several individual standards that relate to substance abuse. Overall these new standards are a significant step embracing knowledge and skills in substance abuse by the counseling profession.

The Future of Substance Abuse Counseling

Given the dramatic impact of substance abuse on our society, you might think that the mental health professions would have been providing encouragement for practitioners to work in this area of need. They have not. There is a need for more substance abuse counselors. The federal government, through the Substance Abuse and Mental Health Services Administration and the Addiction Technology Transfer Program network, has recently begun a recruitment drive for counselors to specialize in working with substance abuse clients. It is clear from this effort that the need for more substance abuse counselors has been recognized. There is every indication that substance abuse counseling will continue to expand in terms of numbers and knowledge base and that it will be an exciting specialty to be a part of.

CONCLUSION

As our society continues to recognize the severity of addiction issues and the impact of alcohol and other drug use and abuse on our society, addiction counselors will be on the forefront of our efforts to combat this devastating problem. Although addiction can be a tenacious problem, we have found that treatment does work and that addicted individuals and their families can be helped to enter recovery and lead normal lives. Addiction counselors have found that to be a part of the recovery process and to witness the enormous positive impact of recovery is a privilege and provides a level of job satisfaction found in few other areas of counseling.

CHAPTER REVIEW

1. The problem of addiction to alcohol and other drugs precedes written history and has affected virtually all cultures. It costs our society billions of dollars each year and the emotional cost is severe. Despite these costs, the problem continues and only a small fraction of addicted individuals receive the counseling and treatment that they need.

2. Addiction is defined and perceived from the perspective of many different models including the *moral model*, the *medical model*, and the *disease model*. These models can significantly impact the way we view and work with addictions.

3. Addiction has a significant negative impact on the addicted individual and the family system. It is important to work with both the individual and the family when dealing with addiction.

4. The development of Substance Abuse Counseling as a counseling specialty has been influenced by many factors including the moral and medical models, Alcoholics Anonymous, the use of recovering addicts as counselors, traditional confrontational treatment models, and Motivational Interviewing. Substance abuse counseling today is both a specialty and a set of skills and knowledge needed by almost all counselors.

REVIEW QUESTIONS

1. In what ways has addiction had an impact on our society?

2. How do the different models of addiction influence how you would work with a substance abusing client?

3. In what ways does addiction impact the individual and the family?

4. What were some of the major influences on the development of substance abuse counseling and treatment?

5. What are some of the main elements contributing to the effectiveness of AA?

6. What are some of the training and career options for counselors who would like to work with addicted clients?

ADDITIONAL RESOURCES

- International Association for Addiction and Offender Counselors (http://www.iaaoc.org/)
- CACREP Specialty Standards for Addiction Counseling (http://67.199.126.156/doc/2009%20Standards.pdf)
- Addiction Technology Transfer Center Network (http://www.attcnetwork.org/index.asp)
- Addiction Technology Transfer Center Network: Imagine Who You Could Save

(An ATTC Network workforce development video; http://www.attcnetwork.org/explore/priorityareas/wfd/index.asp)
• National Association for Alcoholism and Drug Abuse Counselors (http://www.naadac.org/)

• NBCC Master Addictions Counselor Certification (http://nbcc.org/certifications/mac/Default.aspx)

REFERENCES

Alcoholics Anonymous. (2001). *Alcoholics Anonymous* (4th ed.). New York: AA World Services.

American Psychiatric Association. (2000). *Diagnostic and statistical manual of mental disorders* (4th ed., text revision). Washington, DC: Author.

Babor, T. F., De La Fuente, J. R., Saunders, J., & Grant, M. (1992). *AUDIT: The Alcohol Use Disorders Identification Test: Guidelines for use in primary health care.* Geneva, Switzerland: World Health Organization.

Babor, T. F. & Del Boca, F. K. (Eds.). (2002). *Treatment matching in alcoholism.* New York: Cambridge University Press.

Brooks, F. & McHenry, B. (2009). *A contemporary approach to substance abuse and addiction counseling.* Alexandria, VA: American Counseling Association.

Brown, S. (1985) *Treating the alcoholic: A developmental model of recovery.* John Wiley & Sons.

Bureau of Labor Statistics. (2006). Counselors. In *Occupational outlook handbook, 2006–2007.* Retrieved July 16, 2007, from http://www.bls.gov/oco/ocos067.htm.

Center for Substance Abuse Treatment. (1998). *Addiction counseling competencies: The knowledge, skills, and attitudes of professional practice (Technical Assistance Publication Series # 21).* (DHHS Publication No. SMA 98–3171). Rockville, MD: Author.

Center for Substance Abuse Treatment. (1999). *The national treatment improvement evaluation study: Retention analysis.* Rockville, MD: SAMHSA.

Council for Accreditation of Counseling and Related Educational Programs. (2009). *2009 CACREP standards.* Retrieved May 22, 2009, from http://67.199.126.156/doc/2009%20Standards.pdf.

Ewing, J. A. (1984). Detecting alcoholism: The CAGE questionnaire. *Journal of the American Medical Association, 252,* 1905–1907.

Fisher, G. L., & Harrison, T. C. (2005). *Substance abuse: Information for school counselors, social workers, therapists, and counselors* (3rd ed.). Boston: Pearson/Allyn & Bacon.

Fureman, B., Parikh, G., Bragg, A., & McLellan, A. (1990). *Addiction severity index: A guide to training and supervising ASI interviews based on the past ten years* (5th ed.). Philadelphia: University of Pennsylvania/VA Center for Studies of Addiction.

Gorski, T. T. (1993, March/April). Relapse prevention: A state of the art review. *Addiction and Recovery,* pp. 16–17.

Harwood, R., Koenig, L., Siegel, J., Gilani, J., & Chen, Y.-J. (2001, June 18). *Economic benefits of treatment: Preliminary findings from the Persistent Effects of Treatment Studies (PETS)—Cuyahoga.* Paper presented at the meeting of the College on Problems of Drug Dependence, Scottsdale, AZ.

Horgan, C., Skwara, K. C., & Strickler, G. (2001). *Substance abuse: The nation's number one health problem, key indicators for policy.* Prepared by the Schneider Institute for Health Policy, Brandeis University for the Robert Wood Johnson Foundation. Princeton, NJ: RWJF.

Horn, J. L., Wanberg, K. W., & Foster, F. M. (1986). *The alcohol use inventory: Test booklet.* Minneapolis: National Computer Systems.

Johnston, L. D., O'Malley, P. M., Bachman, J. G., & Schulenberg, J. E. (2006). *Teen drug use continues down in 2006, particularly among older teens; but use of prescription-type drugs remains high.* University of Michigan News and Information Services: Ann Arbor, MI. Retrieved July 11, 2007, from http://www.monitoringthefuture.org.

Kurtz, E. (1979). *Not-God: A history of Alcoholics Anonymous.* Center City, MN: Hazelden Educational Materials.

Lewis, D. C. (2000). *Position paper on drug policy.* Physician Leadership on National Drug Policy (PLNDP), National Project Office, Brown University Center for Alcohol and Addiction Studies, Providence, RI. Retrieved July 2, 2007, from http://www.plndp.org/Resources/researchrpt.pdf.

Miller, G. (1985). *The substance abuse subtle screening inventory*. Bloomington, IN: SASSI Institute.

Miller, W. R., & Rollnick, S. (2002). *Motivational Interviewing: Preparing people for change* (2nd ed.). New York: Guilford Press.

Prochaska, J. O., & DiClemente, C. C. (1986). Toward a comprehensive model of change. In W. R. Miller & N. Heather (Eds.), *Treating addictive behaviors: Processes of change* (pp. 3–27). New York: Plenum Press.

Selzer, M. L. (1971). The Michigan Alcoholism Screening Test: The quest for a new diagnostic instrument. *American Journal of Psychiatry, 127,* 1653–1658.

Substance Abuse and Mental Health Services Administration. (1998). *Services research outcomes study*. Rockville, MD: U.S. Department of Health and Human Services.

Substance Abuse and Mental Health Services Administration. (2004). *The confidentiality of alcohol and drug abuse patient records regulation and the HIPAA privacy rule: Implications for alcohol and substance abuse programs*. Rockville, MD: Author.

Retrieved June 28, 2007, from www.hipaa.samhsa.gov/Part2ComparisonClearedTOC.htm.

Substance Abuse and Mental Health Services Administration. (2006). *2005 national survey on drug use & health*. Rockville, MD: Author. Retrieved June 27, 2007, from http://www.oas.samhsa.gov/nsduhLatest.htm.

Substance Abuse and Mental Health Services Administration. (2008a). Intervention summary: All stars. Retrieved May 16, 2008, from http://www.nrepp.samhsa.gov/programfulldetails.asp?PROGRAM_ID=129.

Substance Abuse and Mental Health Services Administration. (2008b). *SAMHSA's national registry of evidence-based programs and practices*. Retrieved May 16, 2008, from http://www.nrepp.samhsa.gov/.

Stevens, P., & Smith, R. L. (2005). *Substance abuse counseling: Theory and practice* (3rd ed.). Upper Saddle River, NJ: Pearson Education.

White, W. L. (1998). *Slaying the dragon: The history of addiction treatment and recovery in America*. Bloomington, IL: Chestnut Health Systems/Lighthouse Institute.

CHAPTER 13

Rehabilitation Counseling

LEARNING OBJECTIVES

After reading this chapter, you should be able to

- gain insight regarding your beliefs and assumptions about people with disabilities;

- understand four different viewpoints regarding the disability experience and how each view impacts personal and professional interactions with people with disabilities;

- understand rehabilitation philosophy as applied to professional practice;

- understand the nature of work performed by rehabilitation counselors, training required to be a Certified Rehabilitation Counselor, and employment opportunities that exist in this field; and

- understand why the field of rehabilitation counseling offers rewarding career opportunities.

CHAPTER OUTLINE

Employment Opportunities for
   Rehabilitation Counselors
Certification

Special Topics in Rehabilitation Counseling

Further Considerations in Rehabilitation Counseling

Conclusion

INTRODUCTION

Before describing the field of rehabilitation counseling, it is important to review basic concepts, terminology, and philosophical underpinnings that influence this profession. In this chapter, I will first provide an overview of the clientele that you are likely to work with and explore four different views of disability. It is important to look at each view because of the ramifications on the professional counseling relationship that you develop with clients who have disabilities. Because of the importance that individual perceptions play in forming this relationship, several learning activities are provided to help you gain greater awareness regarding your perceptions and beliefs toward persons with disabilities. Although there may be a tendency to "skip" or gloss over these learning activities, if you complete them, you will gain a better understanding when working with persons with disabilities. After this foundational information is reviewed, the chapter will explore the nature of work required of rehabilitation counselors, specific training needed to become a rehabilitation counselor, employment settings in which these counselors practice, and information concerning relevant professional certifications. Toward the end of the chapter, I will share a story that hopefully provides some insight on what it means to work as a rehabilitation counselor. I will also outline some important topics and related considerations within the field.

As evident in these chapters, there are many academic disciplines that prepare you to work as a professional counselor. Perhaps at this point in your professional development, you may have a clear idea about the work setting (e.g., school, hospital, community mental health clinic), clientele (e.g., children, adolescents, adults, older adults), type of client problems that you want to address as part of your practice (e.g., anxiety disorders, depression, drug/alcohol abuse, violence), counseling approach (e.g., cognitive-behavioral, person-centered, reality therapy), and/or the counseling system that you want to impact (e.g., individual, family, group, community). Perhaps you do not have a clear idea about these aspects but you know that wanting to help others has always been part of your make-up and is something very satisfying to you. You may be the kind of person that when friends and classmates have problems and concerns, they tend to seek you out and appreciate your ability to listen and understand. These qualities are, in fact, part of any professional counseling discipline, and while there are many paths to choose, in this chapter, you will examine the path that involves working with people with disabilities.

Hopefully, at the end of this chapter, you will have a better understanding of what it means to be a rehabilitation counselor and, regardless of the clarity of your professional identity, the possibility of working as a rehabilitation counselor will have been reaffirmed or perhaps introduced as something you may want to consider more closely. In order to help you understand the professional field of rehabilitation counseling and to gain better insight regarding your beliefs about people with disabilities, let's start with the initial learning activity.

Active Learning Exercise **13.1**

First, write down a list of feeling words, images, and terms that you associate with the term *disability*. Simply write down as many word associations as quickly as you can. Since you will not share this list with anyone, do not worry about what you write down. Do this activity now before reading on.

Second, go through your list and see if you can find any themes that are evident in your word list. Did you notice any clear themes from your list or did your list produce a diversity of ideas or reactions from the word list? Did your word associations tend to be ones that were more related to suffering, pain (emotional and physical), and dependence? Or were they more related to images of overcoming adversity, achievement, or growth and transcendence? What kinds of emotions (if any) were expressed? Did your list tend to focus on one system (individual, family, community, and society at large) or multiple systems? Were images of prejudice, bias, or discrimination contained in your list?

Finally, verbally share your themes with other classmates and discuss which one(s) were similar and which were unique. What might this activity reveal regarding your beliefs concerning persons with disabilities and how you view the "disability" experience?

PERSONS WITH DISABILITIES

The most recent census data provided by the U.S. Department of Commerce reported that about one in five, or 50 million, people reported having at least one disability (U.S. Census Bureau, 2005). Given that data collected for the census are somewhat dated, new medical interventions to save and prolong life have emerged, earlier and more reliable assessments in diagnosing illness and disability are being used, and the recent war casualties inflicted on military personnel means there will be greater numbers of persons with disabilities than ever before, there is a reasonable expectation that disability numbers will continue to climb when the next census is conducted. In terms of what these data suggest to persons interested in any one of the counseling professions, it also means that no matter your professional work setting or preferred age group that you intend to work with, most likely you will eventually work with persons with disabilities. Depending on the client age group that you want to work with, census data reveal that among children between the ages of 6 and 14, about one in eight children have some type of disability, whereas one in two Americans who are 65 years and older has a disability.

In addition, about 12 percent or 32.5 million Americans, have a severe disability (U.S. Census Bureau, 2002). These statistics support the need for professional counselors who have specialized training to work with the variety of disabilities that persons and their families experience.

In terms of types of disabilities, using categories by the 2002 Census Bureau study, persons who are 15 years of age and older can be placed in at least one of several disability domains. The first domain, *communication*, includes functional problems associated with difficulty seeing, hearing, and speaking. The second domain, *physical*, includes individuals who use a wheelchair, cane, crutches, or walker, and experience problems such as lifting objects 10 pounds or heavier, climbing stairs, and getting in/out of bed. This group also includes persons who identified themselves as having one or more conditions such as arthritis; back or spine problems; cancer; cerebral palsy; diabetes; epilepsy; head or spinal cord injury; heart trouble; kidney, lung, stomach/digestive, thyroid, or respiratory problems; missing legs, arms, feet, hands, or fingers; or paralysis and/or stroke.

The third domain, *mental*, includes persons who have a learning disability, mental retardation, or other developmental disability, or any other mental or emotional condition that seriously interferes with everyday activities, such as trouble getting along with others, trouble concentrating, trouble coping with day-to-day stress, and/or difficulty managing money/bills. Persons with mental disabilities also include those who identify as having one or more related conditions, such as Alzheimer's, attention deficit hyperactivity disorder, autism, learning disability, mental or emotional problems, mental retardation, and senility or dementia.

FOUR VIEWS OF DISABILITY

Smart (2004) contends that how we view the disability experience varies according to the purpose, values, and needs of the perceiver as well as the professional discipline of the definer. As she notes, there are a variety of administrative, clinical, cultural, and personal definitions of disabilities that are all based on "invented human assumptions" that ultimately determine how we view and interact with persons with disabilities. According to Smart and Smart (2006), disability assumptions are associated with one of four theoretical models: (1) biomedical, (2) functional, (3) environmental, and (4) sociopolitical.

Biomedical Model

The traditional biomedical model views disability within the context of physical capacities and related functional outcomes. Disability is therefore defined within a comparative framework where the person must achieve tasks in the same way as a "normal" person or, if unable, perform the task using some other accommodation (e.g., allowing more time to complete a task, asking for assistance from another person) or adaptive aide (e.g., hearing aid, wheelchair). The biomedical framework views disability within an individual context of physical and/or mental conditions that through treatment may be corrected or improved. Consequently, persons such as those with mental illness, diabetes, and traumatic brain injury are, by definition, disabled. Embedded in this view is the belief that disability is not something valued but rather perceived as a deviance that the person must correct in order to be accepted by others. The treatment process is something done to the person and therefore requires passivity by the person with the disability, who, in turn, must rely on the expertise and training of other professionals to correct the deficiency. As a result, "the individual with a disability is expected to be resilient, courageous, and to demonstrate self-control and optimism" (Smart, 2004, pp. 34–35). At the same time, the biomedical view maintains the stigma associated with disability through categorization of groups rather than individuals such as "the blind," "quads" (persons with quadriplegia), and/or "the mentally ill." By doing so, it supports the societal view to focus on the disability category as opposed to universal challenges faced by persons with various disabilities.

Functional and Environmental Models

In contrast to the biomedical view, functional and environmental models define *disability* in terms of individual and environmental characteristics. Disability is therefore viewed as an interactional process involving the capabilities of each person as manifested within a specific environment. For example, one's capacity for work is a functional outcome that is largely influenced by environmental factors. A person with a disability may be fully qualified for a specific job but may not have reliable or available transportation to get to the job and, as a result, may require an environmental intervention. As part of rehabilitation practice, the counselor may assist the person in placing a newspaper ad for someone to ride share, contracting with someone to provide transportation, or if needed, encouraging the person to move to another residence where public transportation is readily available. These interventions then can be more complex since they are intended to impact the client's environment.

Sociopolitical or Minority Model

The final and most recent view of disability is expressed through the sociopolitical or minority model of disability. This model recognizes that the major barrier for persons with disabilities is not those associated with architectural or other physical barriers (e.g., unable to get into a restaurant because there is no wheelchair ramp) but something that is more pervasive and, at the same time, less obvious. To better demonstrate this unnamed barrier, imagine you are working as a high school guidance counselor and one of your students with a strong academic record and clear interest in science indicates that he or she wants to pursue medical school. The student comes to you to identify appropriate colleges that offer strong baccalaureate programs in science and pre-medicine. As a secondary school counselor, you work with this student to identify relevant programs, encourage the student to talk with the admissions counselors at schools that are appealing, discuss the advantages and disadvantages of each school, and, if needed, process the information to help the student make a final decision. Now, imagine this same student happens to be blind or Deaf, or has a severe learning disability. Is your response to help the student the same as before, or do you think, "How in the world does this person expect to become a doctor?" Because this career outcome for a person who has one of these disabilities may not be something as part of your personal experience, there may be a tendency to say to the student, "Perhaps you might want to choose another career." Yet, it may come as some surprise to you that there are, in fact, medical doctors with these as well as other disabilities. In fact, one of the earliest known physicians in the United States who was blind was Jacob Bolotin, born in 1888 (Perlman, 2007). Dr. Bolotin's accomplishment as a medical doctor (he taught in three different medical schools) provides testimony to the sociopolitical view that perhaps the most formidable barrier facing persons with disabilities is the attitudes of persons without disabilities. Whether knowingly or unintentionally, our beliefs about others who are different from us (in this case, having a disability) have a tremendous influence on what we perceive people are capable of accomplishing. These beliefs often result because persons without disabilities tend to apply a comparative value of what they believe is "normal" and therefore limit educational, vocational, and social opportunities for those perceived as "less than normal" or different from "the majority" view (see Wright, 1983). In other words, because a person with a disability does not perform the task or social role in the same way that a person without a disability performs it, by assumption, he or she is devalued if it is attempted in a different way or perceived as not possible. As Smart and Smart (2006) note:

> In the past, the disabled role was determined by people who did not have disabilities and therefore had no experience in managing a disability on a day-to-day basis. Individuals with disabilities were expected to learn the rules of this role; to live the rules; and, most important, to believe in the rules. The rules and expectations of this role, although unwritten, were strongly enforced, and individuals who did not comply with these expectations often experienced severe consequences, including lack of services and social isolation. These rules included the following: always be cheerful; face the disability with courage, optimism, and motivations [*sic*]; manage the disability as well as possible (in the view of others); adhere to medical and rehabilitation regimens; request only those accommodations and assistance that others feel are necessary; make others comfortable with the disability; and keep all aspirations at a reasonable level, or stated differently, do not ask for much. (p. 34)

As evident in this statement, the sociopolitical view recognizes that persons must behave in prescribed ways consistent with the expectations of persons without disabilities. Similar to individuals from other minority groups, stereotypical views about disability tend to maintain prejudicial attitudes and stigma associated with disability. These biases, whether intentional or not, often result in limiting or excluding participation in social roles that are automatically assumed for persons without disabilities. A recent example of challenging social roles for persons with disabilities was evident in a national television dance show, *Dancing With the Stars*. As you may recall, in the show there was a contestant who had sustained a leg amputation. In spite of having an artificial limb, Heather Mills not only demonstrated to the world that she could walk but she could also dance quite well! Had most television viewers not seen or read about her, they may have continued to believe that it would be impossible for "someone like her" to participate and perhaps win the dance competition. As this example demonstrates, beliefs regarding one's capacity for employment, independent living, parenthood, sexual and social relationships, and recreation are often greatly influenced by the type and severity of disability and what persons without disabilities perceive is possible or appropriate. As someone interested in working as a professional counselor, you need to address your biases and beliefs regarding disability as well. In order to demonstrate this point further, complete the next learning activity.

Active Learning Exercise **13.2**

Read each of the two lists below. After reading both lists, indicate which disability group you believe is capable of engaging in each of the life activities listed.

Disability Group	Life Activity
Blind	Attend college
Deaf	Drive a car
Learning disability	Go to a movie
Mental illness	Go snow skiing
Mental retardation	Raise a family
Quadriplegia	Play piano

After deciding which group can participate in which activity, read the Herbert (2000) article in the Additional Resources section. Considering the points raised in the article that relate to this learning activity, what might your list indicate concerning your perceptions about specific disabilities? How are your views different from or similar to your classmates' responses?

BECOMING A REHABILITATION COUNSELOR

As someone who intends to work as a professional counselor, you should realize that although many persons you work with have disabilities, it is largely a function of societal values that determines whether a person is "disabled." As a future counselor, you play a key role in helping to challenge this perception by questioning assumptions you make regarding what are acceptable roles to engage in and how they should be pursued by persons with disabilities. Challenging your own beliefs about disability can be difficult, particularly if you have limited social contacts interacting with persons with disabilities. As such, you should actively seek out opportunities by taking elective coursework in rehabilitation counseling, disability studies, or similar academic disciplines as part of graduate study. You might also want to pursue volunteer experiences and supervised clinical fieldwork that includes interactions with people with disabilities. As noted in the earlier statistics cited, if your intention is to work in a helping profession, then you will eventually be working with persons with disabilities.

Although each of the four views provides a context for understanding the disability experience, for most rehabilitation counselors, disability must be understood within the environment where one lives, works, and plays. Rehabilitation services to improve the quality of life for these individuals must therefore occur on several system levels (individual, family, community) and, as it may be implied, include a variety of services that address economic, educational, personal, physical, recreational, social, spiritual, and vocational needs as appropriate to each person. The work of the rehabilitation counselor is therefore multifaceted and offers a unique opportunity to make a difference for persons who, for the most part, have historically been limited by others without disabilities regarding their potential. Although rehabilitation counselors have a specific set of professional skills and knowledge, perhaps more than any single attribute, the quality that sets apart those counselors who are most effective is the ability to focus on each person's worth and how to maximize it. In short, a core belief of professional rehabilitation counselors is to appreciate the inherent value of what each person can do or can learn how to do rather than focus on what the person cannot do.

Philosophy of Rehabilitation Counseling

Recognizing the inherent value of each person, a fundamental rehabilitation belief is that persons with disabilities must be fully involved in the planning, coordination, and delivery of rehabilitation services. These services almost always require an interdisciplinary approach to address the variety and complexity of needs that many persons with disabilities experience. In practice, it requires rehabilitation counselors to view each person holistically rather than in a compartmentalized manner. Counselors cannot simply focus on one life area without addressing other interrelated aspects as well as how these areas have importance within individual, family, and community systems. Although two persons may have the same disability and similar functional abilities, rehabilitation counselors understand how the uniqueness of each individual has tremendous influence on how each person views the disability experience and how their life unfolds. For example, two persons with the same level of spinal cord injury and functional capacities may have totally different reactions regarding the disability experience. As a result of the injury, one person may believe that he or she will have an unfulfilling life full of disappointments, whereas another person may view this injury as a gift, and had it not happened, his or her life would have been unfulfilling and ordinary. This difference between individuals may be attributable not only to unique intrapersonal characteristics but also to a function of situational variables such as age, time since injury, family support network and their reactions to disability, financial status, availability of accessible transportation, and related community resources to support independence. In working to help clients with disabilities achieve equal status with persons without disabilities, as you will see in the next section, rehabilitation counselors ensure that equal access to education, employment, health care, and social services, to name a few, occurs. Ultimately, rehabilitation counselors work toward empowering persons with disabilities to the degree to which they are capable so that they can achieve meaningful and satisfying lives.

Active Learning Exercise **13.3**

As noted in this chapter, each of the four views of disability makes assumptions regarding the role of persons with disability in terms of what rehabilitation services are provided, who makes the decision regarding services, how they are administered, and in what settings. How might these models be different for (a) a newly injured spinal cord injured teenager who has been admitted to a rehabilitation inpatient unit? (b) an adult with long-term mental illness who is in an outpatient community treatment program? or (c) an older person who is blind and seeking employment? Is there value for defining disability from each perspective of biomedical, functional, environmental, and sociopolitical viewpoints in each of these three situations?

Work Performed by Rehabilitation Counselors

Although employment settings and clientele have changed over time, Leahy (2004) contends that most rehabilitation counselors are required to (a) assess client needs, (b) establish an alliance with the client to develop goals and individualized plans to address needs, and (c) procure or provide therapeutic services. These fundamental tasks, though, are perhaps similar to those required of most if not all professional counselors. The difference between these generic tasks and those required of rehabilitation counselors has to do with the specialized knowledge and skills concerning disability and environmental influences that can impede or facilitate clients in reaching their goals in the most integrated settings possible. In fact, a recently accepted definition by a consortium of several professional rehabilitation counseling associations (i.e., American Rehabilitation Counseling Association and the National Rehabilitation Counseling Association), the Commission on Rehabilitation Counselor Certification, and the National Council on Rehabilitation Education states that "a rehabilitation counselor is a counselor who possesses the specialized knowledge, skills, and attitudes needed to collaborate in a professional relationship with persons with disabilities to achieve their personal, social, psychological, and vocational goals" (Maki, 2004). Given this definition, the nature of work requires counselors to evaluate how disability impacts life aspects and provide or procure services intended to improve quality of life.

In studying work tasks that rehabilitation counselors perform, Leahy, Chan, and Saunders (2003) identified 120 different job tasks that comprised seven major job categories. The first major category (43 job tasks) involves vocational counseling and consultation, which consists of providing career counseling (e.g., preparing clients for a job interview), vocational planning (e.g., matching client aptitudes, needs, and reinforcers with job requirements), employer consultation (e.g., consulting with employers regarding compliance with the Americans with Disabilities Act), and job development and placement (e.g., assessing client readiness for employment). The second group, counseling interventions (28 job tasks), includes providing individual, family, and group counseling (e.g., counseling clients regarding sexual concerns related to disability); building client-counselor working relationships (e.g., clarifying mutual expectations with regard to the counseling relationship); and helping clients to adjust to the personal and psychosocial aspects of disability (e.g., counseling clients on identifying emotional reactions to disability). The third set (16 job tasks) consists of using community-based rehabilitation services (e.g., attending team conferences; evaluating and selecting facilities that provide specialized care services for clients). The fourth classification of job tasks (19 tasks) involves case management (e.g., writing case notes, summaries, and reports; coordinating activities of all agencies involved in the rehabilitation plan). The fifth grouping (6 job tasks), applying research to professional practice, involves performing job tasks such as reading professional literature related to business, labor markets, medicine, and rehabilitation, or providing expert opinion or testimony regarding client employability and rehabilitation feasibility. The sixth category (3 job tasks), conducting assessments, involves selecting and administering appropriate tests and determining community services appropriate to individual needs. The final group (3 job tasks), practicing professional advocacy, refers to applying rehabilitation legislation to daily practice, identifying and challenging stereotypes toward persons with disability, and educating clients regarding their rights under federal and state laws. When rehabilitation counselors in the study were asked to rate the relative importance of each job function, the overall categories of case management followed by professional advocacy and counseling interventions were considered the most important of seven categories.

The fact that practicing professional advocacy was the second highest job function reported among rehabilitation counselors should be underscored. This job function provides perhaps another indication of the uniqueness of this profession and how it may be different from other counseling professions. Recalling the negative impact of stereotyping and biases toward persons with disabilities discussed earlier, rehabilitation counselors are often called upon to serve as client advocates. For example, a person with Down syndrome may not have the verbal skills necessary to convince an employer to hire him or her for a specific job. Serving as an advocate, the counselor working in a community-based rehabilitation program would discuss with the employer the unique qualifications of this potential worker, who may not have effective job interview skills but is nevertheless a highly dependable and productive employee. In another instance, the rehabilitation counselor who works in a postsecondary setting may believe that a college professor is not providing reasonable accommodations as guaranteed by the Americans with Disabilities Act of 1990 in supporting a college student with a severe learning disability. The professor believes that giving this student additional time to read a classroom examination is unfair to other students. The counselor may be required to review the legal mandates with the professor, explain the nature of learning disabilities, and/or consult with the appropriate campus office so that the student's rights are protected. And, in a third situation, the rehabilitation counselor in private practice may be asked to conduct awareness training by a local business owner who wants to hire qualified persons with disabilities but is concerned how other workers will react. The counselor may decide to have the employer talk with other employers with whom the counselor has worked where this was a concern that was later resolved. The rehabilitation counselor may also explore employer concerns and fears and provide national employment outcome data of workers with disabilities that specifically addresses this issue. Or, the counselor may decide to conduct on-site employee training that includes discussions about disability, a disability simulation exercise to enhance awareness, and/or a panel of persons with disabilities who talk about common fears that some workers have initially and strategies they can use to address interpersonally stressful work situations.

As these interventions demonstrate, rehabilitation counselors have the potential to work on multiple levels that not only include the person with the disability but their families, other professionals and service providers involved in the rehabilitation process, employers, and the general community at large. Within the context of a "routine day" rehabilitation counselors may (a) provide grief counseling to a group of persons with newly acquired disabilities; (b) attend a team staff conference and report on the progress a client is making in a vocational-technical training program; (c) consult with a psychiatrist regarding the need to change medications for a person with long-term mental illness; (d) arrange for the services of a sex therapist for a couple where one partner has chronic benign pain syndrome; (e) write summary reports on clients who have completed rehabilitation services; (f) make a presentation to employers on available tax incentives for hiring qualified persons with disabilities; (g) conduct a job analysis to ascertain what modifications are needed to accommodate someone with a severe learning disability; (h) administer and interpret vocational aptitude tests to clients; (i) provide clinical supervision to a rehabilitation intern who has a negative bias toward clients with substance abuse problems; (j) use positive confrontation techniques with a client who has fears about returning to work; (k) conduct a transferability skills analysis with a client to assess the diversity of jobs that are currently available based on vocational strengths and interests; (l) consult with an employer on ways to reduce injury at the workplace; and/or (m) testify in a court case as a vocational expert with regard to employment of persons with disabilities. These examples perhaps demonstrate the fact that work as a rehabilitation counselor is anything but routine. Although, like most jobs, there are basic routines one must follow, the scope of practice for rehabilitation counselors is very broad and, perhaps for this reason, an attractive aspect to students thinking about this career path.

Training Needed to Become a Rehabilitation Counselor

Formal academic training in rehabilitation counseling began during the 1940s with programs affiliated with New York University, Ohio State University, and Wayne State University (Leahy, 2004). With the passage of the Vocational Rehabilitation Amendments of 1954, the federal government provided support to universities to develop graduate training programs. As a result of this support, the beginning of a formal academic discipline in rehabilitation counseling was established and remains today (Leahy & Szymanski, 1995). Currently, there are 100 master's level rehabilitation counseling programs accredited by the Council on Rehabilitation Education (CORE, 2009). A CORE-accredited program requires a minimum of 48 semester or 72 quarter hours. An exception to this requirement applies to accredited programs that are also located in states which stipulate a minimum of 60-semester credit hours or 90 quarter hours necessary for counselor licensure. In these instances, accredited university programs must also identify the additional 12 credits or 19 quarter hours for students wanting to pursue licensure (CORE, 2007, p. 18). Programs do not necessarily have to require additional courses, however. The training program must address 10 curriculum domains so that students obtain the essential knowledge, skills, and attitudes needed to work effectively with persons with disabilities including the following:

1. *Professional identify knowledge* examines scope of practice, history and philosophy of rehabilitation, legislation, ethics, professional credentialing, certification, licensure and accreditation, informed consumer choice and consumer empowerment, independent living, assistive technology, public policies, advocacy, systems knowledge of healthcare, education and rehabilitation, and the ecological perspective.
2. *Social and cultural diversity knowledge* addresses family development and dynamics; psychological dynamics related to self-identity, self-advocacy, competency, adjustment, and attitude formation; sociological dynamics related to self-identity, self-advocacy, competency, adjustment, and attitude formation; multicultural awareness and implications for ethical practice; diversity issues including cultural, disability, gender, sexual orientation, and aging issues; current issues and trends in a diverse society; and personal professional development strategies for self-monitoring.
3. *Human growth and development knowledge* examines developmental theories across the life span; behavioral, cognitive, emotional, moral, and physical development; theories of personality development, human sexuality, and disability; spirituality; transition issues related to family, school, employment, aging, and disability; social and learning needs of individuals across the life span; and ethical and legal issues impacting individuals and families related to adjustment and transition.
4. *Employment and career development knowledge* explores disability benefits systems including workers' compensation, long-term disability, and social security; career counseling; job analysis; work site modification and restructuring, including the application of appropriate technology, transferable skill analysis, computer-based assessment tools, vocational planning and assessment, job and employer development, employer consultation, business/corporate human resource concepts and terminology, workplace culture and environment, work conditioning/work hardening, job placement strategies, computer-based job matching systems, follow-up/post-employment services; occupational information, including labor market trends and the importance of meaningful employment with a career focus,

supported employment, job coaching, and natural supports; and ethical issues in employment.

5. *Counseling and consultation knowledge* considers counseling and personality theory; mental health counseling; interviewing and counseling skill development; theories and models for consultation, assistive technologies, vocational consultation, supervision theories, models, and techniques; consumer empowerment and rights; boundaries of confidentiality; ethics in the counseling relationship; multicultural issues in counseling; gender issues in counseling; conflict resolution strategies; computer-based counseling tools; and Internet resources for rehabilitation counseling.

6. *Group work knowledge* includes group dynamics and counseling theory; family dynamics and counseling theory; interdisciplinary teamwork; group leadership styles and techniques; group methods, selection criteria, and evaluation strategies; and group skills development.

7. *Assessment knowledge* involves selecting and administering appropriate assessment method (e.g., standardized tests, situational assessments); obtaining, interpreting, and synthesizing assessment information; conducting ecological assessment; and understanding assessment resources, methods, measurement and statistical concepts, assistive technology, and ethical, legal, and cultural implications in assessment.

8. *Research and program evaluation knowledge* addresses basic statistics and research methods; library resources to identify rehabilitation-related information and clinical literature; and ethical, legal, and cultural issues related to research and evaluation.

9. *Medical, functional, and environmental aspects of disability knowledge* includes the human body system; medical terminology; medical, functional, environmental, and psychosocial aspects of physical disabilities; psychiatric rehabilitation; substance abuse; cognitive disability; sensory disability; developmental disability; assistive technology; dual diagnosis and the workplace; functional capacity; and wellness and illness prevention concepts and strategies.

10. *Rehabilitation services and resources knowledge* includes case and caseload management; vocational rehabilitation; independent living; school-to-work transition services; psychiatric rehabilitation practice; substance abuse treatment and recovery; disability management; employer-based and disability case management practices; design and development of transitional and return-to-work programs; forensic rehabilitation and vocational expert practices; managed care; systems resource information, including funding availability, utilization of community-based rehabilitation and service coordination; consumer advocacy and empowerment; marketing rehabilitation services; life care planning; strategies to develop rapport/referral network; case reporting; professional advocacy; clinical problem-solving skills; case recording and documentation; interdisciplinary consultation; and computer applications and technology for caseload practice.

As part of the curriculum, students are also required to have a supervised rehabilitation counseling practicum of not less than 100 hours, with 40 involving direct service to persons with disabilities. This initial fieldwork experience is intended to increase "awareness and understanding of the differences in values, beliefs, and behaviors of individuals from diverse populations [in order to] promote cultural competence, foster personal growth, and introduce students to counseling approaches and rehabilitation issues that affect service delivery" (CORE, 2007). Similarly, students are also required to complete a 600-hour supervised rehabilitation counseling internship of which 240 hours must involve direct service contact to individuals with disabilities. In addition to promoting cultural competence and personal growth, the internship should be designed so that students are introduced to counseling approaches and rehabilitation issues that impact service delivery (CORE, 2007).

Employment Opportunities for Rehabilitation Counselors

Considering the scope of disability and how it impacts on multiple levels, as you might expect, rehabilitation counselors work in a variety of settings. Given the prevalence of disability within the United States, qualified rehabilitation counselors are employed in state vocational rehabilitation agencies, insurance and proprietary (for profit) rehabilitation companies, community psychosocial programs, drug and alcohol treatment centers, rehabilitation hospitals, psychiatric inpatient and outpatient hospitals and clinics, HIV/AIDS clinics, supported employment programs, sheltered work centers, in-house disability management programs within private businesses, secondary and postsecondary settings, independent living centers, and private practice. Although most graduates work as rehabilitation counselors who serve the broad spectrum of needs of persons with disabilities, many students elect to specialize with respect to a specific disability, work setting, or job function. For example, graduates may work as rehabilitation counselors for the Deaf, mobility and orientation specialists for persons who are blind, mental health counselors for persons with long-term mental illness, or substance abuse counselors for persons recovering from alcohol and drug abuse and dependence. They may also wish to work in a specific work setting providing more specialized services to enhance quality of life for persons with disabilities. In these instances, graduates may want to work as career development counselors, job placement specialists, assistive technology specialists, crisis counselors, disability coordinators, and independent living specialists. Eventually, counselors are often promoted to supervisory and administrative positions that involve clinical and administrative supervision of front-line counselors, program development and evaluation, resource allocation, and facility/agency management.

With respect to career growth, analysis of personnel needs due to retirement and growth clearly indicate that rehabilitation counseling is a growing profession (U.S. Department of Labor and Industry, 2007). For example, within the state vocational rehabilitation system alone, the demand for qualified rehabilitation counselors in the past and in the present far outweighs supply (e.g., Dew & Peters, 2002; Pointer, 2003). The same employment need has been witnessed in other nonprofit and for-profit agencies, clinics, community-based programs, hospitals, schools, and related settings serving persons with disabilities as well (e.g., Ethridge, Rodgers, Roe, & Fabian, 2007). In fact, this continued demand is something that has been documented for the past 40 years (e.g., Bishop & Crystal, 2002; Rasch, Hollingsworth, Saxon, & Thomas, 1984; Sussman & Haug, 1968). In partial response to the lack of qualified rehabilitation counselors, the Rehabilitation Services Administration (RSA) within the U.S. Department of Education has provided federal training grants to support tuition and related costs of master's students intending to work in state vocational rehabilitation agencies and other nonprofit rehabilitation programs. Students interested in this training grant may wish to review the list of accredited rehabilitation programs that is available through the Council on Rehabilitation Education (see Web site information in Learning Activity 13.4 and review the link "Recognized Programs." This link will provide you with a document entitled "COREPrograms101708.doc"). With this list, you can then contact the Program Coordinator from each university program and inquire whether RSA funding is available).

Certification

Perhaps more than any other professional counseling field, rehabilitation counseling has developed a solid research base in establishing its professional scope of practice. For over 45 years, there has been a series of coordinated studies (e.g., Jaques, 1959; Leahy et al., 2003; Rubin et al., 1984) that has helped to identify and refine work roles and functions that rehabilitation counselors perform and, in doing so, has resulted in defining the qualified professional. Operationally, this professional is one who has completed at least a master's degree in rehabilitation counseling or a similar field of training (e.g., counselor education), received certification as a Certified Rehabilitation Counselor (CRC) and, in states that have professional licensure, achieved this credential (e.g., Licensed Professional Counselor or Licensed Mental Health Counselor).

Certification refers to recognition by a professional organization that an individual has received appropriate training (coursework and clinical experience) and demonstrated competence through examination or other evaluation means and therefore is entitled the specific designation. The organization responsible for establishing qualification standards for certification as rehabilitation counselors is the Commission on Rehabilitation Counselor Certification (CRCC). Established in 1974, CRCC is responsible for insuring that professionals meet certain entry-level standards and maintain these standards throughout their careers (CRCC, 2009). In order to qualify as a CRC, an applicant must demonstrate knowledge of the 10 content domains noted earlier by passing a national examination. As noted earlier, while there are various ways to qualify for the examination, the most expedient method is to complete an accredited master's degree program in rehabilitation counseling accredited by the Council on Rehabilitation Education and then register for the national examination. Once the applicant passes the national examination by the CRCC, there is an additional requirement to complete 100 hours of continuing education over a five-year period in order to maintain certification. CRCs are also obliged to follow the professional code of ethics. Currently, there are approximately 16,000 CRCs in the United States (Susan Stark, personal communication, June 17, 2009). The importance of certification not only provides a credential indicating minimal professional competence but, in certain employment sectors such as proprietary rehabilitation companies and public vocational rehabilitation agencies, it is often a condition for employment. The benefit of achieving certification as a rehabilitation counselor may also help to achieve other related professional certifications. For example, rehabilitation counseling graduates who pursue additional coursework and relevant supervised clinical experience may be eligible for certification in alcohol and drug abuse counseling (Master Addiction Counselor or Certified Alcohol and Drug Addiction Counselor), career counseling (Master Career Counselor), insurance rehabilitation (Certified Insurance Rehabilitation Specialist), mental health counseling (Certified Clinical Mental Health Counselor), and general counseling (National Counselor Certification). Finally, if you are considering a career in rehabilitation counseling, you may wonder, "How much do Certified Rehabilitation Counselors earn?" A recent report from the CRCC found that in May 2007, the average salary among 1,700 CRCs was $57,146, with most working in state vocational rehabilitation agencies (CRCC, 2009).

Active Learning Exercise **13.4**

In order to learn more about the field of rehabilitation counseling, you may want to visit Web sites of various professional organizations such as the American Rehabilitation Counseling Association, the National Rehabilitation Counseling Association, and/or the International Association of Rehabilitation Professionals. To gain a more detailed perspective, you might also want to contact rehabilitation counselors in your area and arrange for a telephone interview or perhaps set up some time to visit them at their work sites and ask to job shadow for a day. If you are interested in pursuing graduate studies in rehabilitation counseling, a list of accredited programs is available through the Council on Rehabilitation Education at http://www.core-rehab.org/.

A Day in the Life of a Rehabilitation Counselor

Camping with Tony

It is difficult to capture what a typical "day in the life" of a rehabilitation counselor might look like since, as you can infer in the initial paragraph regarding employment opportunities for rehabilitation counselors, their work days vary as a function of clientele served, settings where they work, and life areas or problems they deal with when working with people with disabilities. For example, rehabilitation counselors may specialize in working with persons with long-term mental illness, but they could work in a community-based setting helping individuals live in a structured group home with other persons to develop effective social and independent living skills. Another rehabilitation counselor who works for the state vocational rehabilitation program might

(continued)

A Day in the Life of a Rehabilitation Counselor *(continued)*

work with these same individuals to help them obtain and maintain satisfying work while another rehabilitation counselor who specializes in alcohol and other drug issues might assist some of these individuals in maintaining sobriety.

Although this example demonstrates the point regarding the diversity of work that rehabilitation counselors perform as applied to just one client population, it doesn't capture the passion that I know many counselors experience every day in working with people with disabilities. While this chapter has provided you with basic information about rehabilitation counselors, it has not conveyed any sense of the unique contribution and potential influence each of you can have in changing the lives of persons with disabilities. In order to hopefully demonstrate this influence, I would like to share a brief story of someone who I worked with years ago—"Tony." I hope sharing this story gives you a snapshot of one of my "days in the life" and perhaps may give you some inkling of why I feel passionate about rehabilitation counseling. Hopefully, after reading this story, it might entice you to learn more about rehabilitation counseling. For students already studying this field, I hope that it affirms your career choice as a rehabilitation counselor.

During one of my earlier sabbaticals as a rehabilitation professor, I had the opportunity to learn about and facilitate therapeutic adventure programs for persons with disabilities (see Herbert, 1996, 1998). Although therapeutic adventure is a lot of fun, it is also a great deal of work that requires careful planning and coordination in taking persons with severe disabilities out in the wilderness that can last from several hours to several weeks at time. As I had very limited skills as an outdoor recreational leader and even less technical skills in outdoor survival, my main role as a rehabilitation counselor was to help facilitate the group process that often becomes a critical part of therapeutic adventure programs. I was simply one of several professional staff who took various groups into the wilderness to learn about the outdoors but more importantly to help persons learn about themselves.

One of our trips at Breckenridge, Colorado (Bear Meadows—to be exact) involved working with a group of young adults with various disabilities who had never been camping, let alone spent a week in the wilderness with all its inherent beauty and challenges that go with it. The "usual" one-week program included various activities such as camping, hiking, whitewater rafting, rappelling, rock climbing, and participating in a universally designed (accessible) high ropes course. After each activity, we always took time to reflect what the activity meant for each person and what it could mean when he or she returned back to his or her homes and communities. One of group members, Tony, was a person with cerebral palsy. Functionally, this meant that Tony had some difficulty walking independently and maintaining balance (throughout each day during the outdoor adventure program, he usually tripped and fell anywhere between 5 and 10 times). When speaking (which was not that often), he had a moderately significant speech impediment. This meant that while you could understand Tony, you had to listen carefully. Also, when speaking, Tony would sometimes drool, which, at times, would cause discomfort among some members, who would remind him to wipe his mouth. Despite these characteristics, it was evident during our trip that Tony had a great deal of determination but he also tended to hold back from talking with others. This situation would sometimes change when Tony would settle in his sleeping bag right before we were all ready to go to sleep. As my sleeping area was next to his, this meant that we would have an opportunity to talk. While I would like to think that his willingness to open up during this night's exchanges was a result of my counseling skills, I think greater credit goes to our unique environment. Sleeping under a night sky with stars that are so bright that you can actually see satellites passing over does something to stir life's big questions and discover even bigger answers.

Up to this point, I thought Tony was a man of few words but I soon discovered that he could be quite talkative, and given our setting and what had happened this particular day, Tony wanted talk. So, for the next hour I listened about what this day meant to him. Initially, Tony started talking about how he had always been afraid of others. How, as a little boy, he always felt different from others and, later growing up, how this awareness resulted in his being very shy and withdrawn. He then talked about how this day in the wilderness was the first time he could ever remember that other people depended on him (many of the activities are designed to develop interdependence and mutual support among group members) rather than him "always having to depend on others." He talked about how being with others in our group gave him a sense of accomplishment that he could never recall feeling before. Eventually, Tony thought about how this experience might impact him when he returned home. He wanted to rethink the kind of work he was currently doing (custodial) and believed that he was capable of more. From this experience, he was now thinking about pursuing vocational technical training to get a more satisfying job. After listening to him and realizing that we were the only two whispering in our camp as all of the others were fast asleep, I asked him if there was anything else he wanted to say before turning in. He waited for a few seconds and, as he was watching the canopy of stars above, he inhaled a deep breath and then said, "This has been the greatest day in my life." I knew from the sincerity in his voice that it was, and after listening to him, all I was able to muster was, "That's great, Tony. I am glad I was here to share it with you." Although my response will not go down in the counseling annals of "Best Empathic Response Ever Made," I felt a deep but quiet joy that I was there with him, and perhaps in some way, all of the people on this one day helped him to take one life step forward to create some new possibilities. In the end, I think it should be a goal for all rehabilitation counselors.

SPECIAL TOPICS IN REHABILITATION COUNSELING

Before offering a list of special topics that you might find of interest, I want to first offer a disclaimer. As I was thinking about what special topics to address in this chapter, I found that I was having some difficulty in identifying them and providing enough information so that you would have an understanding as to why these topics were particularly "special." The fact is that rehabilitation counseling is a broad field where one can find special topics simply on the basis of your individual interests. The literature is replete with journals that have devoted a specific issue on a special topic. For example, I am the editor of *Rehabilitation Education*, and each year we have one issue that addresses a special topic. In 2008, we devoted a special topics issue to master's level training of rehabilitation counselors, including accreditation standards and specifics about the curriculum. Similarly, other rehabilitation journals such as the *Journal of Applied Rehabilitation Counseling*, *Journal of Disability Policy Studies*, *Journal of Rehabilitation*, *Journal of Rehabilitation Administration*, and *Rehabilitation Counseling Bulletin* have published a variety of special topics issues germane to their readership. Consequently, the list of special topics listed here represents my own inclinations and not ones that have been informed by any scientific method. I would invite each of you review the rehabilitation related journals to see what may be important to you.

Given the initial disclaimer, special topics that rehabilitation counselor educators are deeply concerned about include the following:

1. What are best practices in rehabilitation counseling that are based on solid scientific evidence that will improve the quality of life for persons with disabilities?
2. Why, despite the passage of the Americans with Disabilities Act of 1990, have employment outcomes for persons with disabilities not improved?
3. How do we effectively recruit and maintain a professional rehabilitation counseling profession to serve the growing needs of the diverse clientele we serve?
4. Given the current economic problems with funding social service programs, how can we develop more cost-efficient interventions that will reduce poverty among persons with disabilities?
5. What are promising medical and technological advances that will dramatically improve functioning for persons with disabilities?

FURTHER CONSIDERATIONS IN REHABILITATION COUNSELING

Earlier in this chapter, you learned that the greatest obstacle keeping persons with disabilities from participating fully in American society concerns the less than favorable attitudes held by persons without disabilities. In contrast, perhaps the greatest mechanism to promote integration of persons with disabilities in various community settings and social roles is through assistive technology (AT). This concept as defined by the Technology-Related Assistance of Individuals with Disabilities Act of 1988 (Public Law No. 100–407) states that AT is "any item, piece of equipment, or product system, whether acquired commercially off the shelf, modified, or customized, that is used to increase, maintain, or improve functional capabilities of individuals with disabilities." This technology can range from simple devices to improve mobility such as canes, walkers, or motorized wheelchairs to more complex technology such as home environmental units that control room temperature, lighting, security alarms, and other mechanical or electrical devices through voice activated commands. These advances allow persons with disabilities to perform tasks independently and, in essence, exercise greater control in their daily lives. While these technological advances have a profound impact on improving the quality of life for persons with disabilities, the greatest impediment for not using AT more effectively is that, in many instances, the persons who are most likely to benefit from this technology are not involved in the basic decision process, such as what technology should be used and how (Scherer & Sax, 2004).

CONCLUSION

The decision to exclude or minimize the opinions, desires, or input of persons with disabilities as applied to AT, or any rehabilitation intervention for that matter, is inconsistent with a fundamental precept of our profession—the right of consumer choice or self-determinism. As rehabilitation counselors we recognize that each person has the right to decide his or her own course of rehabilitation services. Clearly, there will be times when clients choose a course of action that we might disagree with, such as to not seek alcoholism treatment, to pursue a different vocational training program, to remain living at home with a parent, or to drop out of school. These decisions may be counterproductive to what we believe is in the best interest of our clients but, in the final analysis, we must allow our clients to determine their own futures. Imposing our values and taking a course of action inconsistent with our clients' desires (with the exception of when the client may engage in behaviors injurious to themselves or others—e.g., suicide, child abuse) is incompatible with good rehabilitation practice. As new counselors, it is sometimes difficult to see the wisdom of this core value but, in time, it is one that makes sense both practically and philosophically. Our professional role is to assist in the rehabilitation journey that hopefully improves the quality of life for each person. It is a journey worth taking!

CHAPTER REVIEW

1. Rehabilitation counselors recognize the importance of how individual perceptions regarding capabilities of persons with disabilities are often determined by belief systems held by others. This belief system is strongly influenced by which disability model (biomedical, functional, environmental, and sociopolitical) each counselor adheres to and, as a result, how each person may reach his or her potential in life.

2. While the work performed by rehabilitation counselors varies considerably as a function of clientele served, work setting, and specialty area of practice, the basic professional functions involve (a) assessing client needs, (b) developing a plan to promote an effective working alliance with the clients, and (c) procuring or providing services necessary to improve one's quality of life.

3. Formal training necessary to work as a rehabilitation counselor focuses on 10 content areas that requires supervised field-based experience at the graduate level. The recognized credential required of a

professional rehabilitation counselor is to obtain national certification in this specialty area (i.e., Certified Rehabilitation Counselor).

4. Given the prevalence of disability in the United States, employment opportunities for rehabilitation counselors remains strong. Rehabilitation counselors work in a variety of settings as a function of job function (e.g., adjustment to disability counseling, job placement), interest in working with a particular type of clientele (e.g., Deaf, mental retardation, psychiatric disability, substance abuse) or work setting (e.g., community rehabilitation program, hospital, school).

5. The greatest obstacle confronting persons with disabilities is the attitudes held by others. In contrast, the greatest mechanism for promoting integration of persons with disabilities may be through assistive technology.

REVIEW QUESTIONS

1. What reasons explain why, regardless of your professional practice, you are likely to work with persons with disabilities?

2. Using U.S. census data, disabilities can be broadly defined into one of three categories. Identify these categories and provide an example of a disability within each category.

3. According to Smart and Smart (2006), how we view someone's disability is based on one of four theoretical models. Identify each model and describe a fundamental philosophical belief associated with it.

4. What is the greatest barrier to helping people with disabilities realize their personal, social, and career potential?

5. What is a core belief that effective rehabilitation counselors must adhere to when working with persons with disabilities?

6. How important is client advocacy in the professional practice of rehabilitation counselors?

7. Is the work of a rehabilitation counselor primarily a "routine" job? Why or why not?

8. What does it mean to be a Certified Rehabilitation Counselor?

ADDITIONAL RESOURCES

- To complete Learning Activity 13.2, please read the following article:

   Herbert, J. T. (2000). Simulation as a learning method to facilitate disability awareness. *Journal of Experiential Education, 23*(1), 5–11.

- To complete Learning Activity 13.4, visit the following professional organization Web sites for rehabilitation counselors:

   American Rehabilitation Counseling Association (http://www.arcaweb.org/)

   International Association of Rehabilitation Professionals (http://www.rehabpro.org/)

   National Rehabilitation Counseling Association (http://nrca-net.org/)

- To learn more about accredited rehabilitation counseling graduate programs, visit the National Council on Rehabilitation Education Web site at http://www.core-rehab.org/.

- Students interested in learning more about disability and related rehabilitation counseling topics should visit the National Rehabilitation Information Center at http://www.naric.com/. The Web site provides information on thousands of technical reports, journal articles, and resource information citations—at no cost. If you have to write a paper as part of a class assignment, this Web site is a fantastic resource!

REFERENCES

Bishop, M., & Crystal, R. M. (2002). A human resources perspective on counselor retirement and replacement in the state-federal vocational rehabilitation program: A nationwide concern. *Journal of Rehabilitation Administration, 26*(4), 231–238.

Commission on Rehabilitation Counselor Certification. (2009). Retrieved June 20, 2007, from http://www.crccertification.com/pages/about_crcc/112.php/.

Commission on Rehabilitation Counselor Certification. (2009). *2008 salary report: An update on salaries in the rehabilitation counseling profession.* Retrieved June 15, 2009, from http://www.crccertification.com/aboutCRCC.

Council on Rehabilitation Education. (2007). *Accreditation manual.* Retrieved June 18, 2009, from http://www.core-rehab.org/accrman.html

Council on Rehabilitation Education. (2009). *CORE master's programs in rehabilitation counselor education, 2008–2009 academic year.* Retrieved June 17, 2009, from http://www.core-rehab.org/progrec.html.

Dew, D. & Peters, S. (2002). Survey of master's level rehabilitation counseling programs: Relationship to public vocational rehabilitation recruitment and retention of state vocational rehabilitation counselors. *Rehabilitation Education, 16,* 61–65.

Ethridge, G., Rodgers, R. A., & Fabian, E. S. (2007). Emerging roles, functions, specialty areas, and employment settings for contemporary rehabilitation practice. *Journal of Applied Rehabilitation Counseling, 38*(4), 27–33.

Herbert, J. T. (1996). Use of adventure-based counseling for persons with disabilities. *Journal of Rehabilitation, 62*(4), 3–9.

Herbert, J. T. (1998). Therapeutic effects of participating in an adventure therapy program. *Rehabilitation Counseling Bulletin, 41,* 201–216.

Jaques, M. E. (1959). *Critical counseling behavior in rehabilitation settings.* Iowa City: State University of Iowa, College of Education.

Leahy, M. J. (2004). Qualified providers. In T. F. Riggar and D. R. Maki (Eds.), *Handbook of rehabilitation counseling* (pp. 142–158). New York: Springer Publishing.

Leahy, M. J., Chan, F., & Saunders, J. L. (2003). Job functions and knowledge requirements of certified rehabilitation counselors in the 21st century. *Rehabilitation Counseling Bulletin, 46,* 66–81.

Leahy, M. J., & Szymanski, E. M. (1995). Rehabilitation counseling: Evolution and current status. *Journal of Counseling & Development, 74,* 163–166.

Maki, D. R. (2004). CORE president's report. CORE strategic position 2004–2009. Retrieved November 17, 2009, from http://www.core-rehab.org/Newsletters.html.

Perlman, R. (2007). *The blind doctor: The Jacob Bolotin story.* Santa Barbara, CA: Blue Point Books.

Pointer, M. (2003). Characteristics and leadership styles of state administrators of vocational rehabilitation. *Journal of Rehabilitation Administration, 27,* 83–93.

Rasch, J. D., Hollingsworth, D. K., Saxon, J. P., & Thomas, K. R. (1984). Student recruitment issues in the 1980s. *Rehabilitation Counseling Bulletin, 28,* 46–49.

Rubin, S. E., Matkin, R. E., Ashley, J., Beardsley, M. M., May, V. R., Onstott, K., et al. (1984). Roles and functions of certified rehabilitation counselors. *Rehabilitation Counseling Bulletin, 27,* 199–224.

Scherer, M. J., & Sax, C. L. (2004). Technology. In T. F. Riggar and D. R. Maki (Eds.), *Handbook of rehabilitation counseling* (pp. 271–288). New York: Springer Publishing.

Smart, J. (2004). Models of disability: The juxtaposition of biology and social construction. In T. F. Riggar and D. R. Maki (Eds.), *Handbook of rehabilitation counseling* (pp. 25–49). New York: Springer Publishing.

Smart, J. F., & Smart, D. W. (2006). Models of disability: Implications for the counseling profession. *Journal of Counseling & Development, 84,* 29–40.

Sussman, M. B., & Haug, M. R. (1968). Rehabilitation counselor recruits. *Journal of Counseling Psychology, 15*(3), 250–256.

U.S. Census Bureau. (2005). Americans with disabilities: 2005. Retrieved November 17, 2009, from http://www.census.gov/hhes/www/disability/sipp/disable05.html.

U.S. Department of Labor and Industry. (2007). Counselors. In *Occupational outlook handbook, 2008–2009 edition.* Retrieved May 8, 2009, from http://stats.bls.gov/oco/ocos067.htm#outlook.

Wright, B. A. (1983). *Physical disability—A psychosocial approach.* New York: Harper & Row.

CHAPTER 14

Couple and Family Counseling

LEARNING OBJECTIVES

After reading this chapter, you should be able to

- understand families from systemic and developmental perspectives;
- describe the history and development of couples and family counseling;
- identify the characteristics of well-functioning families and common patterns of family dysfunction;
- discuss the various approaches to couple and family counseling;
- describe the training and credentialing of couple and family counselors;
- appreciate couple and family counseling as a career path; and
- understand ethical issues unique to couple and family counseling.

CHAPTER OUTLINE

Introduction

The Family: Systemic and Developmental Perspectives
A Systemic Perspective
A Developmental Perspective

The History and Development of Family Counseling

Perspectives on Family Functioning
Characteristics of Well-Functioning Families
Common Patterns of Family Dysfunction

Approaches to Family Counseling

Family Systems Therapy
Structural Family Therapy
Strategic Family Therapy
The Human Validation Process Approach
Experiential Family Therapy
Narrative Therapy
Solution-Focused Brief Therapy

Ethical Issues in Couple and Family Counseling

A Career as a Marriage and Family Counselor/Therapist

Work Locations and Income for Couple
and Family Counselors/Therapists
The Job Outlook for Couple and Family
Counselors/Therapists

Training and Credentialing of Couple and Family Counselors/Therapists

Professional Associations for Couple and
Family Counselors/Therapists

IAMFC Training Standards
AAMFT Training Standards
State Licensure
The Reciprocal Nature of State Licensure
and Association Membership

Special Topics and Further Considerations

Systems Counseling Approaches in School
Settings
Online Couple and Family Counseling

Conclusion

CHAPTER REVIEW
REVIEW QUESTIONS
ADDITIONAL RESOURCES
REFERENCES

INTRODUCTION

Couple and family counseling/therapy has grown significantly since the official beginning of the family therapy movement in the 1950s. Although Alfred Adler and Rudolf Dreikurs originally proposed and demonstrated the efficacy of working with the family as a unit in the 1920s (Carlson, Watts, & Maniacci, 2006; Sherman & Dinkmeyer, 1987), it was not until the last quarter of the 20th century that family counseling attained universal acceptance within the mental health profession (Gladding, 2007; Goldenberg & Goldenberg, 2008).

Historically, most counselors were trained to view clients as individuals, ignoring the role of the family and societal influences in the development and continuation of psychological problems. In recent decades, however, mental health professionals have recognized that counseling with individuals without consideration, and often inclusion, of the family unit is frequently detrimental to maintenance of successful outcomes in counseling.

The diversity of couple and family systems and the demands upon today's couples and families is greater than ever before. You may have noticed the phrase *marriage and family* in your past readings on this topic. Our usage, instead, of the *couples and family* language is partly in response to this diversity, recognizing that all couples may not fit a legal definition of "marriage," yet, for counseling purposes, may share some or all of the same issues. Due to the increasing demands and accompanying levels of stress experienced by couples and families today, mental health professionals need to be prepared to work with clients' counseling issues within a family context. The purpose of this chapter is to provide a brief introduction to the field of couple and family counseling in hopes of whetting your appetite for intense study and practice of counseling couples and families. We begin by discussing the characteristics of the family from a systemic and developmental perspective. Next we address the history of the couple and family counseling movement. In the following section, we address characteristics of well-functioning families and family dysfunction. We then overview several widely recognized approaches to couple and family counseling. Next we briefly address ethical issues that are largely unique to couple and family counseling. In the next to last section, we present career information, training, and credentialing of couple and family counselors. We conclude by addressing special topics and further considerations regarding couple and family counseling.

Active Learning Exercise **14.1**

How do *you* define *family*? What personal influences or information guides your definition? What are some other ways that *family* might be defined?

THE FAMILY: SYSTEMIC AND DEVELOPMENTAL PERSPECTIVES

What is a family? Every person has basic emotional and physical needs. Although the physical needs are fairly obvious, the emotional ones are much less easily recognized. According to Foley (1989), the emotional needs can be reduced to three dimensions: intimacy, power, and meaning. Humans have a need to belong, to be in close relationship with others. They have a need for self-expression, to be unique. Lastly, people have a need to find meaning and purpose in their lives. One might argue that fulfillment of these needs is possible without involvement in a family unit. Foley argued, however, that the possibility of meeting these needs apart from a family—in some form or fashion—is remote. Thus, one definition of a family is the social unit in which people by mutual consent attempt to fulfill their needs for intimacy, self-expression, and meaning and purposefulness.

Although the preceding definition is good as far as it goes, it does not adequately address (or even allude to) the many contextual factors that influence the family as a whole or the individual persons that make up the family system. A more encompassing definition of the family, and one that integrates easily with the definition in the previous paragraph, is offered by Goldenberg and Goldenberg (2008):

> A family is a natural social system that occurs in a diversity of forms today and represents a diversity of cultural heritages. Embedded in society at large, it is shaped by a multitude of factors, such as its place and time in history, race,

ethnicity, social class membership, religious affiliation, and number of generations in this country. The way it functions—establishes rules, communicates, and negotiates differences between members—has numerous implications for the development and well-being of its members. Families display a recurring pattern of interactional sequences in which all members participate. (p. 23)

A Systemic Perspective

A system is comprised of sets of different parts that are interconnected, interdependent, and related in a stable manner over time. The family is systemic in nature. Whether it is well functioning or not, the family is a system that consists of a number of persons in relationships over a period of time. Although there are various therapeutic approaches to couple and family counseling with differing ideas about how families improve their functioning, there is general agreement among almost all of the approaches that the family is conceptualized as an integrated system comprised of members whose interactions with one another influence the family experience for all its members. This idea, a basic tenet of general systems theory, provides the conceptual framework for understanding interrelationships within the family and shifts the focus of a family member's problem(s) from an intrapersonal focus to an interpersonal one. This nonlinear framing of problem behaviors shifts ownership of the problem to the entire family unit (Gladding, 2007; Goldenberg & Goldenberg, 2008).

> Picture the family as a decorative mobile handing by a string from the ceiling. The string is connected to a long thin stick and there are other strings hanging down from each end of the stick. Each one has something else dangling down from it. A normal mobile is carefully balanced and has a certain equilibrium to it. If you come to it and push on one little element on the mobile, what happens? It affects the whole system. As the mobile settles down after having been touched, it regains equilibrium. Suppose you cut one of the dangling objects off. What is that going to do to the system? It's going to change and be lopsided. This pictures the family as a system and how the family can be dysfunctional. There are interlocking parts to the system.... Interacting components that co-vary such that each element in the family is dependent on the functioning of the other elements in the family. (Rekers, 1988, p. 38)

Other basic characteristics of viewing the family from a systemic perspective include the following:

1. The family as a whole is greater than the sum of its parts taken separately. The family maintains a collective identity that is different from the individual identities of each of its members.
2. Why behavior occurs within the family is not the focus of a counselor working within a systems framework; the focus is on what, how, and when the behavior occurs. All behavior is communication, and communication is continuously occurring. It is important to attend to the two functions of interpersonal messages: content (factual information) and relationship (how the message is understood). The *what* of a message is conveyed by how it is delivered (Gladding, 2007). Counselors practicing within a systems context view the transactional patterns occurring within the family as the primary focus of counseling.

3. The family is viewed as a system in which any change within one member affects the system as a whole and, reciprocally, affects each individual member. This idea, referred to as circular causality, indicates that events with a relationship context occur in a circular manner rather than a linear one.

4. A family commonly contains a number of coexisting subsystems. Subsystems are those parts of the overall system assigned to carry out particular functions or processes within the system as a whole. The marital or partner dyad constitutes a subsystem, as do the mother-child, father-child, and child-child dyads (Goldenberg & Goldenberg, 2008).

5. The ability of the family to modify its functioning to meet the changing demands of internal and external factors is known as morphogenesis. Morphogenesis usually requires a second-order change (the ability to make an entirely new response) rather than a first-order change (continuing to do more of the same things that have—or have not—worked previously) (Watzlawick, Weakland, & Fisch, 1974).

6. The family attempts to maintain stability and resist change through the process of homeostasis. When the balance of the system is disturbed, family members will seek to return to the previous level of balance or homeostasis by using internal and ongoing interactional mechanisms that maintain a balance of relationships. According to Goldenberg and Goldenberg (2008), homeostasis is the family self-regulation efforts that result in a steady state, but the process of homeostasis is hardly a static one. Families may have to create a new balance by renegotiating relationships and altering existing family structures in order to accommodate family members' growth and change over time.

A Developmental Perspective

When thinking about developmental tasks within a life cycle perspective, one may think of the growth and maturation of the individual. The human life cycle literature views life as a series of developmental tasks whereby individuals negotiate various challenges of a particular phase of life and then move on to the next. Life is change and the cycle of human life, although usually proceeding in an orderly manner, does not progress in a fluid, continuous fashion.

Families also have life cycles. According to the family life cycle perspective (see Carter & McGoldrick, 1999), the family is a social system that faces a series of developmental tasks that require mastery at each phase of the cycle. Continuity and change are both characteristics of the family system as it moves through time. In both cases, a shift or transformation is required in the system's organization. A key to adaptive functioning through the family life cycle is the recognition of the need for system reorganization and the system's flexibility to accomplish it. In well-functioning families, boundaries and alignments are sufficiently flexible to be readjusted to accommodate needed changes in the life cycle of the family (e.g., children moving from childhood to adolescence). The appearance of symptomatic behaviors in a family member at transition points in the family life cycle, however, may indicate the family is having difficulty in negotiating the transition.

Over the past 40-plus years there have been dramatic changes in family life cycle patterns resulting from changing birth rate patterns, the changing role of women, the rapid rise of divorce and remarriage, and the diversity of domestic partnerships and living arrangements, to name a few. Despite such significant changes (and concomitant limitations), the family life cycle approach is, nevertheless, a helpful organizing framework for viewing families as a system in movement through time. Carter and McGoldrick (1999) and their associates addressed these significant changes and how they impact and are impacted by the developmental changes of the family life cycle. It is beyond the scope of this brief chapter to address the many variations on a theme, and readers are encouraged to examine the work of Carter and McGoldrick.

In addition to the life cycle development issues just addressed, a number of other influences on families need to be considered in order to gain a fuller understanding of the family development process. These include gender issues, ethnic and cultural ground, and socioeconomic considerations.

To understand family development, counselors must consider the fact that men and women experience life differently, both in their families of origin and in the families formed via marriage or partnerships. Men and women are reared espousing different role expectations, beliefs, values, goals, and opportunities. These gender divergences are influential on later adult relational interactions.

It is also crucial for counselors to include the role of the impact of ethnicity and culture on family development. Ethnicity and culture are fundamental influences for how families define what constitutes a family, how they view life cycle phases and developmental tasks, how families establish and reinforce acceptable values and behaviors, and which traditions, rituals, and ceremonies they develop to mark transitions in the life cycle. A person's ethnic and cultural background influences how he or she thinks, feels, and acts in both individual and family contexts. It is essential, therefore, that counselors consider how culture and ethnicity impacts family development for each client family. Furthermore, counselors need to be aware of their own ethnic and cultural values in order to avoid, as much as possible, imposing their beliefs and values on to their clients and client families.

Historically, family life cycle developmental models are based on middle-class or upper-middle-class socioeconomic considerations. The developmental patterns in poor families, however, may vary significantly from the aforementioned paradigm. Financially impoverished environments tend to create different family structures and organizations. For example, life cycle progress in poor families is often accelerated by early and often unwed pregnancies. These groups of persons often create multi-parent families that join together in reciprocal relationships to share their limited financial resources (Goldenberg & Goldenberg, 2008).

THE HISTORY AND DEVELOPMENT OF FAMILY COUNSELING

Gladding (2007) identified three major trends in history contributing to the development of family counseling: (1) a rise in the divorce rate after World War II, (2) the changing role of women in social status and employment opportunities, and (3) an increased life span for both men and women in the United States. These social changes along with the acceptance of counseling as a viable process for problem-solving and decision-making created a need for increased training and research in working with families.

Major events in the early development of family counseling included the beginning of marriage and premarital counseling, the child guidance movement, the early use of group dynamics or processes in counseling, and research studies on the role of the family in the development of schizophrenia (Goldenberg & Goldenberg, 2008). As early as the 1920s and 1930s, professionals in a variety of settings developed and used marriage interventions and premarital counseling programs; however, the focus was largely intrapsychic rather than interpersonal and remained so for several decades thereafter. The child guidance movement, founded by Adler in Vienna in the early 1900s, strongly influenced practitioners working with families, and Dreikurs in the United States expanded the notion of intervening in child problems by working with the entire family. Also, early in the 1900s, Jacob Moreno developed psychodrama within the context of group therapy and helped participants work through interpersonal situations that produced distress and dysfunction. Beginning in the late 1930s and early 1940s, researchers and practitioners worked with schizophrenic patients in hospital settings attempting to determine the relationship between family dynamics and schizophrenia. Pioneers like Nathan Ackerman, James Framo, and Murray Bowen integrated systemic ideas into their practices and developed new theoretical perspectives of mental illness (Framo, 1996).

The 1950s is generally considered the official beginning of family counseling and therapy. No one person, however, may be singled out as the first to adopt a systemic approach for working with families. At this time, several practitioners across the United States were meeting with families and viewing symptoms of identified patients as a function of family interactional patterns, and they began to learn about each others' work. In 1956, the Palo Alto Group—including Gregory Bateson, Don Jackson, Jay Haley, and John Weakland—wrote their seminal paper on the double-bind, describing a theory of the relationship between family communication patterns and schizophrenia (Gladding, 2007; Goldenberg & Goldenberg, 2008).

Beels (2002) notes that the 1960s was a time of family-centeredness and group welfare that contributed to the evolution of family therapy. During this decade family counseling became a recognized topic at professional meetings, and the 1960s was a very productive period for persons working from a systems perspective. In 1962, Don Jackson and Nathan Ackerman founded the first family therapy journal, *Family Process*, and Virginia Satir published her book *Conjoint Family Therapy*. In the 1960s and early 1970s, the work of Jay Haley (strategic family therapy), Salvador Minuchin (structural family therapy), and Carl Whitaker (experiential family therapy) emerged in the literature (Gladding, 2007; Goldenberg & Goldenberg, 2008).

The 1970s and 1980s continued the productivity established in the 1960s. During this time significant expansion to the traditional systems perspective occurred. Leading these changes that argued for a more circular understanding of family counseling were the Milan group, led by Maria Selvini-Palazzoli, Harry Goolishan, Harlene Anderson of the Houston Galveston Family Institute, and Karl Tomm from the University of Calgary. Also, during this time Michael White and David Epston in Australia began developing their narrative therapy approach to helping families. According to Kaslow (2000), the feminist movement in the 1980s brought the emphasis of gender sensitivity and the role of gender in family dynamics to family counseling. Also in the 1980s, family counselors examined the role and impact of cultural and ethnic diversity on family functioning and family counseling.

Family counselors in the 1990s responded to managed care constraints with brief and solution-focused perspectives in their work with couples and families. The late Steve de Shazer, William O'Hanlon, and Michelle Weiner-Davis published numerous journal articles and books presenting their brief, solution-focused (or solution-oriented) methods that emphasized solutions and possibilities rather problems (Goldenberg & Goldenberg, 2008).

Contemporary issues in family counseling continue to center on the changing role and understanding of the family and family process in a multicultural and pluralistic society and changing perspectives regarding family counseling. These changes may be seen in (a) the movement away from strict adherence to one particular theoretical perspective or school of thought and the movement toward integration; (b) the increasing interest in and appreciation of constructivist and constructionist ways of helping families; (c) the changing patterns of family counseling within the constraints of managed care, including the use of evidence-based interventions; and (d) the ever-increasing attention paid to the role of gender and cultural issues, societal oppression, and spirituality and religious values in the lives of clients and client families.

PERSPECTIVES ON FAMILY FUNCTIONING

Until the 1980s, family research literature focused primarily on characteristics and symptoms of dysfunctional families. Addressing only negative aspects of family functioning, however, provides a myopic perspective.

> I would not dream of teaching someone to play tennis by only telling them how *not* to do it: "Now you do *not* hold a racket this way. You do *not* do a backstroke this way." A coach would not succeed if he (or she) only made remarks like, "This is wrong, don't stand like this, this is terrible," while never telling the person how to stand right and how to hold the tennis racket correctly. But to a large extent we have done this in the area of family life. For example, we've told people what families of delinquents or runaways are like, and we've said, "Now don't let your family be like that." We have not used the positive model approach. We have not said, "Here's what a strong family is like and your family can work on these positive qualities. (Stinnett, 1985, p. 37)

In this section we address characteristics of well-functioning families and family dysfunction.

Active Learning Exercise **14.2**

Before you read the next section, make a list of what you think are key characteristics of well-functioning families. How do the characteristics on your list contribute to well family functioning?

Characteristics of Well-Functioning Families

Beginning in the late 1970s, some family researchers began focusing on the characteristics of strong, well-functioning families. This research has continued over the recent decades (Beavers & Hampson, 1990, 2003; Curran, 1983; Epstein, Bishop, & Baldwin, 1982; Epstein, Ryan, Bishop, Miller, & Keitner, 2003; Stinnett, Chesser, & DeFrain, 1979; Stinnett, DeFrain, King, Knaub, & Rowe, 1981; Walsh, 2003; Watts, Trusty, & Lim, 1996). The following characteristics of well-functioning families were the ones most commonly mentioned in the literature. Ancillary characteristics were often discussed in the literature as being part of or subsumed under these core characteristics.

- Commitment
  - Members of the marital or partner couple are committed to each other.
  - There is a high level of trust and security in the relationship.
  - The parent(s) is/are consciously committed to the development and well-being of the family.
  - There is a high level of trust and security within the family as a whole.

- Communication
  - Family members strive to actively listen and empathize with one another.
  - Members strive to be honest and genuine when attempting to communicate.
  - Members feel permission to appropriately express their own thoughts and feelings.
  - Conflict and negotiation is considered a normal part of family process. When faced with divergent opinions, members choose to respond in a respectful and constructive manner rather than in a condemnatory and destructive one.

- Clear boundaries
  - The marital/partnership couple is affectionate and intimate, consistently sets aside time apart from children for the dyadic relationship, and has other couples as friends.
  - Parent(s) meet(s) intimacy and social needs through their relationships with adults rather than their children.
  - Families are part of a social network of families that provide enjoyment, support, and a sense of *community* for family members.

- Positive family atmosphere
  - The family atmosphere is encouraging, affirming, and optimistic.
  - The family environment allows members to freely express appreciation and love for each other.
  - Family members seek to support one another and express their love in an unconditional manner by being caring, compassionate, respectful, and accepting of individual differences.
  - Families have a sense of humor, but not at the expense of one another. Members are able to see and appreciate the humor in everyday living and can readily laugh at themselves.

- Connectedness
  - Members share a feeling of belongingness. They enjoy one another and purposefully spend time together in both planned and spontaneous activities; they make spending both *quality* and *quantity* time together a priority.
  - Time is divided into time for the marital dyad, parent and child interactions, and the family as a whole.
  - Families seek to create and continue family traditions. Parents attempt to instill/pass on cultural and family heritage to their children.

- Adaptibility
  - Families have sufficient adaptability to constructively address and take responsibility for problem prevention and/or resolution.
  - Individual and family developmental transitions are handled in a flexible manner.
  - When families are faced with a crisis beyond their capacity to cope, they will readily admit problems and seek help outside the family.

- Spirituality
  - Family members have meaning and purpose to life that is often, but not always, evidenced by some form of organized, formal religious commitment.
  - Spirituality in these families influences the moral development of members and the development of relationship-enhancing qualities such as love, patience, kindness, support, and altruism.

Active Learning Exercise **14.3**

How might a counselor usefully employ the preceding list of characteristics in counseling couples and families? What concerns do you have about using such a list in couple and family counseling? How might you employ the list *and* address your concerns?

When working with couples and families, it is important that counselors look at strengths and assets and not merely limitations and liabilities. The characteristics of well-functioning families can help counselors and families identify family strengths and serve as *points for dialogue* to address areas for growth. Counselors also need to understand these characteristics as a process across a continuum. That is, families will never completely or perfectly manifest all the well-functioning characteristics.

Common Patterns of Family Dysfunction

There are many patterns of family dysfunction discussed in the literature. Due to space limitations, we discuss three patterns of family dysfunction commonly addressed in the literature: dysfunctional boundaries, dysfunctional communication, and dysfunctional family structure.

Dysfunctional Boundaries

Boundaries within a family are the means by which family members perceive their function within the system and the subsystems contained therein. A crucial task of the marital/couple subsystem is the development of boundaries that allow for the satisfaction of the dyad's needs but protect the subsystem from the intrusion of in-laws, children, and others. Boundaries between other subsystems within the family system are equally necessary. There must be a clear hierarchy of power with parents leading the family in a unified manner. Parents must avoid interfering with sibling conflicts, adolescents must not expect or be expected to take on parental or spousal responsibilities, and extended family members (e.g., in-laws) must not be involved with the conflicts of a family subsystem (Minuchin, 1974; Minuchin & Fishman, 1981; Nichols, 1988).

Minuchin (1974) delineates three basic types of boundaries: clear, enmeshed, and disengaged. Strong, well-functioning families have clear boundaries. In other words, family members experience both personal autonomy *and* belonging and togetherness. Clear boundaries are flexible, allowing for readjustment of subsystem functioning as the family system develops. *Enmeshment*, or enmeshed boundaries, describes the chaotic and tightly interconnected manner in which a family acts. Family members may become overdependent or overinvolved in each others' lives, and personal autonomy is sacrificed as the individuality of members is lost. The subsystem boundaries become so blurred that there are no clear lines of responsibility and authority. Consequently, members do not understand their proper role and function within the family system. *Disengagement*, or disengaged boundaries, describes families that have extremely rigid boundaries with a resultant lack of closeness. Family members are isolated and often appear unrelated. Disengaged families offer very little nurturance, support, and guidance for its members. Personal autonomy is at a high level but at the sacrifice of a sense of family closeness. Family members often have difficulty forming relationships outside the family due to the lack of relational experiencing within the family.

It is important to note that all families may have some degree of enmeshment or disengagement, and these relational styles do not, in themselves, imply dysfunction. Some cultures value family closeness to a greater extent than personal autonomy. Counselors working with culturally diverse couples and families should carefully explore the meaning of boundaries in the cultural context prior to assuming that a family's boundaries are dysfunctional.

Dysfunctional Communication

In surveying over 500 family professionals, Curran (1983) discovered that healthy communication was the number one response regarding traits of healthy families. The importance of healthy communication to the healthy functioning of families is well documented in the research literature (e.g., Beavers & Hampson, 2003; Curran, 1983; Epstein et al., 2003; Stinnett et al., 1979; Stinnett et al., 1981; Walsh, 2003; Watts et al., 1996).

Communication is more is more than one person speaking and another listening. All communications have two different levels or functions: report and command. The report (or content) level is the information conveyed by the words we use. The command (or metacommunication) level communicates how the report level is to be understood and provides a commentary on the nature of the relationship. The metacommunication level is the more powerful influence on human relationships, albeit the more difficult to notice and understand (Nichols, 1988; Watzlawick, Beavin, & Jackson, 1967).

Dysfunctional couples and families exhibit deficits in the ability to constructively express thoughts and feelings and actively listen to one another. Communication dysfunction occurs when communication is *incongruent*; that is, when the verbal (report or content) and nonverbal (command or metacommunication) levels of communication do not agree. Examples of nonverbal communication include body position or posture, breathing rhythm, facial expression, muscle constriction or relaxation, and vocal tone and intensity (Satir, 1983). In well-functioning families, there is agreement or *congruence* between the verbal and nonverbal aspects of communication.

Dysfunctional Family Structure

A family's structure is the invisible set of functional demands that organizes family relations. The structure represents the rules the family has developed for relational patterns between family members indicating how, when, with whom, and in what manner members relate. In other words, family rules are the process by which the family operates and gets things done. Stated and unstated rules exist in all families and may, or may not, be understood by all family members. Rules indicate beliefs and values. Rules are expressive of the belief system whereby the family operates and are based primarily on the beliefs and values of the parental subsystem. Each family has its own unique set of rules because each family has its own unique beliefs and values (Minuchin, 1974; Satir, 1972).

Family rules also delineate family *roles*. The term *role* refers to the socially expected behavior for a person occupying a place in a particular family system. In all families there are both formal and informal roles. Formal or traditional roles are assigned and certain role-congruent behaviors are expected. Informal roles, conversely, are assigned to members so that a family's social and emotional needs may be met. Family members are typically unaware of the role-assignment process but may be able to identify their role(s) if questioned about the family's rules and roles. Family roles are not necessarily dysfunctional, however, and the performance of roles is a significant indication of how a family is functioning. In well-functioning families, roles are flexible, easily interchanged, and family stressors are handled creatively. Roles in dysfunctional families, however, are rigidly inflexible and family stressors are handled by rigid, inflexible, and cyclical patterns of behavior (Minuchin, 1974; Satir, 1972).

Many dysfunctional families unconsciously assign the role of *scapegoat* or *identified patient* to one member of the family (often a child). The scapegoat is one of the most common reasons families seek counseling; he or she is the one the family wants "fixed." According to Satir (1983), the scapegoating process most often occurs due to poor marital intimacy and interaction. Bowen (1978) states that when stress levels are elevated in the marital dyad, a vulnerable person outside the dyad—usually a child—will be *triangulated* to generate a common bond between the parents; specifically, the problematic behavior of the triangulated person.

In assessing the rules and role enactment of a family system, counselors must pay careful attention to the ethnic and cultural norms of the culturally diverse families with whom they work. Knowledge of different values, customs, and traditions—and understanding of how these elements impact the family's understanding of rules and roles—are crucial for culturally sensitive counseling with diverse families.

APPROACHES TO FAMILY COUNSELING

There are numerous models of family counseling addressed in the literature. In addition, many of the traditional individual-focused approaches have developed couple and family applications (e.g., cognitive-behavioral couple and family therapy; Watts, 2001). Discussing the various approaches to couple and family counseling is beyond the scope of this brief chapter. Therefore, this section briefly summarizes seven prominent theories that inform the work of clinicians practicing within a family counseling framework. These theories include Bowenian family systems, structural, strategic, human validation process, experiential, narrative, and solution-focused therapies.

Family Systems Therapy

Bowen family systems therapy, developed by Murray Bowen in the 1950s, is among the first systemically based approaches for working with families (Gladding, 2007). This therapy, sometimes referred to as transgenerational family therapy, conceptualizes the family as an emotional unit, a network of interlocking relationships, best understood when analyzed within a multigenerational framework (Goldenberg & Goldenberg, 2008). Through the Bowenian lens, dysfunction in the family results when members of the marital dyad have poor differentiation of self and are emotionally stuck together with their families of origin. An individual's level of differentiation or fusion with his or her family of origin can best be observed when the individual experiences anxiety-producing family situations. As a primary technique, a Bowenian family systems therapist would guide the family in constructing a multigenerational genogram with the purpose of helping family members understand mutigenerational patterns and influences from their families of origin. A genogram is a graphic layout that provides a visual picture of a family tree (Goldenberg & Goldenberg, 2008). Becvar and Becvar (2006) suggested that the genogram provides a visual mapping that may help family members see patterns and relationships in a new light, creating a more objective assessment of their families of origin. Although not a technique-focused approach to therapy, some other techniques of this theoretical approach include detriangulation (whereby the counselor helps clients to be both in contact with and emotionally separate from their families) and the therapist as coach (whereby the counselor serves as an active expert who asks factual questions, helps family members clarify their the roles and relationships in the family, and helps family members in defusing emotions and avoiding blame).

Structural Family Therapy

Structural family therapy, one of the most influential theories of the 1970s, originated with the work of Salvador Minuchin at the Philadelphia Child Guidance Clinic. The foundational constructs of structural family therapy emphasize that an individual's symptoms are best understood as rooted in the context of family transactional patterns and that a change in family organization or structure must take place before the symptoms are relieved (Goldenberg & Goldenberg, 2008). As noted earlier, family members relate to each other according to certain structures that, according to Minuchin (1974), form an "invisible set of functional demands that organizes the ways in which family members interact" (p. 51). Symptoms within the family are believed to arise when family structures are inflexible, whether enmeshed or disengaged, and appropriate structural adjustments are not made. In addition, when boundaries, which are the unwritten rules that help define roles and functions of family members, become rigid or confused within or between subsystems, family dysfunction occurs. Working from a structural family therapy perspective, the therapist must provide a directive leadership role in changing the structure or context in which the symptom is embedded. According to Goldenberg and Goldenberg (2008), the major focus of the structural therapist is to "actively and directly challenge the family's patterns of interaction, forcing the members to look beyond the symptoms of the identified patient in order to view all of their behavior within the context of family structures" (p. 224). To help the family accomplish this, the structural therapist would use the technique of reframing, or changing a perception by explaining a situation from a different and often more positive context (Gladding, 2007). Additional techniques include engaging clients in enactments (a procedure whereby family members role-play the family conflict rather than merely talk about it, thus giving the counselor an opportunity see the family dysfunction), and structural family maps (a procedure whereby the counselor draws a map indicating the family structure, including boundaries and subsystem relationships within the family).

Strategic Family Therapy

Jay Haley, strongly influenced by the work of Gregory Bateson and Milton Erickson, is credited with the development of the strategic approach to family therapy (Carlson, 2002). Haley used the term *problem-solving therapy* to describe his approach to family therapy. He contended that current interactions of the family, rather than historical events or family of origin issues, create family problems. When problems or symptoms surface, they are not successfully resolved within the family because family members cannot change as they are locked in repetitive and nonproductive communication patterns (Nugent & Jones, 2005). Family problems can be solved under the direction of an innovative, active, and directive therapist, who will challenge the power and unspoken rules that govern many of the behaviors of family members. Strategic therapists view themselves as experts in therapy and take responsibility for directly influencing the family with concrete actions and strategies that bring about change and resolution of the presenting problem. The therapist may use the strategies of reframing or relabeling (whereby problem behaviors are more positively interpreted), directives (whereby clients are given homework or outside assignments to encourage family members to behave differently), and paradoxical intervention or prescribing the symptom (whereby clients are encouraged to continue or increase the presenting problem; compliance demonstrates they have at lease some control of the problem, noncompliance usually results in significant lessening or cessation of the problem).

The Human Validation Process Approach

Developed by Virginia Satir, the human validation process approach to family therapy views dysfunctional families as consisting of persons whose freedom to grow and develop has been blocked. Dysfunctional behavior results from the interplay of low self-esteem, incongruent communication, and dysfunctional rules and roles (Gladding, 2007; Goldenberg & Goldenberg, 2008; Satir, 1972, 1983). The approach has three overarching goals. First, family members will grow in understanding of self and in the ability to communicate congruently. Second, family members will develop increased respect for the uniqueness of each member. Last, family members will view individual uniqueness as an opportunity for growth (Gladding, 2007; Goldenberg & Goldenberg, 2008). In the human validation process approach, the family therapist is a facilitator, a resource person, an observer, a detective, and a teacher/model of congruent communication, warmth, and empathy. The therapist is highly active, personally involved in the system, yet able to confront when necessary. Typically, the marital or couple dyad is seen first and then conjoint family therapy is convened. The approach is humanistic and highly experiential, using techniques such as the family life fact chronology (a chronology of significant events in the life of the family—and the extended family—typically obtained at the beginning of counseling); family sculpting (whereby one or more family members, during a counseling session, physically place family members in positions that signify their role or position in the family); and family reconstruction (in this procedure, typically done in group settings, a family member enlists persons to role-play family members and enact significant family events) (Gladding, 2007; Goldenberg & Goldenberg, 2008; Satir, 1972, 1983).

Experiential Family Therapy

Experiential family therapy, developed by Carl Whitaker, characterizes family dysfunction in terms of interactional rigidity and emotional deadness. The specific presenting problem is often related to preestablished roles for—and collusions between—family members. Symptoms often serve to maintain the status quo (Goldenberg & Goldenberg, 2008). The primary goal of experiential therapy is growth and creativity, rather than mere symptom reduction, because individual growth and creative freedom will reduce the need for the symptom. According to this approach, growth occurs when family members are able to experience the present moment and communicate that experience with other family members. Experiential family therapists focus on *being* fully with the client family and to use themselves to help family members fully express what they are experiencing. Typically working with a co-therapist, experiential family therapists are very active but usually not very directive, serving as a coach or surrogate grandparent. Using a conjoint family therapy framework, the therapeutic relationship—or *therapist as a person*—is the primary technique. Additional techniques include reframing (e.g., the therapist suggests that presenting problems are attempts at growth); modeling fantasy alternatives (e.g., role-playing behavioral possibilities), the therapeutic use of self (whereby therapists share fantasies, images, and personal metaphors from their lives); and "as if" situations (whereby family members enact new roles and experience new perspectives) (Gladding, 2007; Goldenberg & Goldenberg, 2008).

Narrative Therapy

Narrative therapy, developed by Michael White and David Epston, deviates from traditional systems thinking. According to this approach, a family is a microsystem embedded in a cultural macrosystem. The family does have its own belief and value system, but it is significantly influenced by beliefs and values of the larger cultural system. According to narrative therapy, dysfunction stems from oppressive forces external to families that generate family problems. Families fail to recognize their strengths and abilities and develop personal and family *narratives* that are centered on the problem and are failure oriented. The goal of narrative therapy is to help the family *re-story* the problem-saturated narrative, thereby *authoring* a new and ongoing narrative of success and empowerment. Narrative therapists make extensive use of reflection-oriented questions to help the family (a) assess the problem; (b) externalize the problem (e.g., How does *anger* try to control your interactions?); (c) find strengths by discovering *unique outcomes* (times when the problem is not present or distressing; e.g., Tell me about a time when *anger* tried to take control and you did not let it. What was different about this time?); (d) discover *preferred outcomes* (e.g., What will your relationship look like when you are consistently not letting *anger* take control?); and (e) create a new story (clients liberate themselves from their problem-saturated narrative and create a new story about themselves that reenvisions their past, present, and future). The therapist serves as editor, reader, and publisher of the family's new story (with the family's permission) (Freedman & Combs, 1996; Gladding, 2007; Goldenberg & Goldenberg, 2008; Watts, 2003; West, Watts, Trepal, Wester, & Lewis, 2001).

Solution-Focused Brief Therapy

Originally developed by Steve de Shazer, solution-focused brief therapy (SFBT) also deviates from traditional systems thinking and shares with narrative therapy the notion that knowledge is chronologically and culturally embedded. According to this approach, clients and client families *language* their realities, and their realities can be changed by *doing* and *viewing* things differently (O'Hanlon & Weiner-Davis, 2003). Clients and client families present for counseling because they develop ongoing, recurring patterns of problem-solving that do not work, and consequently, they become demoralized and discouraged. The fundamental goal of SFBT is to assist families in the process of restoring patterns of hope (Littrell, 1998). The client-counselor relationship in SFBT is cooperative, collaborative, optimistic, and respectful. SFBT counselors seek to help clients change family members' behavior and attitudes from a problem/failure focus to a focus on solutions and success and to discover latent assets, resources, and strengths that may have been overlooked as family members focus primarily on problems and liabilities (Watts & Pietrzak, 2000). Similar to narrative therapists, SFBT counselors make extensive use of reflection-oriented questions as they work with clients and client families. Techniques commonly used in SFBT include the pre-session change question (e.g., Between the time you made the appointment and right now, have you made any movement toward a solution to your problem?); the miracle question (e.g., If a miracle occurred tonight and you awoke tomorrow and the problem was gone, what would be different in you life that would indicate the problem was solved?); the *first sign* question (e.g., What would be the first indication to you that the miracle had occurred? What can you start doing right now to begin making some of this miracle occur?); exception finding questions (e.g., Are there times when the problems does not occur? How are things different at those times?); scaling questions (e.g., On a scale of 1 to 10, how committed are you to solving this problem? If I asked your wife, how would she answer?); and cheerleading (e.g., Wow, that's great. How were you able to do that?) (DeJong & Berg, 1998; Littrell, 1998; O'Hanlon & Weiner-Davis, 2003; Watts, 2003; West et al., 2001).

ETHICAL ISSUES IN COUPLE AND FAMILY COUNSELING

Every professional mental health discipline and association has a code of ethics, and all of the codes address issues such as client welfare, confidentiality, counselor competence, and dual relationships. We would be remiss in failing to address, albeit briefly, some ethical issues that are typically not addressed in individual- and group-oriented ethical guidelines. In an excellent text addressing ethical, legal, and professional issues in couple and family counseling, Wilcoxon, Remley, Gladding, and Huber (2007, p. 122) delineate, in the form of questions, a number of ethical issues unique to couple and family counseling that merit careful reflection.

- *Defining problems.* "Can therapists automatically assume the right to define couples' and families' presenting problems in terms of their own therapeutic orientation?"
- *Convening counseling.* "How much concerted effort (or pressure) can therapists exert in convening all significant familial and extrafamilial members for therapy sessions?" Furthermore, "Should willing individual marital partners or several family members seeking assistance go untreated because one individual refuses to participate?"
- *Facilitating change.* "Should therapists impose their control on couples and families? If so, to what extent should they impose it in seeking change in the relationship system?" In addition, "How much intrasystem stress should be engendered or allowed to materialize in the pursuit of change?"
- *Employing paradox.* "What are the ethical implications inherent in employing paradoxical procedures?"
- *Considering context.* "How can the impact of working with couples and families within the larger context of service agency impingements be ethically pursued." Furthermore, "What other nontraditional family structures and dynamics exist to present unique ethical concerns for marriage and family therapists?" (Wilcoxon et al., 2007, p. 122)

Professional ethical codes cannot address every possible situation and, therefore, serve as guidelines for reasonable and prudent ethical decision-making. Ethical codes are not static documents and are periodically revised due to changing community standards and situations as well as developing technologies. As Wilcoxon et al. (2007) indicate,

> [Ethical codes are] finite document[s] that can cover only a limited number of issues. To a large extent, historical factors influence what is incorporated into any code of ethics. Significant changes in society can result in a code that omits issues of current concern or contains gaps in its discussion of those issues. (p. 173)

For example, Wilcoxon et al. identify four complex contemporary ethical issues that may have significant impact on both counselors and client systems. These include the use of technology in couple and family counseling, the implications of diagnosis—the *Diagnostic and Statistical Manual* and its use in couple and family counseling—managed mental health care considerations, conflicts arising from dual or multiple relationships, AIDS and the counselor's duty to protect, and publication and research ethical considerations.

A CAREER AS A MARRIAGE AND FAMILY COUNSELOR/THERAPIST

Although there are numerous graduate programs preparing marriage and family counselors/therapists (MFC/Ts), there is still concern that there will not be enough mental health workers to serve our nation's needs in the future. The report of the Annapolis Coalition on the Behavioral Health Workforce expresses concerns that there is "an anemic pipeline of new recruits to meet the complex behavioral needs" of our population (Hoge et al., 2007, p. 2). Many MFC/T graduates like to stay close to larger cities, where most mental health workers are concentrated, leaving rural areas underserved (Hogg Foundation for Mental Health, 2007; Center for Health Statistics: Health Professions Resource Center, 2006). Another issue is the aging of MFC/Ts. Nationally, the average age of MFC/Ts is 54 (Northey, 2004).

Work Locations and Income for Couple and Family Counselors/Therapists

Employment sites for MFC/Ts include community mental health agencies, private practice, inpatient facilities and hospitals, social service agencies, churches, universities and research centers, courts and prisons, business and consulting companies, employee assistance programs, and health maintenance organizations (American Association for Marriage and Family Therapy [AAMFT], 2007a). In a 2002 survey with 252 clinical members responding, AAMFT found that private practitioners averaged $58,787 per year, while MFC/Ts working in agency or organizational settings averaged $46,850 (AAMFT, 2007b). In another study, Northey (2004) found that the mean MFC/T salary in 2004 was $46,573 compared to the mean national income of slightly over $43,000. Career InfoNet cited the median yearly wages for MFC/Ts in 2005 to be $42,300 (America's Career InfoNet, 2007b).

The Job Outlook for Couple and Family Counselors/Therapists

The U.S. Department of Labor predicts that the number of MFC/Ts in the United States will change from 24,000 in 2004 to 30,000 in 2014, an increase of 25 percent (America's Career InfoNet, 2007a). The growth for MFC/Ts is projected to be faster than average, nationally (O*NET OnLine, 2007).

A Day in the Life of a Couple and Family Counselor

A Day in the Life of a Marriage and Family Therapist in Private Practice

My name is Sara and I am a master's level Licensed Marriage and Family Therapist in private practice working in a small county seat city. I work full-time with as many as 32 client hours scheduled each week, although with cancelations and schedule changes I typically see only 28–30 face-to-face hours each week. Additionally, I am licensed as both a professional counselor and a social worker.

I've have 32 years of professional experience, starting as a therapist in a long-term adolescent treatment program, followed by several years as a community mental health worker in a major city. Three years into my career, I added a part-time private practice. Following a move to the small city, I developed contacts within the community, focusing on marketing my practice to physicians, ministers, and social service agencies in the community. Today I carry the lease for a multi-office suite, subletting space to a psychologist (full-time), and one part-time marriage and family therapist. I hire and train one part-time receptionist and one part-time billing clerk. I pay bills, clean toilets, call exterminators, buy computer equipment, and make sure the office has adequate office supplies. Since time management is crucial to profitability, I frequently use the hours freed by cancelations to attend to record keeping, case follow-up, bill paying, supply purchases, and catching a bite to eat. There are other tasks to attend to between client sessions. Insurance companies must be called requesting additional sessions, 30-page packets must be filled in each year for re-credentialing with each provider panel (I'm on over 20 panels). Client-permitted calls are made to school personnel, physicians, and other mental health care personnel for purposes of planning treatment, consultation, and exchanging records. Other spare moments are used to consult with my colleagues or to supervise the work of my employees. Since some insurance companies require electronic submission, I carefully select office software, billing formats, and attend to HIPPA requirements. In order to maintain my licenses, I obtain Continuing Education Units at state, regional, and sometimes national conferences, although I am keenly aware that if I don't work, I don't get paid.

I highly value the freedom to set my own schedule and to manage my own practice. I typically start my week with a 10 hour day followed by three 8 hour days and a 6 hour day, starting and ending at different times during the day. I don't work weekends, but work four evenings per week (my children are grown and my husband works several evenings per week). My self-imposed limit is five hours of clients in a row. Although I often see couples and families on a cash only basis, my practice is primarily insurance work, seeing individuals of all ages. I sustain a strong referral base with physicians due to regularly spending 5–10 minutes consulting with the families of my insurance clients. I supplement talk therapy with sand tray and creative arts/activity therapy, trading off the cost of the additional office space needed for those modalities for the flexibility of moving to rooms specifically set up for those modalities, and the benefits each provide in working with children and adolescents especially. Because time is such a premium, I take some notes during session and then quickly complete the notes before the next session starts. I use a laptop computer in my office to look up resources for clients during sessions; I've become adroit at googling for client resources.

I prevent burnout by taking care of myself. I arrange my work week to allow personal time for exercise, good nutrition, and time with my family. My wellness focus includes attending to my spiritual needs, maintaining pets and plants, and enjoying recreational reading. I leave my work at the office.

TRAINING AND CREDENTIALING OF COUPLE AND FAMILY COUNSELORS/THERAPISTS

Couple and family counselors have been sharing information and informally training potential colleagues since the late 1950s. Some of the early training was provided through workshops at national meetings for the American Association of Marriage Counselors and the American Orthopsychiatric Association, through workshops held at various agencies and through research projects focusing on families across the country. Throughout the 1960s and into the 1970s, education in the field came through workshops, conferences, and staff training through organizations. This tradition continues and expands as current and potential MFC/Ts seek workshops, conferences, training programs and graduate course work.

Professional Associations for Couple and Family Counselors/Therapists

By the late 1970s, the American Association for Marriage and Family Counselors (AAMFC) set standards for student, associate, and clinical memberships. In 1978 AAMFC changed its name to the American Association for Marriage and Family Therapy. Other professional associations have influenced the direction of training of MFC/Ts (Gladding, 2007). A group of practitioners created the American Family Therapy Academy in 1977. In 1986, Division 43 (Family Psychology) of the American Psychological Association was formed. The American Counseling Association (ACA) also has a division for marriage and family counselors. The International Association of Marriage and Family Counselors (IAMFC) was formed in 1986 and affiliated with the American Association for Counseling and Development (now known as the American Counseling Association) in 1990 (Smith, Carlson, Stevens-Smith, & Dennison, 1995). Each association created standards for membership, which in turn have been codified into specific graduate course work and training programs. The most influential organizations for couple and family counselors and therapists are IAMFC and AAMFT. Please see Additional Resources at the end of this chapter for Internet links to the aforementioned associations.

IAMFC Training Standards

The IAMFC worked closely with the Council for Accreditation of Counseling and Related Educational Programs (CACREP) to establish standards for training marriage and family counselors. Programs demonstrating the ability to meet those standards receive CACREP accreditation for "marital, couple and family counseling/therapy." Currently there are 32 CACREP-accredited marital, couple, and family counseling/therapy master's level programs.

Marital, couple, and family counseling/therapy programs carrying CACREP accreditation must meet common CACREP core curriculum standards (CACREP, 2009), as well as specific curricular experiences and demonstrated knowledge and skills in the following areas:

- Foundations of marital, couple, and family counseling/therapy (history, epistemological philosophy, professional orientation and roles, ethical issues related to working with couples and families, diversity training, and applications)
- Contextual dimensions of marital, couple, and family counseling/therapy (dynamics of couples and families, human sexuality and applications for MFC/Ts, societal trends, and diversity issues impacting practice)
- Knowledge and skill requirements for marital, couple, and family counseling/therapy (application of theory to practice with couples,

families, and individuals; interviewing, assessing, and intervention skills; preventative approaches; specific problems that impede progress with families; and applications of research and technology)
- Clinical instruction (600-hour internship, with 240 hours of direct service defined as work with families, couples, and individuals from a systemic perspective). (CACREP, 2009)

AAMFT Training Standards

The graduate coursework guidelines for AAMFT are divided into five categories, including 11 specific master's level courses and practicum experiences. The curriculum categories include marriage and family studies, marriage and family therapy, human development, professional ethics, and research. Clinical experience is provided in a one-year, 300-hour clinical practicum at the graduate level followed by at least two years postgraduate clinical work experience (1,000 hours minimum) under the supervision of an AAMFT-approved supervisor (minimum 200 hours of supervision).

An accreditation commission was established by AAMFC in the late 1970s to establish standards for accreditation of both universities and free-standing institutes. For example, in 1978, there were three universities accredited by AAMFT: East Texas State University, the University of Southern California, and Brigham Young University. In addition, AAMFT accredited free-standing institutes such as Milwaukee Family Service and the Philadelphia Child Guidance Clinic. The Commission on Accreditation for Marriage and Family Therapy Education (COAMFTE) now sets standards and accredits programs meeting academic and clinical preparation standards for clinical membership in AAMFT. Today, there are 60 master's level and 23 doctoral level COAMFTE-accredited university programs in the United States and Canada. Additionally, COAMFTE accredits 16 free-standing institutes.

State Licensure

Both ACA and AAMFT have worked with state level counseling and MFT organizations to seek licensure in states for MFC/Ts. All 50 states and the District of Columbia have licensure for MFC/Ts. Each state has its own standards for academic preparation and post-degree supervised internships. The AAMFT Web site (www.aamft.org) offers a handy reference listing contact information for each state in the United States and each province in Canada. As states have achieved licensure of MFC/Ts, university programs have adjusted curriculum to prepare program graduates to meet the academic and clinical experience requirements for licensure in their respective states or provinces.

The Reciprocal Nature of State Licensure and Association Membership

The two national associations speaking for MFC/Ts, IAMFC and AAMFT, have adapted their certification and clinical membership standards, respectively, to accept MFC/T licensees. For example, the National Credentialing Academy (2007) certifies state-licensed MFC/Ts in good standing, who show no injunctions or malpractice judgments or pending actions. The academy also certifies National Board Certified Counselors with acceptable MFC/T coursework, postgraduate supervision, and letters of reference; CACREP and COAMFTE graduates with letters of endorsement; AAMFT Clinical Members; and master's level graduates in the behavioral sciences with evidence of appropriate training, supervision, and endorsements (National Credentialing Academy, 2007).

The AAMFT will grant clinical membership to applicants with a license to practice as a MFC/T or to applicants with an appropriate master's or doctoral degree; successful completion of specified courses in marriage and family studies, marriage and family therapy, human development, professional ethics, and research; a one-year, 300-hour clinical practicum; and a minimum of two years postgraduate clinical work experience (1,000 hours minimum) under the supervision of a AAMFT-approved supervisor (minimum 200 hours of supervision).

SPECIAL TOPICS AND FURTHER CONSIDERATIONS

Systems Counseling Approaches in School Settings

Since the 1980s family counselors have recognized the influence that society's larger systems have on family systems. Lusterman (1988) introduced the idea of adopting an ecosystemic approach to working with families presenting with a child who is having school problems. In this approach, the family counselor must have knowledge of both the family system and the school system and how the interaction of those two systems may impede or enhance the child's progress. The family counselor will "map the ecosystem" (Lusterman) to decide who to include in the treatment plan and how to invite change in a way that does not blame either system for the problem, but rather encourages both systems to work toward a solution that will benefit the child. In this role, the counselor becomes a sort of systems consultant who facilitates a family-school collaboration leading to systemic change (Wynne, McDaniel, & Weber, 1986).

More recently, experts in the fields of both school counseling and family counseling have suggested that professional school counselors would benefit from training in family counseling and systems theory in order to better serve students in schools (Davis, 2005; Holcomb-McCoy, 2004; Kraus, 1998). Since the inception of the vocational school counseling model of the 1950s, school counseling has been viewed from an individual perspective. The growing shift from an individual focus in counseling to a systems approach has impacted schools as well as other counseling settings. Schools and families are the primary socializers of children; therefore, school counselors who have the training and ability to work within a systemic approach are able to assist their clients in attaining both educational and family goals.

Online Couple and Family Counseling

The use of the Internet to deliver counseling services to clients who are unable to be in face-to-face meetings with a counselor are becoming more commonplace and acceptable. The ACA established norms and guidelines for counseling over the Internet in *Ethical Standards for Internet Counseling*. This ethical code has been subsequently incorporated and updated in the new ACA *Code of Ethics* (ACA, 2005; Kaplan, 2006). Some of the Internet tools available for online counseling are e-mail consultation, text-based chat rooms, and videoconferencing (Jencius & Sager, 2001). Although the idea of being able to provide services to families who live in remote areas or are confined to their homes because of illness is appealing to family counselors, many issues relevant to Internet counseling need to be addressed (Pollock, 2006; Jencius & Sager). Family counselors must consider the implications of the following: (a) the inability to guarantee confidentiality in online counseling; (b) the problem of setting clear boundaries when the Internet is available 24 hours a day, every day; (c) the problem of counseling over the Internet across state lines and the inconsistency of licensure and regulations from state to state; (d) the refusal of many insurance companies to cover Internet counseling; and (e) the risks of not being able to clearly discern the facial expressions, body language, and other dispositions of the clients, which may lead to overlooking serious pertinent information about clients. Clearly the availability and increasingly more *therapy-friendly* modalities of Internet counseling will continue to increase, and thus, couples and family counselors need to engage in rigorous research regarding the efficacy and ethical implications of this new field.

CONCLUSION

Family configurations have changed significantly in recent decades and today's counselors work with diverse family structures and dynamics. Counselors working with couples and families face significant challenges and must be knowledgeable and well trained in the theory and practice of couple and family counseling and the professional issues involved with the discipline. This chapter was merely an overview of the couple and family counseling field. Persons interested in working with couples and families should actively pursue training and supervision in couple and family counseling both during and after their formal counseling education.

CHAPTER REVIEW

1. Some basic characteristics of the family as a system include holism, communication, circular causality, coexisting subsystems, morphogenesis, and homeostasis.
2. Just as individuals must negotiate various developmental tasks throughout the human life cycle, so also families must negotiate developmental tasks throughout various family life cycles.
3. Although Adler and Dreikurs began working with the family as a unit in the 1920s, it

was not until much later in the 20th century that family counseling received universal acceptance within the mental health profession. Further, the profession of couple and family counseling has evolved significantly the past three decades, largely due to significant societal and economic changes.

4. Characteristics of well-functioning families most commonly mentioned in the literature include commitment, communication, clear boundaries, positive family

atmosphere, connectedness, adaptability, and spirituality. Three commonly discussed characteristics of family dysfunction include dysfunctional boundaries, dysfunctional communication, and dysfunctional family structure.

5. There are numerous approaches to family counseling, and many of the traditional individual-focused approaches have developed couple and family applications. Seven of the most prominent approaches specific to family counseling include Bowenian family therapy, structural family therapy, strategic family therapy, the human validation process approach, experiential family therapy, narrative therapy, and solution-focused brief therapy.

6. Ethical issues unique to couple and family counseling include how problems are defined, determining who should attend counseling sessions, therapist use of power to facilitate systemic change, therapist use of paradoxical interventions in family counseling, and the importance of considering numerous contextual issues when working with couples and families.

7. The two most influential associations for couple and family counselors/therapists are the International Association of Marriage and Family Counselors and the American Association for Marriage and Family Therapy.

8. Couple and family therapists can be credentialed via professional certification and state licensure.

REVIEW QUESTIONS

1. Define and explain the family from a systemic and developmental perspective.
2. Discuss how couple and family counseling has developed as a profession.
3. Describe the differences between well-functioning families and those struggling with family dysfunction.
4. Discuss similarities among the various approaches to family counseling. What differences do you see?

5. What aspects of training and credentialing are unique to couple and family counseling when compared to the requirements of the National Certified Counselor credential or your state's professional counseling license?
6. What ethical issues unique to couple and family counseling appear to be the most problematic to you?

ADDITIONAL RESOURCES

- International Association of Marriage and Family Counselors (http://www.iamfc.com)
- American Association for Marriage and Family Therapy (www.aamft.org)
- American Family Therapy Academy (http://www.afta.org)

- American Psychological Association Division 43 (Family Psychology; http://www.apa.org/divisions/div43)
- International Family Therapy Association (http://www.ifta-familytherapy.org/home.html)

REFERENCES

American Association for Marriage and Family Therapy. (2007a). *A career as a marriage and family therapist*. Washington, DC: Author. Retrieved May 20, 2007, from http://www.aamft.org/resources/Career_PracticeInformation/career.htm.

American Association for Marriage and Family Therapy. (2007b). *What MFTs get paid*. Washington, DC: Author. Retrieved May 20, 2007, from http://www.aamft.org/resources/Career_PracticeInformation/MFTSalaries.asp.

Americas Career InfoNet. (2007a). *Occupation information: Employment trends by occupation across states: Marriage and family therapists*. Washington, DC: Department of Labor. Retrieved May, 20, 2007, from http://www.acinet.org/acinet/occ_rep.asp?id=&level=BAplus&optstatus=101000000&nodeid=2&soccode=211013&stfips=18.

Americas Career InfoNet. (2007b). *Occupation information: Marriage and family therapists: Texas*. Washington, DC: U.S. Department of Labor. Retrieved May 20, 2007, from http://www.acinet.org/acinet/occ_rep.asp?level=&optstatus=101000000&id=&nodeid=2&soccode=211013&stfips=48.

American Counseling Association. (2005). *Code of ethics*. Retrieved November 16, 2009 from http://www.counseling.org/Resources/CodeOfEthics/TP/Home/CT2.aspx.

Beavers, W. R., & Hampson, R. B. (1990). *Successful families*. New York: W. W. Norton.

Beavers, W. R., & Hampson, R. B. (2003). Measuring family competence: The Beavers systems model. In F. Walsh (Ed.), *Normal family processes* (3rd ed., 549–580). New York: Guilford.

Becvar, D. S., & Becvar, R. (2006). *Family therapy: A systemic integration* (6th ed.). Boston: Allyn & Bacon.

Beels, C. (2002). Notes for a cultural history of family therapy. *Family Process, 41*, 67–82.

Bowen, M. (1978). *Family therapy in clinical practice*. New York: Aronson.

Carlson, J. (2002). Strategic family therapy. In J. Carlson & D. Kjos (Eds.), *Theories and strategies of family therapy* (pp. 80–97). Boston: Allyn & Bacon.

Carlson, J., Watts, R. E., & Maniacci, M. (2006). *Adlerian therapy: Theory and practice*. Washington, DC: American Psychological Association.

Carter, B., & McGoldrick, M. (Eds.). (1999). *The extended family life cycle: Individual, family, and social perspectives* (3rd ed.). Boston: Allyn & Bacon.

Center for Health Statistics: Health Professions Resource Center. (2006, February). *Highlights: The supply of mental health professionals in Texas—2005* (Publication No. 25–12347). Austin, TX: Author.

Council for Accreditation of Counseling and Related Educational Programs.(2009). *2009 standards*. Alexandria, VA: Author. Retrieved November 16, 2009 from http://67.199.126.156/doc/2009%20Standards.pdf.

Curran, D. (1983). *Traits of healthy family*. New York: Winston.

Davis, K. M., & Lambie, G. W. (2005). Family engagement: A collaborative, systemic approach for middle school counselors. *Professional School Counseling, 9*, 144–151.

DeJong, P., & Berg, I. K. (1998). *Interviewing for solutions*. Pacific Grove, CA: Brooks/Cole.

Epstein, N. B., Bishop, D. S., & Baldwin, L. M. (1982). The McMaster model: A view of healthy family functioning. In F. Walsh (Ed.), *Normal family processes* (pp. 115–141). New York: Guilford.

Epstein, N. B., Ryan, C. E., Bishop, D. S., Miller, I. W., & Keitner, G. I. (2003). The McMaster model: A view of healthy family functioning. In F. Walsh (Ed.), *Normal family processes* (3rd ed., 581–607). New York: Guilford.

Foley, V. D. (1989). *Family therapy*. In R. J. Corsini & D. Wedding (Eds.), *Current psychotherapies* (4th ed., pp. 455–500). Itasca, IL: Peacock.

Framo, J. (1996). A personal retrospective of the family therapy field: Then and now. *Journal of Marital and Family Therapy, 22*, 289–316.

Freedman, J., & Combs, G. (1996). *Narrative therapy: The social construction of preferred realities*. New York: Norton.

Gladding, S. T. (2007). *Family therapy: History, theory, and practice* (4th ed.). Upper Saddle River, NJ: Merrill Prentice Hall.

Goldenberg, H., & Goldenberg, I. (2008). *Family therapy: An overview* (7th ed.). Belmont, CA: Thompson Brooks/Cole.

Hoge, M., Morris, J., Daniels, A., Stuart, G., Huey, L., & Adams, N. (2007). *An action plan on behavioral health workforce development*. Cincinnati, OH: Annapolis Coalition on the Behavioral Health Workforce.

Hogg Foundation for Mental Health. (2007). *The mental health workforce in Texas: A snapshot of the issues*. Austin, TX: Author.

Holcomb-McCoy, C. (2004). Using the family autobiography in school counselor preparation: An introduction to a systemic perspective. *The Family Journal, 12*, 21–25.

Jencius, M., & Sager, D. (2001). The practice of marriage and family counseling in cyberspace. *The Family Journal, 9*, 295–301.

Kaplan, D. (2006). Ethical use of technology in counseling. Retrieved November 16, 2009, from http://www.counseling.org/Publications/CounselingTodayArticles.aspx?AGuid=421e99b9-ec6c-4f46-a6c4-4f8b6101275a.

Kaslow, F. (2000). Continued evolution of family therapy: The last twenty years. *Contemporary Family Therapy, 22,* 357–386.

Kraus, I. (1998). A fresh look at school counseling: A family-systems approach. *Professional School Counseling, 1,* 12–17.

Littrell, J. M. (1998). *Brief counseling in action.* New York: W. W. Norton.

Lusterman, D. D. (1988). Family therapy and schools: An ecosystemic approach. *Family Therapy Today, 3,* 1–3.

Minuchin, S. (1974). *Families and family therapy.* Cambridge, MA: Harvard University Press.

Minuchin, S., & Fishman, H. C. (1981). *Family therapy techniques.* Cambridge, MA: Harvard University Press.

National Credentialing Academy. (2007, May). *National credentialing academy for family therapist standards.* Corpus Christi, TX: Author. Retrieved May 20, 2007, from http://www.natlacad.4t.com/standards.html.

Nichols, M. P. (1988). *The power of the family.* New York: Fireside.

Northey, Jr., W. (2004, November/December). Who are marriage and family therapists? *Family Therapy Magazine, 3,* 10–13.

Nugent, F. A., & Jones, K. D. (2005). *Introduction to the profession of counseling* (4th ed.). Upper Saddle River, NJ: Merrill Prentice Hall.

O'Hanlon, B., & Weiner-Davis, M. (2003). *In search of solutions* (rev. ed.). New York: W. W. Norton.

O*NET OnLine. (2007, May). Summary report for: 21–1013.00 Marriage and family therapists. Washington, DC: U.S. Department of Labor. Retrieved May 20, 2007, from http://online.onetcenter.org/link/summary/21–1013.00.

Pollock, S. L. (2006). Internet counseling and its feasibility for marriage and family counseling. *The Family Journal, 14,* 65–70.

Rekers, G. A. (1988). *Counseling families.* Dallas: Word.

Satir, V. (1972). *Peoplemaking.* Palo Alto, CA: Science and Behavior Books.

Satir, V. (1983). *Conjoint family therapy* (3rd ed.). Palo Alto, CA: Science and Behavior Books.

Sherman, R., & Dinkmeyer, D. (1987). *Systems of family therapy: An Adlerian integration.* New York: Brunner/Mazel.

Smith, R. L., Carlson, J., Stevens-Smith, P., & Dennison, M. (1995). Marriage and family counseling. *Journal of Counseling and Development, 74,* 154–157.

Stinnett, N. (1985). Six qualities that make families strong. In G. A. Rekers (Ed.), *Family building: Six qualities of a strong family* (pp. 35–50). Ventura, CA: Regal.

Stinnett, N., Chesser, B., & DeFrain, J. (Eds.). (1979). *Building family strengths.* Lincoln: University of Nebraska Press.

Stinnett, N., DeFrain, J., King, K., & Knaub, P. (Eds.). (1981). *Building family strengths 3: Roots of well-being.* Lincoln: University of Nebraska Press.

Walsh, F. (Ed.) (2003). *Normal family processes* (3rd ed.). New York: Guilford.

Watts, R. E. (2001). Integrating cognitive and systemic perspectives: An interview with Frank M. Dattilo. *The Family Journal, 9,* 472–476.

Watts, R. E. (2003). Selecting family interventions. In D. Kaplan (Ed.), *Family counseling for all counselors* (pp. 121–160). Greensboro, NC: ERIC/CAPS.

Watts, R. E., & Pietrzak, D. (2000). Adlerian "encouragement" and the therapeutic process of solution-focused brief therapy. *Journal of Counseling and Development, 78,* 442–447.

Watts, R. E., Trusty, J., & Lim, M. G. (1996). Characteristics of healthy families as a model of social interest. *Canadian Journal of Adlerian Psychology, 26,* 1–12.

Watzlawick, P., Beavin, J. H., & Jackson, D. D. (1967). *Pragmatics of human communication.* New York: Norton.

Watzlawick, P., Weakland, J. H., & Fisch, R. (1974). *Change: Principles of problem formation and problem resolution.* New York: W. W. Norton.

West, J. D., Watts, R. E., Trepal, H. C., Wester, K. L., & Lewis, T. F. (2001). Opening space for client reflection: A postmodern consideration. *The Family Journal: Counseling and Therapy for Couples and Families, 9,* 431–437.

Wilcoxon, S. A., Remley, T. P., Jr., Gladding, S. T., & Huber, C. H. (2007). *Ethical, legal, and professional issues in the practice of marriage and family therapy* (4th ed.). Upper Saddle River, NJ: Merrill Prentice Hall.

Wynne, L. C., McDaniel, S. H., & Weber, T. T. (1986). *Systems consultation: A new perspective for family therapy.* New York: Guilford.

PART 4

Developing a Personal and Professional Counselor Identity

CHAPTER 15

Considering the Counselor as a Person

LEARNING OBJECTIVES

After reading this chapter, you should be able to

- understand how your characteristics will influence your development as a counseling professional;

- understand how aspects of the profession will impact you personally and professionally;

- realize the influence that your biases can have on your success as a professional counselor;

- describe how to validate the qualities of others and gain validation for yourself; and

- discuss the aspects of yourself that require continuing attention for your health and the growth of your clients.

CHAPTER OUTLINE

Introduction

A Great Profession—If It Fits You

Reasons for Becoming a Professional Counselor

Facing the Challenges of Professional Counseling
Understanding Counselor Vulnerability
Dealing with Difficult Clients
Coping with Pressures for Results

INTRODUCTION

Professional counselors come in all shapes, sizes, colors, and views of the world. They enter counselor training, not as blank slates, but instead with all the unique characteristics that genes, parents, relatives, friends, enemies, and the whole of their environment have produced. The already complex people who begin training then go through many more changes before they become professional counselors (Hazler & Kottler, 2005). It is a different person, not just a more knowledgeable one, who is successful in counselor training, and the transition is filled with unexpected obstacles to overcome.

Counseling is a deeply personal relationship in which the complexities of the client, counselor, and environment challenge the beliefs, skills, knowledge, and reactions of each person involved. Preparing for multiple relationships like these requires much more than information and skill acquisition. Extensive self-examination of each counselor's personal values, biases, emotional triggers, and beliefs about people who are different from them is essential. This personalized learning process demands motivation, energy, and personal risk-taking in order to seek and integrate the information into the new person that graduates from a counselor education program.

This chapter will help you recognize the circumstances and pressures that require professional counselors to do extensive self-examination of their motivations, biases, values, and beliefs about people. It will also demonstrate how this self-examination is connected to the characteristics needed to become a successful professional counselor and remain so without burning out. Throughout the chapter you will find ways to initiate, follow through, and integrate this personal development. You should emerge from the chapter with a better understanding of how the person you are matches what is needed to be a professional counselor, the challenges to be faced, and how to maintain the many aspects of your health in the growing process.

A GREAT PROFESSION—IF IT FITS YOU

How are you going to know if this profession will be the right fit for you? There is no simple answer and even the complex answers change as you grow as a person and professional. So what does it feel like when someone has been in the profession for years? Perhaps a way to begin is to get a sense of our experiences.

I (RH) can pretty much identify the time and place where it hit me that I might want to be a counselor. The place was an elementary school classroom where I was teaching. The students and I had just had a great discussion about the lives of the students, life, and how to get the most from it. Then we went back to the next lesson and the realization hit that I didn't want to leave the personal discussion for a science lesson. I wanted more of this personal involvement with these students. The kind of involvement I could get as a counselor.

During the almost 40 years since that day in the classroom, I have counseled in the military, a prison, schools, universities, and private practice. Many of those years also involved research and training counselors. It sounds like I couldn't hold a job, but fortunately that was not the case. As I continued to learn more about different people and myself, I kept changing. The changes brought about new doubts, desires, and opportunities to meet new challenges that I never dreamed were there. It has been the best of times.

The years have also seen the worst of times from the stress of the work and the changes in myself. It never crossed my mind when I started this career path that I would get bored with it at times, fail with clients, or see individuals and groups of people being hurt and feel helpless to fix it. What do you do when people you work with fail to improve, commit a crime, or suicide? How much of that is because I didn't do all I could? These times produce reactions that raise doubts about who I really am, what I really know, my actual value, and whether I can be a better person. The doubts bring challenges that are not the pleasant ones we might choose to face.

As far as I (KBW) can remember, I have always enjoyed being with people and helping people get over hurdles to make themselves better. The past 23 years in the counselor profession have taken me to several higher education institutions including small, private, historically black colleges and universities; small, private, historically European American colleges and universities; church-affiliated schools; and large public institutions. The experiences have taught me that I not only like what I do, but I would not change it for anything in the world. All of my professional life has been in higher education as staff, faculty, or administrator. The experiences of being able to help people overcome barriers have also facilitated changes in me as I recognize parts of myself in clients. These insights keep me from being too hard on myself when frustrated with the vocational, social, and home challenges that we all undergo as a matter of life and growth.

Personal growth has been the positive residual from the problems experienced in day-to-day dealing with clients, colleagues, families, and friends. The helping profession is lined with challenges to be encountered in every walk of life that have taught me to live to "fight another day," for not only those I serve, but for myself as well. Approaching senior member status in the profession, I am reminded that I used to take myself too seriously. Now, I only take what I do seriously, recognizing that all the other distractions are just background noise that can get in the way of current success and future progress.

Several opportunities have presented themselves to do other things and make more money in corporate America. But it has been private practice, teaching, training students, and researching that have proved to be my enduring loves. The experiences have confirmed that a vocation that is natural to a person will continue to hold value even into retirement just for the love and enjoyment of the profession. Many people can do the counseling *job* and never really reach their potential as helpers or even fully enjoy the work. Only when it really fits you will you love it as a vocation and profession over your entire career.

We are all going to get tired and need recuperation from time to time throughout the year, both for ourselves and also for the benefit of those we serve. It is this reality that new human service providers must learn with time, patience, and eventual understanding of the circle of life that brings multiple challenges and opportunities. I never planned on being a college professor, but along the way I took advantage of the experiences that arose from the confidence others had in me. Most of these people had more confidence in me than I did in myself. It is taking these chances that has enhanced my growing potential and has allowed me to give back to clients, students, and peers in ways that I could never have envisioned. The right cognitive and behavioral map for your future is dynamic and not static; it includes many challenges of just being alive and being open to new people and experiences. Listening and observing for new ways to be are the great elements for helping others and yourself through this lifelong journey.

Many people choose the counseling profession and drop out long before we have. The enthusiasm and ability to cope with the daily struggles of others wears on a person, so it is essential that you recognize yourself for what you are right now, actively seek and look forward to who you will continue becoming, and take good care of yourself along the way. The process starts with examining the real reasons why you want to become a professional counselor. Next you need to consider what aspects of the counselor are most critical and how they need to be developed and maintained when problems arise. It all adds up to dealing with yourself in the wellness model that the counseling profession espouses for clients, rather than only dealing with yourself after your health becomes debilitating. An overview of those concepts comprises the remainder of this chapter.

REASONS FOR BECOMING A PROFESSIONAL COUNSELOR

Why do people enter the counseling profession? There are as many combinations of reasons as there are people, but all the publicly stated reasons are often combined with others that are not so easily admitted. Table 15.1 shows just a few examples.

The differences between the two types of reasons along with the willingness to recognize both sides are important parts of the struggles experienced by counselors-in-training and professional counselors. The desire to serve can

TABLE **15.1**

Reasons for Becoming a Counselor

Stated Reasons	What Mostly Goes Unsaid
"I want to make a difference in people's lives."	I want to feel needed.
"I admire the counselor who helped me."	I want to be admired.
"A counselor can change people's lives."	I want the power to change people's lives.
"People and their lives are so interesting."	Figuring people out makes me feel intelligent.
"Caring for others is important to society."	I want to feel cared for in relationships with clients and colleagues.
"I want to help people understand themselves and feel better about their lives."	I'll understand myself and like my life better by understanding and helping others.
"I want to do the best I can for people."	I want to be respected as a professional.
"I want to learn to help people who need it."	This degree and work will make me a success.
"People deserve a good life."	My life should be the way I envision it.

be strong, but we also need personally valued rewards to have a sense of balance in our lives (Hazler & Kottler, 2005). Spending too much time doing for others at the neglect of your own needs can lead to dysfunction (Skovholt, Grier, & Hanson, 2001; Stebnicki, 2008). We do people disservice when we give up so much of ourselves that we can no longer be effectively there for others. Counselors-in-training need to recognize both their socially admired aspects and also their more self-centered aspects (Roach & Young, 2007). These characteristics are both part of being human, so they will be present in counselors as well as those to be served.

Clients are asked to work with both the strengths of which they are proud, and also those aspects of themselves that are harder to accept. We try to convince clients that improvement in their lives will come from attending to and working with both sides. It is vitally important that counselors do no less of this self-assessment work than we ask of clients. Many aspects of counselor training will direct you to do exactly that. The tasks will not show up on multiple-choice tests, but they will be among the most challenging aspects of the program and the profession.

Active Learning Exercise **15.1**

Make a list of your reasons for becoming a professional counselor. Of which reasons are you less proud? What are the ones that you like to share with others? Share your list with others to begin your professional counselor self-exploration.

FACING THE CHALLENGES OF PROFESSIONAL COUNSELING

Whatever the specific reasons for people entering the counseling profession, there are stressors built in that demand attention if counselors are to maintain enthusiasm and commitment. The professional portion of a counselor is expected to be strong, empathic, caring, knowledgeable, and ethical in ways that always put client needs first. The trick for counselors is to recognize the potentially debilitating aspects of the work while developing these productive characteristics that will benefit others.

Understanding Counselor Vulnerability

Empathy and caring for others are key examples of what good counselors have, but these are the same qualities that create vulnerability to distress (Stebnicki, 2008; Yassen, 1995). The more empathy we have with clients, the more we become invested in their struggles and suffering. It is not easy to walk away from client experiences after a session without it taking a toll on the counselor. Potential results are compounded by counselor recognition of their responsibility for creating positive client outcomes. The fact that clients, loved ones, and other stake holders frequently have unrealistic expectations for these outcomes only adds to the pressure and potential for seeing counseling as having failed. In combination, such factors produce enormous personal pressure to solve problems that may never be satisfactorily resolved for client stakeholders or counselors themselves. Clients do have the ultimate responsibility for whether they change or remain stagnate in their ability to modify behaviors, but counselors who care about clients and are doing their best to help will still feel great personal pressure to see clients through to success.

Dealing with Difficult Clients

Counselor trainees quickly find out that clients do not always react in the ways that theories might lead one to expect. Clients can be noncommunicative, irrational, demanding, or deceitful. When things don't go their way, clients can take out their anger and frustration on the person most likely to not strike back at them—the counselor. Some of this has to do with the fact that trainees are new to the profession with a lesser degree of knowledge and skill development, but clients can be just as hard on experienced counselors. Difficult clients are simply part of the real world of counseling that must be handled effectively to experience a continuing joy and enthusiasm for the work (Kottler, 1992, 2000). Counseling can be very rewarding, but no one will tell you that counseling is easy. After all, it is only because clients are having difficulty that we have this profession.

Coping with Pressures for Results

We are in a results-oriented time. The government, HMOs (health maintenance organizations), schools, and agencies want definitive results to justify funds spent. Clients, and those who care about clients, are less interested in the funding, but adamant about results being visible in a better existence (Carney & Hazler, 2005; Cypres, Landsberg, & Spellmann, 1997). Everyone wants the results to be clear, to be specific, and to happen quickly. Agency counselors need to meet quotas for clients seen no matter how many clients don't show up for services, so the 40-hour week is often only a figment of a professional's imagination. School counselors need to deal with the most needy students, provide guidance to all, serve as support to the teachers, and then justify how it adds up to student educational progress. Mixed in the middle of it all is a pile of paperwork so that everything done and accomplished can be verified. The pressures are great and counselors need to lead personally and professionally organized lives in order to meet them. Being a professional counselor is more than therapeutically talking with clients; personal organization is a critical component of counseling success and survival.

Avoiding Burnout

The result of these and other pressures can produce numerous problematic outcomes for counselors, with burnout being the most commonly mentioned (Lawson, 2007; Stebnicki, 2008). *Burnout* is a general term describing a diminished motivation and capacity to perform at a consistently high professional level in reaction to the pressures of counseling work (Maslach, 2003). Common symptoms are decreased empathy, deteriorating professional behaviors, and increasingly unhealthy personal behaviors. Counselors who are less self-aware or give less attention to potential supporters allow the problems to continue until professional, legal, ethical, and personal problems can result. Self-aware counselors recognize the signs in themselves, or they accept the input of colleagues, supervisors, and loved ones who often see the signs first. Only when you know what is actually happening to you can you take actions to make your life better.

Active Learning Exercise **15.2**

Make a list of tasks, situations, and types of people that stress you. For each task, situation, or type of person you listed, write down what it is that causes the stress for you. How do you imagine handling or not effectively handling these types of stressors as a counselor?

Finding Support in Professional Relationships

The influence of the professionals surrounding the counselor can be highly supportive, nonexistent, or counterproductive (Hazler & Kottler, 2005). They may be professionals, but they are also people just like you with unique personalities, styles, cultural influences, and changing life situations. When life is going well they react one way, and when things are going poorly they react in other ways that can be less pleasing to colleagues. Professionalism is a key to minimizing these changes, but it doesn't eliminate them. The pressures counselors feel to be successful in stressful situations often cause them to treat colleagues worse than clients, family, or friends. Thus, it is important for counselors to take care of themselves by not internalizing the many challenges that are inherent in the profession.

The tendency is to treat professional colleagues as people who are the helpers and therefore don't need support. The results can be feeling less close to colleagues than clients and leaving colleagues sometimes resenting a perceived lack of concern for their welfare. It may sound counterintuitive, but counselors need to give similar quality attention to colleagues, supervisors, and consultants as they do to clients, or they can become professionally isolated from all the support and assistance that is available (Hazler, 2008). The effective counselor is one who consistently benefits from consultation and support from colleagues and supervisors, so it is critical to use skills with them that will promote maintenance of strong relationships.

UNDERSTANDING YOUR BIASES AND BECOMING CULTURALLY COMPETENT

We all have unique ways of looking at the world. Growing up poor in a rural community or an urban environment creates different perceptions of the world than growing up with sufficient wealth to virtually eliminate worry about heat, cold, and hunger. Minorities view society's opportunities as more limited than those from the majority culture. Religion, race, gender, and many other culturally relevant factors interact with personal dimensions to create multiple views of the world that differ between groups and also between individuals within groups. Each of these factors influences behaviors, how behaviors are perceived, and how people react to those perceptions. Cultural variations are limitless, so anyone desiring to help individuals or groups must continually seek understanding of the specific worldview being encountered and how it interacts with one's own. Understanding yourself and how others view you is the first of several steps in becoming aware and increasing ability and satisfaction.

Culture refers to patterns of human behavior and the symbolic structures that give activities meaning. It also refers to theoretical bases for understanding and evaluating human behaviors and activities ("Culture," n.d.). Discrimination in its many forms (e.g., race, sexual orientation, disability status) is often connected with the norms and biases within cultures. Bias occurs when we have inadequate understanding of culture and personality factors in others and ourselves or when we fail to act appropriately, based on what we do correctly understand. Each of us will always have biases based on our culture, and those will change as we experience different people and ways of life. The task is to become consciously aware of these biases, revise them based on new experiences and information, and realize that they are often no more or no less legitimate than those of others.

Biases include a host of prejudices, isms (e.g., racism, genderism), and things learned from home, church, school, and other institutions of social and political influence. Success as a counselor begins with admitting our biases and prejudices that have the potential to harm the people we serve (Sue & Sue, 2008). We must also recognize that people who are not part of the majority group in a country, city, or school have been and continue to be mentally and physically damaged either consciously or unconsciously by people lacking sufficient awareness needed to facilitate rapport building. *The majority rules* statement may communicate a sense of democratic action, but it can also communicate disrespect, pain, and suffering to those consistently in the minority. Finally, we must recognize and demonstrate respect for the many differences in people we contact through professional duties and social interactions. Whether those differences are large or small, and how well you recognize and deal with them, will make a huge difference in your value to others and the appreciation they have for you and your work.

It is only when we understand the importance and quality of another person's culture and realize how it compares to our own that we can stop ourselves from the type of thinking, talking, or behaving communicated in the following common statements:

- "We are all human and I do not see the gender of females when I talk to female clients and students."
- "I don't see the race and/or ethnicity of the person so I can't be biased."

These are the types of concepts that devalue the uniqueness of others, eliminating the special nature of what each individual brings to a relationship. The explicit result is that persons with one worldview will not be very successful in helping others unlike themselves. They will never really know others and will consistently misjudge the people they are serving. The differences between us are just as important to understand as the things we have in common.

Consider the example of how culture becomes important with a simple handshake. A firm handshake by North American citizens communicates competence and a strong sense of being. On the other hand, there are cultures in which people grow up learning that a firm handshake indicates aggression. What is welcomed as strength and confidence to some will be received as aggressive and threatening to others. A residual from a less than firm handshake could be a person not getting a job because of perceived weakness and lack of self-confidence. How do you react to different handshakes? First impressions of a client by a counselor often begin with a handshake, so counselors who are not fully aware of their own cultural views and are not open to alternate clients mannerisms can immediately begin making inappropriate judgments and diagnoses of clients.

Another example is handholding. Some cultures outside of the United States both permit and encourage males holding hands to display friendship and affection among heterosexual males. Many people observing males holding hands in the United States may perceive this show of affection as an inappropriate act that breaks social norms for males, while others will draw incorrect conclusions about the sexual preference or the morality of the hand holders. Our emotional reactions are less controlled than our logic and will be heavily based on the characteristics of our given cultures. Only by understanding and recognizing our cultural biases, remaining open to alternate ways of being, and continually seeking greater understanding of other people from their perspectives are we able to avoid making inappropriate judgments, statements, and decisions about others.

People do not need to come from another country or even from another area to have widely different views on what are appropriate behaviors and beliefs. We all differ, and it is up to individual counselors to recognize the differences between their own views and those they serve. Without this starting place, counselors are immediately in danger of committing at least two major ethical violations. The first is being likely to harm the other person and the second is having little likelihood of being a positive influence.

Active Learning Exercise **15.3**

Identify three to five of your beliefs about people learned from family, school, religion, and so forth. What people would disagree with you about these three to five beliefs? Seek out people who would disagree with you and take time to understand how they acquired those beliefs. Remember that this is about *their* beliefs and not your own. Share the differences with fellow students, faculty, and others to further explore who you are in comparison to others and how those differences can affect your relationships.

PROVIDING VALIDATION FOR OTHERS AND FOR YOURSELF

People can and will accept constructive feedback from friends or superiors if they feel validated by others. Two definitions of validation are uniquely tailored for human service professionals. One outlined in Wikipedia ("Validation," n.d.) views validation as a way to make legal and confirm data or information. Another version refers to the communication of respect for a person through explicitly acknowledging the experiences, opinion, and thoughts of that person as legitimate. The combined definitions describe validation as an affirming and confirming action, not about being right or wrong.

Clients come seeking validation for who they are and the lives they live, and counselors hope to find their own professional validation through the progress of clients. When clients affirm that the validation process is working, counselors too feel validated for their efforts to positively support clients' lives, feelings, struggles, and thoughts. The validation process is viewed as a way of assisting clients who in turn facilitate confidence and growth in the counselor through verbal or nonverbal communication of "a job well-done" (Wilson, 2006). An important implicit part of the validation definition is that it has nothing to do with whether you agree with the person or the issues being presented (Wilson, 2006). Right and wrong is not the issue, but affirming the experiences of others from their personal worldview is the key.

We strive to be the best possible counselors, coaches, moms, dads, or friends that can facilitate rapport building and understanding in those whose views or perceptions of the world may vary greatly from our own. The validation process can be used by anyone desiring to facilitate growth and understanding. Terms like *counselor* and *client* may predominate in this chapter, but substituting nouns like *mom, dad, teacher,* and others fit this concept equally well. Validation is a life-supporting skill in any context. Simply put, validation is the process that will let people know that you are listening and not judging (Wilson, 2006).

Positively supporting the experiences of others is the way we continue building relational capital between individuals or groups as we continue learning about ourselves and others through the validation process. Validation is also a tool to increase a greater understanding in the human condition that we call life. Accurately grasping and employing the validation concept may improve the lives of both the person being validated and the person doing the validation (Wilson, 2006).

Sometimes those we serve will view our interactions as negative and hostile, leaving them feeling isolated, misunderstood, and marginalized by an individual or system that is rigid and myopic to minority views and perceptions. Positively acknowledging these situations does not mean one has to agree or have similar experiences, but it does demonstrate valuing, understanding, and acceptance of different perspectives. For example, some may think that in order validate the experiences of people who are African American, one has to be African American or have experiences similar to African Americans. This is not true! African Americans and European Americans do view progress around racial discrimination in distinctly different ways (Smith, 2006), but when European Americans can verbally and nonverbally reflect and seek greater understanding of what most African Americans experience, European Americans can provide good space for open communication and relationship building. Cognitively relieving oneself from the need to determine who is right or wrong and replacing it with exploration and understanding of another person or group is a key to increasing rapport. The following example illustrates the difference in someone's reaction when trying to help the person to see a view you believe is more reasonable versus validating the individual's views based on their experiences.

> Mike (male career counselor) was discussing vocational options with Beth (female client) who is seeking advice on how to enter the male-dominated field of engineering. She would like to become an engineer, but is concerned about experiencing sexism (conscious or unconscious) as she enrolls in more engineering classes and eventually graduates with a master's degree. One example of the experiences she reported was that when enrolled in an introductory engineering class as an undergraduate, the male professor did not call on her several times when her hand was raised first to answer a question. This was in contradiction to what she observed when male students raised their hands. Beth also found that many of her male peers avoided her and would not let her join their study groups after several attempts and weeks of classes.
>
> After hearing Beth's (female client) experiences in the engineering class as an undergraduate, Mike (career counselor) might respond in more or less validating ways that would create corresponding reactions from Beth.
>
> *Non-validating response by Mike*—"I am not sure I understand your concerns about possible sexism in the engineering class. Is it possible that you misinterpreted and were not really being ignored in class? Could you have done something to agitate your peers or the professor? One possibility could be that the professor may not have seen your hand raised the times you had your hand raised."

Beth's thought as she hears the non-validating statement—"Another male just doesn't get it. Why did I think this might be any different?"

Validating response by Mike—"You describe having experienced discrimination by males in several ways including the sexism encountered in college. It is disturbing, and particularly so if it were to carry over into the engineering job market after graduation. You see the unfairness of it all have real worries about the problems it can cause for you in your career."

Beth's thought as she hears the validating statement—"Right! Someone who understands. Maybe he can help me think about what to do."

The aforementioned gender example briefly highlights the validation process here, though a multitude of variables (e.g., race, ethnicity, sexual orientation) could make the same point. The ultimate way to validate someone is to put your views and opinions on the back burner and give credit to the other person's experience. Validation is not about your views and opinions, but about positively acknowledging people's experiences from their perspective. Validating the feelings of others facilitates rapport building (Wilson, 2006) and provides the basis for you to be validated by clients and others. It is also vital to watch the nonverbals that might be sending non-validating messages to your clients. While validating your client's experiences is important to increasing rapport, being aware of nonverbal behavior is another critical component for sending the right message to the people that we serve.

Active Learning Exercise **15.4**

Identify two people with whom you have great trust. Under each person's name make a list of five personally important things each would know about you and another list of what you imagine they believe about each of those five things. (You should see that the people you trust are those who you believe validate important aspects of you.)

Now identify two people with whom you have little trust. Under each person's name make a list of five important things they know about you and another list of what you imagine they believe about each of those five things. (You should see that the people who you trust less are those who do not accept or understand important aspects of you.)

Think about a discussion you observed between individuals or groups that had a less than satisfying ending for all parties. Note how many times they directly validated the other's opinions and how many times comments only promoted their own opinions (non-validating).

Now think about a discussion you observed between individuals or groups that had a highly satisfying ending for all parties. Note how many times they directly validated the other's opinions and how many times comments only promoted their own opinions (non-validating).

Compare the number of validating and non-validating comments in the discussions that ended in joint satisfaction versus those that ended with less satisfaction to see the difference that validating comments can make in relationship satisfaction.

PERSONAL CHARACTERISTICS OF THE SUCCESSFUL COUNSELOR

The successful counselor needs much more than information and counseling techniques to be effective. The pressures on a counselor to help clients require personal characteristics to maintain the highest quality work over time. People come to the counseling profession with varying degrees of these personal characteristics, and the most successful ones learn to recognize how to foster the development and maintenance of both their stronger and weaker characteristics.

Energy and Stamina

It is common for non-counselors to question the difficulty of this work. "How taxing can counseling with adults or children be? Sitting in a chair with an adult or on the floor with a child for less than an hour at a time doesn't sound so bad to a construction worker."

What counselors soon find out is that the concentration it takes to closely attend to each of the clients, parents, consultants, consultees, and supervisors you see each day takes an enormous amount of mental, emotional, and physical energy (Stebnicki, 2008). Students are commonly surprised at how tired they are after a few counseling sessions and start imagining what that is like when you do it all day on a regular basis. It takes high energy to be effective each day and the stamina to maintain that energy level over time. It is no easy task, which is the reason that counselor training programs are concerned about attention to student and counselor wellness (Roach & Young, 2007; Witmer & Granello, 2005). Maintaining your health over time is essential to your success, satisfaction, and enjoyment of work as a counselor.

Personal Growth Orientation

The orientation toward the personal growth aspect of Maslow's self-actualizing person has increased in importance in modern society because of rapid changes in people, societies, and amounts of information. To stay exactly as you are means that you will quickly be out of step with the world going on around you. Those who are excited to seek new relationships, information, insights, and abilities so that they can change their lives for the better are the ones who feel fulfilled and appreciate their successes.

Counseling does more than only bring new insights to clients. Self-aware counselors also gain understanding about people and life that they can apply to themselves. Close attention to yourself and those around you will continue to bring new insights that promote greater understanding of others and yourself if you are open to them (Hazler & Kottler, 2005). The best counselors are continually growing and improving as they learn from their lives, work, and studies. This growth is critical to professional development and keeping a sense of enthusiasm. It is also essential to the counselors' personal lives where changes in loved ones, friends, colleagues, employers, and themselves demand adjustments in relationships.

Tolerance for Ambiguity

A counselor once shared the following about her hobby:

> I like to make simple wood furniture on my free time. I know from the start what it is to look like, then carefully make it, and the result is a great finished product. I'm in complete control. It is my way to balance the ambiguity of counseling.

There are no simple answers in counseling and no truly finished products. Growth and development simply do not work as cleanly as this counselor's carpentry weekends. Sometimes answers appear to be so simple that both client and counselor ought to be saying, "Just stop doing that and do it this better way," but that is just wishful thinking.

The answer seems so clear, but still it doesn't work. This is how counseling with live people differs from reading about a problem and identifying a solution. People and society are more complex than that. Counselors never really know the whole story of a person and even as clients actually live the story they don't recognize all the problem permutations. Even when great progress is made and one problem is solved, a life rarely remains all one wants it to be. The product is never complete, and the counselor must be able to accept the ambiguity and lack of positive finality that is inherent in the job (Levitt & Jacques, 2005; Skovholt et al., 2001).

Capacity for Intimacy

Quality counseling is an experience where aspects of a person that are rarely if ever shared can come into the open. People select special individuals and private places to do this kind of highly personal self-exposure. In return, they expect and deserve a similar intimate interaction from the counselor. The relationship includes highly personal understanding, acceptance, exploration, and caring confrontation. Counselors must be ready to be full participants in the middle of these intimate relationships.

Intimacy requires a great deal of risk. How will you react if your views, ideas, or words are rejected or even deemed hurtful by a client? What will you do when the client's situation and pain is too close to a personal struggle of your own? What problem or level of someone's pain might cause you to shut yourself off from the person, seek escape to another topic, or begin focusing more on yourself than the client? Intimacy leads to strong emotions and counselors need to be ready for this experience, while at the same time be able to control their reactions within the relationship. It is a balancing act for which you need to be emotionally capable and prepared for unexpected reactions from both the client and yourself (Venart, Vassos, & Pitcher-Heft, 2007).

Desire to Learn About the Complexities of People

Counseling is more complex than traditional teaching because there is no specific set of information or skills that can be communicated to achieve a given person's goals. Helping a client to gain understanding and take personal action demands first learning about the person and their issues in some depth. The individual whose motivation is to tell clients what to do will be neither successful nor satisfied with their counseling work. Success and satisfaction come to counselors who are more excited about learning than they are about telling and explaining. It is the enthusiasm for exploring people's thinking, emotions, behaviors, and cultural influences that is the valuable counselor characteristic (American Counseling Association, 2005; Sue & Sue, 2008).

Consider the common difficulty people have with losing weight as an example of why the counselor's desire to learn is so important. The physical formula for losing weight is quite simple for most people: eat less and exercise more. There are billions of dollars worth of books bought each year to explain how to make it happen. People generally know what to do, but most are unsuccessful the vast majority of the time. The problem is not in the models for losing weight, but instead the complex interactions of physical, mental, emotional, social, and cultural factors that make a person unique. What works for one person will not work for another, so the counselor's task is to learn as much as possible about the interaction of all the different aspects of an individual. Counselors who seek the challenge of continually learning more about all the factors interacting on a person will be the ones able to devise and revise plans to help clients find success and acceptance in place of past failures.

Risk-Taking

Counseling is an exciting vocation filled with the exploration of people's lives and the adventure of seeking an unknown future along with them. The excitement and adventure don't come cheap, since they are connected to substantial risk as both client and counselor step out of their comfort zones. The potential for growth requires an uncomfortable stretching of our knowledge into unfamiliar mental territories that at times makes us afraid. This type of risk-taking is essential to counselors' personal and professional growth. Counselor risk-taking is equally important for clients who need us risking and growing if we are to have a place in the traumas of their existence and treat them as a unique entity rather than as standard model into which we simply plug in old responses (Cory, Cory, & Cory, 2006).

Risk-taking is what increases understanding, the tools we use, and the number of people we are able to help. When counselors find themselves being bored with their work, it is not because the work is boring, but because the counselor has reduced risk to the point where the adventure and excitement are no longer there. Willingness to take chances in order to increase your helpfulness will make you a better counselor, colleague, and friend.

The pressures of counselor training have similarities to the counselor's daily work. Self-examination, learning, and taking actions to support and improve oneself is essential work. The summarizing Table 15.2 may help in that identification and action taking process.

Active Learning Exercise **15.5**

Describe yourself in relation to your strengths and challenges in relation to the characteristics listed in this section. Now ask a fellow student and a friend to assess you on the same characteristics and see how well they match. How close is your perception of your characteristics in comparison to how others see you? What plans can you develop to continue in the development of each characteristic over time?

TABLE **15.2**

Summary of a Counselor's Personal Characteristics

Characteristic	Pressures Creating Need for Characteristic
Energy and stamina	The physical and emotional demands of counseling are unexpectedly high for people entering the field and require fitness of body as well as mind.
Personal growth orientation	Rapid changes in clients and society require continual evaluation and implementation of counselor personal beliefs and behaviors.
Tolerance for ambiguity	Client and societal problems are never fully solved and constantly changing so that counselors must focus on progress and not cures.
Capacity for intimacy	Clients exploring their most private and painful aspects have expectations that counselors can be comfortable and companionate partners in the exploration.
Desire to learn about the complexities of people	The unlimited diversity of problems, people, and cultures requires counselors to be continuously enthusiastic about learning new aspects of individuals and groups to make themselves valuable to increasingly more people and society.
Risk-taking	Exploring the confusion and complexity of client situations causes growth and the counseling process to be filled with misunderstandings, unexpected outcomes, and wrong turns that take bravery from both client and counselor to seek and overcome.

MAINTAINING PERSONAL WELLNESS

The personal rewards of helping people overcome problems and trauma are enormous, leaving counselors feeling wonderful about themselves and the profession. The other side of the equation is that the stresses inherent in the profession can have just as powerful a pull toward a sense of exhaustion, defeat, and powerlessness. The task of counselors is to be prepared to do their best possible work, and that includes taking sufficient care of themselves in order to weather the stresses and get maximum joy from the career.

The scholarship of wellness and its application to counseling has received increasing emphasis since the 1990s. Most of that emphasis has been on clients and the general population, but the same concepts are directly applicable to the professional culture of counselors (Lawson, Venart, Hazler, & Kottler, 2007). There is an ongoing need to balance the trauma we deal with on a regular basis with a healthy lifestyle to maintain personal wellness (Venart et al., 2007).

Myers and Sweeney (2005) provide a comprehensive model and assessment tool for evaluating and maintaining wellness that can be used as a more extensive evaluation and personal planning guide. Many aspects of the model touched upon in previous sections of this chapter are connected to the model's five primary factors. Your answers to some questions related to the five factors will change throughout your life, reflecting all the expected and unexpected experiences, new information, physical passages, and emotional fluctuations that are a natural part of life. The key is to have an accurate understanding of your answers at any given time and then to act on them accordingly.

Active Learning Exercise **15.6**

Answer the questions under each heading.

1. *Creative self*
   - What do you do to create opportunities to explore new ideas, experiences, and ways to thinking?
   - How do you maintain awareness of the emotional and other changes going within and around you?
   - How do you create opportunities for self-expression in your work?

2. *Coping self*
   - What are the ways you deal with stress and how healthy are those methods?
   - How do you deal with work or life events that challenge your beliefs and self-worth?
   - How do you use leisure activities to gain joy and maintain balance in your life?

3. *Social self*
   - How well do you foster the supportive relationships that are or could be available to you?
   - Are you adequately promoting relationships in which you can both give and receive the intimate, caring, honest, and loving attention that everyone deserves?
   - What are the efforts you make to feel part of positive work and life communities?

4. *Essential self*
   - Do you give time to express and explore the spiritual aspects of yourself that encompass your key values and beliefs?
   - How close is the physical, personal, social, and emotional person you are to the one you have the potential to be?
   - Do you take as much care of your safety, health, and well-being as you would have loved ones do for themselves?

5. *Physical self*
   - How much of what you eat and drink strengthens your body and increases the stamina needed for the most productive and enjoyable existence?
   - To what extent do you perform the type and amount of exercise that continually supports and strengthens your body for the riggers of a long life and career?
   - Are you adequately attending to the needs for physical rest and renewal?

CONCLUSION

Working your way through this chapter has provided both the reasons to explore aspects of yourself and some initial means to begin that exploration in order to become a quality professional counselor. Your journey begins with knowing your reasons for wanting to enter the profession and realizing that you may be proud of some reasons, while others will require further examination as to how to deal with them. Training for and then practicing in such an interpersonally intimate profession with people who are culturally very different from you is accompanied by many stressors that you will need to recognize and learn to deal with effectively. Identifying the personal characteristics necessary to deal with the stresses, strengthening them, and developing a wellness model to keep you performing at maximum potential will be the keys to a successful program and career.

CHAPTER REVIEW

1. Many of the reasons people have for wanting to be professional counselors are altruistic, but others are related to the needs and wishes of the potential counselor. It is important to explore all the reasons you would like to become a counselor in order to recognize aspects of your own needs that could influence your work positively or negatively.
2. Counseling is a stressful profession due to the nature of intimate relationships with clients and colleagues, along with pressures to obtain successful results in the shortest possible period of time.
3. All counselors have biases that will influence the ways they treat clients and colleagues. Learning what they are and how to revise and/or work with them in order to validate others and yourself is essential to success.
4. Having success with the greatest diversity of people and maintaining that over time requires understanding of personal characteristics that counselors need and a wellness model to foster them and avoid burnout.

REVIEW QUESTIONS

1. Why do people seek to become professional counselors, and how should their reasons for seeking this work influence their choice?
2. What are the personal and work stresses that counselors face on a regular basis?
3. What are the biases that counselors bring to clients and colleagues that arise from their cultural experiences?
4. In what ways can counselors validate the experiences of their clients?
5. What are the personal characteristics that are needed by counselors and how can they be strengthened?
6. What are the multiple dimensions of wellness that counselors need to continually utilize in order to deal with the stresses and pressures of the work?

ADDITIONAL RESOURCES

- American Counseling Association's Task Force on Counselor Wellness and Impairment (http://www.counseling.org/wellness_taskforce/tf_wellness_strategies.htm)
- American Counseling Association *Code of Ethics* (http://www.counseling.org/Resources/CodeOfEthics/TP/Home/CT2.aspx)
- Association for Multicultural Counseling and Development: Multicultural Competencies and Standards (http://www.counseling.org/Resources/)
- Family Insights Blog (http://www.familyinsights.net/about
- Self-Care for Outreach Workers (Curriculum developed by National Health Care for the Homeless Council and based in part on the work of Pearlman, Saakvitne, and the Staff of Traumatic Stress Institute: Center for Adult and Adolescent Psychotherapy; www.nhchc.org/Curriculum/module2/module2B/module2b.htm)

REFERENCES

American Counseling Association. (2005). *ACA code of ethics*. Alexandria, VA: Author.

Carney, J. V., & Hazler, R. J. (2005). Wellness counseling in community mental health agencies. In J. E. Myers & T. J. Sweeney (Eds.), *Counseling for wellness: Theory, research, and practice* (pp. 235–244). Alexandria, VA: American Counseling Association.

Cory, M. S., Cory, G., & Cory, C. (2006). *Groups: Process and practice* (8th ed.). Belmont, CA: Brooks/Cole.

Culture. (n.d.). *Wikipedia.* Retrieved May 14, 2007, from http://en.wikipedia.org/wiki/Culture.

Cypres, A., Landsberg., G., & Spellmann, M. (1997). The impact of managed care on community mental health outpatient services in New York State. *Administration and Policy in Mental Health, 24,* 509–521.

Hazler, R. J. (2008). *Helping in the hallways: Expanding your influence potential* (2nd ed.). Thousand Oaks, CA: Corwin.

Hazler, R. J., & Kottler, J. A. (2005). *The emerging professional counselor: Student dreams to professional realities* (2nd ed.). Alexandria, VA: American Counseling Association.

Kottler, J. A. (1992). *Compassionate therapy: Working with difficult clients.* San Francisco, CA: Jossey-Bass.

Kottler, J. A. (2000). *Doing good: Passion, and commitment to helping others.* Philadelphia, PA: Brunner-Routledge.

Lawson, G. (2007). Counselor wellness and impairment: A national survey. *Journal of Counseling, Education and Development, 46*(1), 20–34.

Lawson, G., Venart, E., Hazler, R. J., & Kottler, J. A. (2007). Toward a culture of wellness. *Journal of Counseling, Education, and Development, 46*(1), 5–19.

Levitt, D. H., & Jacques, J. D. (2005). Promoting tolerance for ambiguity in counselor training programs. *Journal of Humanistic Counseling, Education and Development, 44,* 46–54.

Maslach, C. (2003). *Burnout: The cost of caring.* Cambridge, MA: Malor Books.

Myers, J. E., & Sweeney, T. J. (2005). *Counseling for wellness: Theory, research, and practice.* Alexandria, VA: American Counseling Association.

Roach, L. F., & Young, M. E. (2007). Do counselor education programs promote wellness in their students? *Counselor Education and Supervision, 47,* 28–42.

Skovholt, T. M., Grier, T. L., & Hanson, M. R. (2001). Career counseling for longevity: Self-care and burnout prevention strategies for counselor resilience. *Journal of Career Development, 27*(3), 167–176.

Smith, T. W. (2006). *Taking America's pulse III: Intergroup relations in contemporary America.* The National Conference for Community and Justice, National Opinion Research Center, University of Chicago.

Stebnicki, M. A. (2008). *Empathy fatigue: Healing the mind, body, and spirit of professional counselors.* New York: Springer.

Sue, D., & Sue, D. M. (2008). *Foundations of counseling and psychotherapy.* Hoboken, NJ: John Wiley & Sons.

Validation. (n.d.). *Wikipedia*. Retrieved May 9, 2007, from http://en.wikipedia.org/wiki/Validate.

Venart, E., Vassos, S., & Pitcher-Heft, H. (2007). What individual counselors can do to sustain wellness. *Journal of Counseling, Education, and Development, 46*(1), 50–65.

Wilson, K. B. (2006, July). *Vocational rehabilitation outcomes and phenotypes: Can you tell I am a minority?* Paper presented at the meeting of the National Association of Multicultural Rehabilitation Concerns, Detroit, MI.

Witmer, J. M., & Granello, P. F. (2005). Wellness in counselor education and supervision. In J. E. Myers & T. J. Sweeney (Eds.), *Counselor for wellness: Theory, research and practice* (pp. 342–362). Alexandria, VA: American Counseling Association.

Yassen, J. (1995). Preventing secondary traumatic stress disorder. In C. R. Figley (Ed.), *Compassion fatigue: Coping with secondary traumatic stress disorder in those who treat the traumatized* (pp. 178–208). New York: Brunner/Mazel.

CHAPTER 16

Developing and Maintaining a Professional Identity

LEARNING OBJECTIVES

After reading this chapter, you should be able to

- discuss the development of the counseling profession;
- identify the key factors in defining a profession and how they relate to your professional identity;
- know about the divisions contained within the American Counseling Association;
- be aware of the need for program accreditation and certification/licensure; and
- understand the importance of ethical codes, competency statements, and advocacy for developing and maintaining your professional identity.

CHAPTER OUTLINE

INTRODUCTION

Counseling has developed as a profession over the past six decades. It began as a limited collaboration of focused groups, primarily interested in vocational guidance, to now encompass many specialty areas with a shared identity. The evolution of groups interested in providing assistance to our society expanded because of the rapid growth of the United States. As the country grew so did the counseling profession. However, this progress did not occur without challenges and growth pains. It has been argued that the increase of specialty areas within the counseling profession has created diversity but has not contributed to a collective professional identity (Gale & Austin, 2003). However, Goldberg believes all helping professions "are interested in changing human behavior" (Goldberg, 1998, p. 352, as cited in Gale & Austin, 2003). In addition, many leading educators and practitioners today argue that specializations are contrived barriers and firmly believe in a common base of knowledge that includes counseling theories and knowledge of human development to facilitate changes in human behavior (Gale, 1998, as cited in Gale & Austin).

DEVELOPMENT OF THE COUNSELING PROFESSION

Klatt (1967) outlined the steps in defining a profession. The steps include developing a systematic body of knowledge requiring specific training; emphasizing service to others and the creation of a code of ethics; having an experimental attitude toward information; and forming an organization that establishes a course of training and examination, which then becomes a condition for entry into the profession. The counseling profession has taken these steps toward professionalization. For example, as counseling professionals we recognize that the title of *professional* requires a certain degree of skill. This recognition includes a *fiduciary duty* wherein the duty of utmost good faith, trust, confidence, honesty, and loyalty is owed by the professional to the client. Fiduciary duty is recognized as fidelity. For counseling professionals, fidelity and fiduciary duty are one in the same. Fiduciary duty implies counselors are accountable for client welfare and client rights (Stauffer & Kurpius, 2005). Professional bodies within the mental health profession adhere to ethical codes as a prerequisite for use of the title *professional counselor* and for the practice of counseling. Ethical codes for counseling professionals are further evidence of the professional status of counselors.

Klatt (1967) proposed that the body of knowledge required for a profession must be distinct and specific. The practice of professional counseling involves the application of mental health, psychological, and human development principles through cognitive, affective, and behavioral strategies. The counseling profession is oriented toward health and wellness rather than psychopathology and mental illness. Counseling professionals are equipped to help clients address issues from a wellness perspective, which is one of the distinguishing and singular characteristics of counseling (National Board of Certified Counselors [NBCC], 1993).

Klatt (1967) also stated that an experimental attitude toward information is necessary for the development of a profession. Skovholt and Ronnestad (1992) agreed that professionals' growth and development is a process. Through experience we gain knowledge. Professional development can be influenced by multiple sources (e.g., supervisors, professors, mentors, therapist, experts, peers, and colleagues). The development of a profession and the professional has been described as a long, slow, changeable process wherein the professional base is built, expanded, and individualized. A changeable process allows for growth. Professional counselors uphold this standard by adopting an attitude of lifelong continuing education as evidenced by the commitment of our professional associations and as required by our credentialing organizations. The seeds for such growth were sown early in the 20th century.

Indeed, the historical organizational roots of the counseling profession are deep. The United States Constitution, with the Bill of Rights, was ratified in 1791 and guaranteed the right of association, *the right of the people peaceably to assemble.* This important right was first used by counseling associations in 1913 with the formation of the National Vocational Guidance Association (NVGA), which changed its name in 1985 to the National Career Development Association (NCDA) to reflect changes in society and in customary terminology. In 1952, NVGA joined with three other organizations, now known as the Association for Counselor Education and Supervision (ACES), the Counseling Association for Humanistic Education and Development (C-AHEAD), and the American College Personnel Association (ACPA). These four independent associations convened a joint convention in Los Angeles, California, in 1952 and out of this came the American Counseling Association (ACA), originally known as the American Personnel and Guidance Association. Although ACPA is now an independent organization, the others are still active divisions of ACA.

Through the years, other divisions of ACA formed representing professional counselors' diverse work settings, areas of expertise, and special interests (e.g., school settings, assessment techniques, multicultural counseling, religious and values issues), bringing the total to 19 divisions. Although counselors may have interests that lead them to join other associations—for example, the American Society for Training and Development, the American Psychological Association, or American Art Therapy Association—the focus of this chapter will be on ACA because it is the one association that represents all professional counselors, regardless of area of specialization.

In the following sections we describe counseling's professional association, ACA; discuss professional credentialing; and describe program accreditation for professional counselor training programs. With regard to professional associations, please note that most states have parallel organizations that include some, but not always all, of the ACA divisions. In some states there are separate divisional organizations; in some they are part of a unified association; in some there is a mixture.

THE AMERICAN COUNSELING ASSOCIATION AND ITS RELATED DIVISIONS

The mission of ACA is "to enhance the quality of life in society by promoting the development of professional counselors, advancing the counseling profession, and using the profession and practice of counseling to promote respect for human dignity and diversity" (ACA, 2008). These three components—development of counselors, advancing the profession, and promoting human dignity and diversity—form the core of the association's activities. The divisions of ACA work together to provide opportunities for continuing education, leadership training, and publications to help "counseling professionals develop their skills and expand their knowledge base" (ACA, 2009).

In 1992, the American Association for Counseling and Development, formerly the American Personnel and Guidance Association, changed its name to the American Counseling Association, which was seen by the leaders at the time to better reflect the primary focus of the members of the association and to assist in helping the public understand the unity of the profession. The divisions represent areas of practice (e.g., school or college); modalities (e.g., groupwork or creativity); and interests that cut across all areas (e.g., creativity or social justice). The association's 19 divisions are each described briefly here:

1. *Association for Assessment in Counseling and Education (AACE)*— AACE was founded in 1965 as the Association for Measurement and Evaluation in Guidance. It focuses on the use of assessment in counseling, including improving student and client testing and program evaluation.
2. *Association for Adult Development and Aging (AADA)*—AADA, founded in 1986, as its name implies, considers issues related to adult development and aging. The division advocates for attention to life span issues, both within and outside of the counseling profession.
3. *Association for Creativity in Counseling (ACC)*—ACC is the newest of ACA's divisions. It was formed to be a home for counselors interested in creative approaches to helping, including the use of creative arts by counselors, counselor educators, and students.
4. *American College Counseling Association (ACCA)*—ACCA was formed to help its members, foster student development through counseling and related activities. Many of its members work in colleges, universities, and community colleges.
5. *Association for Counselors and Educators in Government (ACEG)*—This small division meets the needs of counselors who work in government- and military-related agencies. Many of ACEG's members work in Europe or in other countries outside of the United States.

6. *Association for Counselor Education and Supervision (ACES)*—ACES was one of the founding divisions of ACA. This division provides its members with information and support to better educate students and supervise counselors in all work settings.
7. *Association for Lesbian, Gay, Bisexual, and Transgender Issues in Counseling (ALGBTIC)*—ALGBTIC sees its role as one of education for all counselors about stereotypical thinking and homoprejudice. In addition, it focuses on client identity development.
8. *Association for Multicultural Counseling and Development (AMCD)*—In an earlier time in history, multicultural meant non-White. This division, originally the Association of Non-White Concerns in Personnel and Guidance, has expanded its mission to promote all multicultural interests in counseling.
9. *American Mental Health Counselors Association (AMHCA)*—Counseling as a profession has expanded its reach in the last 30 years, and AMHCA is both a cause and an effect of this expansion. With the growth of licensure for counselors, AMHCA has become even more important as it represents counselors engaged within the health care industry.
10. *American Rehabilitation Counseling Association (ARCA)*—Rehabilitation counseling is the center of ARCA's mission. They focus on improving counseling practice to enhance development of people with disabilities.
11. *American School Counselor Association (ASCA)*—Professional school counselors make up the membership of this division. The division promotes the personal academic and career development of students through program planning and evaluation. Like several other divisions, ASCA collaborates with ACA, NBCC, and others on the legislative front.
12. *Association for Spiritual, Ethical, and Religious Values in Counseling (ASERVIC)*—The growing appreciation in counseling of the spiritual needs of our clients can be fostered through involvement in this division. Originally the National Catholic Guidance Conference, ASERVIC has broadened its reach to include a diverse group of individuals who care about this mission.
13. *Association for Specialists in Group Work (ASGW)*—ASGW provides a professional home for counselors interested in using groups in their counseling practice. It is committed to setting and maintaining training standards in group counseling.
14. *Counseling Association for Humanistic Education and Development (C-AHEAD)*—C-AHEAD was one of the founding associations of ACA in 1952. Its focus is on human development and potential, as achieved through the application of humanistic principles.
15. *Counselors for Social Justice (CSJ)*—Describing itself as a community of counselors, this division seeks an end to oppression and injustice through advocacy and equity.
16. *International Association of Addiction and Offender Counselors (IAAOC)*—Public offenders and others with substance abuse problems and other addictions are the clientele served by members of this division. IAAOC advocates for effective counseling and rehabilitation programs for this population.

17. *International Association of Marriage and Family Counselors (IAMFC)*—IAMFC advocates for using a systems approach in counseling families. This division concentrates on prevention, education, and therapy.

18. *National Career Development Association (NCDA)*—Another founding division of ACA, NCDA promotes life span career development locally, nationally, and internationally. It provides training for professionals and paraprofessionals through publications and conferences.

19. *National Employment Counseling Association (NECA)*—NECA was formed to support those in counseling and related occupations who work with clients in employment settings.

For further information about ACA's divisions, see http://www.counseling.org/AboutUs/DivisionsBranchesAndRegions/TP/Divisions/CT2.aspx.

Active Learning Exercise 16.1

Picture yourself as a newly graduated counselor, ready to embark on your career. Choose three areas of special interest that connect to ACA's divisions—one a setting, one a practice modality, one of general interest. Find out what kinds of help ACA and each of these divisions can provide to you as a new professional.

DEVELOPMENT OF PROFESSIONAL IDENTITY THROUGH ACCREDITATION

Another step in the development of the profession included the establishment of an organization defining the training of professional counselors. The Council for Accreditation of Counseling and Related Educational Programs, more commonly known by its acronym CACREP and now independent of ACA, accredits counselor education programs at the masters and doctoral level. CACREP's program accreditations include career, college, community, gerontological, mental health, and school counseling; marital, couple, and family counseling/therapy; student affairs; and counselor education and supervision. Accreditation of counselor education programs was an important step in the development of the profession because it defined the specialized training necessary for a professional counselor, thereby enhancing the professional "identity" of counselors by defining a specialized body of knowledge and training needed.

The mission of CACREP is to promote the professional competence of counseling and related practitioners through the

• development of preparation standards,
• encouragement of excellence in program development, and
• accreditation of professional preparation programs.

For over 25 years, CACREP has maintained high standards for the training of counselors and related practitioners through accreditation of counselor education programs. Program accreditation is a sign of quality and demonstrates the willingness of a counselor education program to voluntarily meet high standards for training counselors. Accreditation assures graduates of a quality education providing a solid foundation for the practice of counseling.

DEVELOPMENT OF PROFESSIONAL IDENTITY THROUGH CERTIFICATION AND LICENSURE

In 1982, ACA (then known as the American Personnel and Guidance Association) created a Special Committee on Registry Efforts. This committee led to the formation of the NBCC. Mentioned earlier, Klatt's (1967) ideas about development of a profession include the creation of an examination, which would serve as a condition for entry into the profession. And thus began the work of NBCC in creating a professional certification based on certain criteria such as a national examination, a code of ethics, and continuing education requirements. The work of NBCC was based on the profession's efforts to strengthen the professional identity of counselors through an effective certification process based on the highest professional standards.

NBCC recognizes individuals who have met rigorous standards in their training, experience, and successful completion of an examination through credentialing. NBCC was formed before state licensure in order to create a certification process clearly reflective of the practice of counseling maintaining the highest standards. The initial certification process allowed counselors to demonstrate their willingness to meet these high standards. The NBCC Web site (http://www.nbcc.org) describes it as follows:

> NBCC was initially created after the work of a committee of the American Counseling Association (ACA). The committee created NBCC to be an independent credentialing body. NBCC and ACA have strong historical ties and work together to further the profession of counseling. However, the two organizations are completely separate entities with different goals.
>
> ACA concentrates on membership association activities such as conferences, professional development, publications, and government relations.
>
> NBCC focuses on promoting quality counseling through certification. NBCC's mission is to promote quality assurance in counseling practice; promote the value of counseling; promote public awareness of quality counseling practice; promote professionalism in counseling; and finally to promote leadership in credentialing The National Board for Certified Counselors promotes professional counseling to private and government organizations through advocacy efforts. NBCC's flagship credential is the National Certified Counselor (NCC). NBCC also offers specialty certification in several areas:
>
> - School counseling—The National Certified School Counselor (NCSC)
> - Clinical mental health counseling—The Certified Clinical Mental Health Counselor (CCMHC)
> - Addictions counseling—The Master Addictions Counselor (MAC)
>
> The NCC is a prerequisite or co-requisite for the specialty credentials. (NBCC, 2009)

Active Learning Exercise **16.2**

Visit the homepage of the NBCC (http://www.nbcc.org). Review the pages related to certifications, certification versus licensure, and the National Certified Counselor (NCC) credential, as well as information about the National Counselor Exam. As you review these pages, look for differences between certification and licensure, and for the eligibility requirements for the NCC credential. Also review each of the specialty credentials to determine what specific skills and knowledge are needed to achieve these credentials. Contrast and compare each credential and the educational requirements needed for each based on your particular program of study. Develop a plan for your future and career goals to achieve the necessary skills, knowledge and education that might be required for any specialization in your counseling practice.

Another way that counseling associations uphold standards is through accrediting service delivery. A pioneering approach to this was taken in 2007 by NCDA when they announced the following:

Center of Career Development Excellence (CoE) Accreditation
Center for Credentialing and Education's (CCE) Center of Career Development Excellence (CoE) accreditation will identify career and workforce development programs that have met specified excellence benchmarks and professional standards. Holding this accreditation will provide a valuable mark of distinction when working with funding sources, as well when marketing to individuals and businesses seeking career and job development services. (NCDA, 2007)

DEVELOPMENT OF PROFESSIONAL IDENTITY THROUGH ETHICAL CODES

Professional identity can be enhanced and developed through ethical codes and professional competency statements. Learning opportunities such as conferences and conventions, journals and newsletters—paper and online—stand-alone workshops, online learning, and traditional publications like books are provided by ACA, as well as other counseling organizations and entities that enhance knowledge and practice of professional counselors. The importance of ethical codes are recognized by many regulatory boards, and specialized continuing education is often required by these entities.

Additionally, and extremely importantly, many counseling organizations provide ethical codes that govern the conduct of members and provide the public with information about expected standards of care. In 2005 ACA adopted their new *Code of Ethics*. There are five purposes of the code, including the following statement from the code itself: "The *Code* serves as an ethical guide designed to assist members in constructing a professional course of action that best serves those utilizing counseling services and best promotes the values of the counseling profession" (ACA, 2005). The 2005 revised ACA ethics code can be viewed at http://www.counseling.org/Resources/CodeOfEthics/TP/Home/CT2.aspx.

In the following we will list each section of the *ACA Code of Ethics* and give a sample criterion.

A. *The Counseling Relationship: A.1.a. Primary Responsibility.* "The primary responsibility of counselors is to respect the dignity and to promote the welfare of clients." This counseling version of the Hippocratic Oath can be seen as the touchstone on which all other sections of the code rely.

B. *Confidentiality, Privileged Communication, and Privacy: B.6.c. Permission to Observe.* Of particular importance to students, this section of the code underscores the rights of clients to confidentiality. This means that clients must give permission for others, including faculty, supervisors, and peers, to observe a session, view recordings, or read session transcripts.

C. *Professional Responsibility*: Although all sections of the code are important, we consider Section C as absolutely essential. We include two examples to illustrate its delineated responsibilities.

- *C.2.f. Continuing Education.* There is a reason that graduation ceremonies are called commencement. Not only are they the beginning of a new life for the graduate, but they are also the beginning of a life committed to ongoing learning. This is especially important when the new graduate's work can seriously affect the lives of others, for good or ill. This section of the ethics code requires that counselors keep current with scientific knowledge and the evidence base in their area of practice as well as learning about the cultures of the people with whom they work.

- *C.2.g. Impairment.* "Counselors are alert to the signs of impairment from their own physical, mental, or emotional problems and refrain from offering or providing professional services when such impairment is likely to harm a client or others." Counselors are human beings, subject to the same illnesses, frailties, and addictions as others, and perhaps because of the nature of their work, subject to greater stress. This section of the code reminds us of this and requires us not only to seek help when we need it but also to assist our colleagues, students, and supervisors in recognizing impairments and seeking help. Turning a blind eye to colleagues' troubles is unacceptable to an ethical practitioner.

D. *Relationship with Other Professionals: D.1.a. Different Approaches.* In a training program, counselors are exposed primarily to other counselors. Once working, counselors almost always have to interact with other members of the mental health professions. Furthermore, even among counselors there is a wide variety of approaches, modalities, belief systems, and so forth. This section of the ethics code reminds us that we do not own the truth.

E. *Evaluation, Assessment, and Interpretation: E.2.c. Decisions Based on Results.* "It is important that counselors interpreting assessment results have a thorough understanding of measurement criteria, including such concepts as validity and reliability." Counselors, especially in schools, are often the expert—sometimes the only expert—in the use and interpretation of assessments. Thus, it is important that they keep current in this arena.

F. *Supervision, Training, and Teaching: F.2.a. Supervisor Preparation.* Some state licensing laws require supervisors to have demonstrated competence; others do not. Nonetheless, the ethical guidelines require such competence. This means that supervisors should have specific training in supervision. Having experienced supervision oneself is not considered adequate training!

G. *Research and Publication: G.5.f. Student Research.* If the field of counseling is to continue to advance its knowledge and skills, its practitioners must be involved in research. Students are to be encouraged to begin this aspect of their work while in graduate school. When they do so, credit should be appropriately given. This means that they should be listed as first author when the work is essentially theirs.

H. *Resolving Ethical Issues: H.1.a. Knowledge.* It is the obligation of every counselor to be familiar with the *Code of Ethics* and to consult with peers and supervisors when in doubt. An inadequate understanding or inaccurate interpretation of the code is not considered an acceptable defense of ethical misconduct. To paraphrase the first statement in the ethics code, the underlying message is, "First, do no harm."

In the case of professional counselors who hold voluntary credentials from an organization with a code of ethics, such as NBCC, there is usually a process for examining possible violations of the ethical standards. An investigation of the claims made may be conducted and disciplinary action taken if needed, and there is usually an appeal process for the parties involved. The NBCC code of ethics provides a minimal ethical standard for the professional behavior of all NCCs. This code provides an expectation of and assurance for the ethical practice for the general public who use the professional services of an NCC. The code also provides an enforceable standard for all NCCs and assures the general public recourse in case of a perceived ethical violation (NBCC, 2009).

The development of a code of ethics is again a part of the evolutionary progress of a profession (Klatt, 1967). Client welfare is part of the counseling profession and is mandated by our professional membership organization as well as the largest counselor certification organization in the world. Professional counselors must be accountable for client welfare and client rights. It is incumbent as professional counselors to uphold our fiduciary responsibility to our clients (Stauffer & Kurpius, 2005).

DEVELOPING A PROFESSIONAL IDENTITY THROUGH COMPETENCY STATEMENTS

Another area that provides assistance to counselors is through the development of competencies. These have been developed by ACA and by its divisions and include multicultural; gay, lesbian, bisexual, and transgendered; group work; career development; and advocacy competencies. In addition there are position papers available to members on a variety of topics.

Neophyte and experienced counselors can use these competency statements as a check list to identify needed areas of growth. Ongoing learning is the hallmark of a competent and ethical counselor. Indeed, NBCC and most states require evidence of continuing education for continuing certification or licensure. Furthermore, ACA's *Code of Ethics* require the same attention. Using competency statements as self-diagnostic tools is an excellent way to do this. Two examples from the multicultural competencies serve to further explicate this point. The former is from the knowledge section, the latter from the skills section.

> Culturally skilled counselors are aware of how their own cultural background and experiences, attitudes, and values and biases influence psychological processes.

> Culturally skilled counselors become actively involved with minority individuals outside the counseling setting (community events, social and political functions, celebrations, friendships, neighborhood groups, and so forth) so that their perspective of minorities is more than an academic or helping exercise. (Sue, Arredondo, & McDavis, 1992, p. 482)

To achieve these competencies is probably a lifetime goal. Effective counselors will commit time to the challenge of meeting them.

Another example may be taken from the career development competencies developed by NCDA. Included in the individual/group assessment section is the following statement: "Assess personal characteristics such as aptitude, achievement, interests, values, and personality traits. Assess leisure interests, learning style, life roles, self-concept, career maturity, vocational identity, career indecision, work environment preference (e.g., work satisfaction), and other related life style/development issues" (NCDA, 1997). As new instruments and modalities become available, counselors must learn to use them if they are to offer their clients the best help available. The move to expanded use of narrative in career counseling, for example, requires assessment techniques quite different from those offered through computerized career decision-making programs. The effective counselor must, according to these competency statements, know how to use both.

The professional development role of associations is the one most visible to members. As stated earlier, associations put on conferences and other meetings and offer online learning opportunities. They also distribute newsletters, magazines, and journals that come periodically to each member—in the case of some divisions electronically, but for the most part in hard copy. ACA also publishes books, manuals, and video tapes/DVDs. Web-based resources are extensive and are updated regularly. This allows the association to have timely information for members and the public. This resource becomes particularly important in times of crisis when both counselors and those they serve are in need of information and often referrals. Furthermore, many of these publications and other professional development activities provide ways for counselors to meet the continuing education requirements (CEUs) of their licensure or certification. Each month the ACA newsletter, *Counseling Today*, offers readers an opportunity to earn CEUs by reading certain articles and taking a test on the content.

DEVELOPMENT OF PROFESSIONAL IDENTITY THROUGH ADVOCACY

Advocacy for the counseling profession reaches into several areas. Specifically, our profession grew from a need to provide services and help individuals achieve wellness using human development principles and counseling theories. Advocacy for the counseling profession is still evolving. The need for licensure advocacy, legislative advocacy, and public advocacy is growing. Legislative advocacy is imperative for the counseling profession to have a voice in the health care debate and reform of the 21st century. Public advocacy is also important to ensure that consumers understand the capabilities of professional counselors. All advocacy efforts ultimately have the effect of helping counselors better meet the needs of their clients. Advocacy helps counselors achieve higher levels of professional identity and a voice in many venues.

Licensure Advocacy or Professional Practice Advocacy

Of primary importance to all counselors is their ability to practice their profession. Professional counselor licensure is rooted in the early 13th-century guilds with the first practice act in the medical field. The first practice act in essence set forth the requirements for practice as well as acceptable training standards. Guilds also protected the practitioners from competition from non-members, that is, those that had not met the training standards. State licensure efforts have been joint activities of state associations and ACA, as well as NBCC. As of this writing, 49 states and the District of Columbia have licensure laws that protect the right of counselors to practice and prevent noncredentialed people from calling themselves professional counselors and conducting professional counseling activities. This major accomplishment lays the groundwork for ongoing protection of specific activities.

ACA, NBCC, AMHCA, and the Fair Access Coalition on Testing have been very active assisting individuals and state branches in protecting the right to practice from legislation that might limit that right, and they support counselors in their quest to continue the use of certain tests and inventories on which they have been trained, as was the case recently in Indiana. Practice protection is an ongoing necessity. Maintaining legislative and lobbying staffs, training volunteers, and providing ongoing education and training to legislators and their aides at the state and national level will continue to be a priority for professional counseling organizations such as ACA, NBCC, and AHMCA. Term limits enacted in many states have made this process more complicated and time consuming, because legislatures are always occupied by new members.

Legislative Advocacy

Many state associations have an annual Day on the Hill, as does the national association. These times provide a focus for educational activities, but the education must be undertaken throughout the year. Another service provided by ACA is the annual Legislative Training Institute, run by the public policy and legislation committee and the professional staff, to which members are invited to apply. Financial support for this training is provided by ACA, the individuals involved, the states sending them, and the ACA Foundation.

The health care system under which most counselors (except for school counselors) practice is one where third-party payments are critical to one's ability to provide care for clients. Getting counselors on health care panels and keeping them there is another example of the kinds of advocacy with which counseling organizations help. They can also influence legislation so as to make sure it includes professional counselors in the list of people qualified to offer and receive reimbursement for services. This function relates to working on assuring that counselors receive salary and equity with other mental health professions, including the right to third-party payments and to work independently. For example, lobbying efforts have led to counselors being included as service providers in legislation that provides funding for veterans and for government employees. Other counseling organizations like NBCC have hired a full-time lobbyist to work on legislative issues surrounding counseling issues.

Public Advocacy

A criticism that has been leveled at counselors and counseling is that the general public does not have a clear idea of who we are, what we do, where we work, and how we fit in the array of mental health services. (One past ACA president said that she would know we had "arrived" when ACA was an answer in the New York Times Crossword Puzzle; J. Breasure, personal communication, March 1996). To address that issue several divisions of ACA, and ACA itself, have engaged in public awareness campaigns. These include proclamations and activities around for example School Counselor Week and National Career Development Month, as well as events like Depression Screening Day, entered into in collaboration with other mental health specialties. These kinds of activities allow local counselors to piggyback with proclamations and activities of their own and provide opportunities to educate the public as well as lawmakers. *Counseling Corner*, a series of articles written for lay people, appears weekly in free newspapers reaching millions of readers. This project is currently funded by the ACA Foundation and includes columns on such topics as speaking with your teenager, dealing with low vision, or recognizing signs of depression.

Advocating for a Client

Another advocacy role of professional associations is to help counselors better serve their clienteles. Indeed, the *ACA Code of Ethics* states, "A. 6. a. When appropriate, counselors advocate at individual, group, institutional, and societal levels to examine [and work toward removal of] potential barriers and obstacles that inhibit access and/or the growth and development of clients" (ACA, 2005).

The ACA advocacy competencies (Lewis, Arnold, House, & Toporek, 2002) describe this process in a three-dimensional model. To be effective, advocacy efforts must take place at the micro and macro levels, in client/student, community, and public arenas. In other words, counselors must act locally to assist their own clientele, work with institutions to effect policies that assist their clientele, and attempt to influence state and national legislation in such a way as to assist their clientele. In each of these arenas they propose an empowerment model where one acts for one's clients as needed and also empowers one's clients to act on their own behalf.

As an example, in the section on individual empowerment, Lewis and colleagues (2002) state, "Counselors can: identify strengths, help individuals identify external barriers, and recognize the signs that an individual's behaviors and concerns reflect responses to systemic or internalized oppression."

Goodman uses the metaphor elsewhere (Goodman, 2009) of starfish, salmon, and whales to represent these three levels of advocacy. Sea stars—the proper name for starfish—represent individuals. There is a story about an individual on a beach throwing stranded starfish into the ocean. Questioned by a passerby as to how, given the number of starfish, it could possibly matter, the person throws another back and replies, "It matters to this starfish." Is this analogous to what happens in individual counseling? That is, is it an important activity but one that does not address issues systemically?

The community arena can be represented by salmon. In the Pacific Northwest these fish are declining in numbers due to ecological degradation of their environment. Helping one salmon, even though it matters to that salmon, is not enough. We need to advocate at the community level to remove dams, reduce logging, and require power plants to cool outflow before discharging it. Only by advocating more broadly will we be successful.

The public arena can be represented by whales, which migrate throughout the world. Several species of whales are endangered because there is not worldwide agreement to ban killing, among other issues. Thus, if we want to save the whales, we must advocate beyond our borders, analogous to the public arena of the ACA advocacy competencies.

And finally, counseling organizations can address the third part of the mission, promoting respect for human dignity and diversity, by directly assisting those in times of special need. ACA members have partnered with the Red Cross in responding to disasters. Hundreds of counselors provided help to those affected by the events of September 11, 2001; hurricanes in the Gulf of Mexico; the shootings at Virginia Tech; and other disasters.

TWO JOURNEYS IN THE QUEST FOR PROFESSIONAL IDENTITY

Both authors of this chapter share a firm commitment to professional identity and both believe in the development and importance of professional identity throughout a counselor's lifetime. In the following, we share our respective journeys with our readers.

Let me (Goodman) tell you my story as it relates to my evolving professional identify. I first joined my state counseling association and ACA as a graduate student. I believed it was a professional privilege and responsibility, and I loved getting those journals right in my own mailbox. I joined different divisions each year as I explored different areas of specialization within counseling. After receiving my master's degree, I got involved in a minor way in a state division, eventually becoming president of that division, president of the state association, president of a national division, and then, president of

ACA. Along the way I spent many hours at board meetings, with committee assignments, and following up on responsibilities. When asked why (or why on earth!) I would spend so much time and sometimes money in association work my reply was always that I got much more than I gave. So, what did I get? Lifelong friends for one—associations are how I met my husband! As a result of memberships and involvement, I gained enormous learning about leadership, about counseling, and about how to more effectively help my clients. Networking helped me get all of the jobs I have had since completing my degree. Opportunities to speak, write, travel, develop new ideas, and follow up on the ideas of others. So, being an active involved member of professional associations is both a right and a privilege. And even during times when life does not permit active involvement, I believe that it is important to support the activities of an association that protects and furthers your rights and the rights of your clients and students to receive counseling services. Paying dues to maintain our profession's growth and health seems to me to be a small price to pay.

Although we each have our own particular stories to tell related to developing and maintaining our professional identities, my story is similar to those of others. My hope is that my story will encourage you to consider how you are intentionally developing your professional identity. What steps are you taking to connect with the profession and its professional association/divisions? If your journey is like mine, then I am confident that with each step you take and each commitment you make to the profession, the rewards will be much greater than the costs. As you strengthen your professional identity, you will need to know important facts about our professional association and its related divisions.

My professional journey (Foster) also began as a master's level student. The university I attended had a very active Chi Sigma Iota International Honor Society chapter (Zeta), which began my interest in professional development and identity. Membership in the state ACA also promoted a desire to be involved at a state and national level. As I finished my master's degree and began to practice, I saw the need for continuing education to develop and hone my counseling skills. As my thirst for knowledge developed, I went back to school, pursuing more graduate studies and eventually completing a doctoral degree. Along my professional journey, I discovered licensure and certification, and the importance of voluntary certification. Through my doctoral studies, I began my involvement with NBCC. As a result of my initial work with NBCC, I was fortunate to work on committees to revise school counselor certification standards, and the development of a new national school counselor certification examination. NBCC elected me to the board of directors because of my belief in the importance of standards and certification. During my tenure as a board member, I had the opportunity to be involved nationally and internationally in promoting standards and certification of counselors. My journey began in my hometown, but then took me all over the world advocating for professional counseling standards and certification. My career has included private practice, working in elementary, middle, and high schools—but my passion lies in credentialing. As a result, I now have a position with NBCC where I can continue working to promote standards and certification of professional counselors worldwide.

I agree with my coauthor that it is a right and a privilege to be involved in our profession whether it is through associational work, continuing education, certification and licensure efforts, or through advocacy for the profession. While membership associations (ACA), accreditation organizations (CACREP) and certifying organizations (NBCC) have different objectives, these groups share the common thread of promoting the professional identity of counselors.

CONCLUSION

Professional identity is achieved in many ways and as a result of different influences. We have shared our respective developmental journeys shaping our collective and individual professional identity. It begins with a strong belief in importance of a common base of knowledge achieved through rigorous educational standards. Other shared elements such as professional associations, certification and licensure, and competency standards add to our professional identity foundation. As professional counselors, we adhere to a code of ethics that stands to protect the public—our clients. Our professional identity is still growing, and as a result of our advocacy and legislative efforts, the public will gain a more defined concept of counselors and the counseling profession.

We both began our commitment to professional identity early in our respective careers, but for both of us, it continues as a lifelong learning and sharing experience. We hope it will be for you as well.

CHAPTER REVIEW

1. Counseling associations provide a professional base for counselors.
2. The American Counseling Association, which is the one organization that represents all counseling specialties, assists its members through providing professional development opportunities, fostering and maintaining professionalism through licensure and other legislative and lobbying efforts, and coordinating advocacy efforts that directly and indirectly help students and clients achieve human dignity.
3. The National Board for Certified Counselors recognizes the professional identity of counselors worldwide, who have met rigorous standards of the profession through education and passed a national exam. These professional counselors continue to meet the high standards of our profession

through adherence to a code of ethics and continuing education to enhance their counseling skills resulting in helping our clients to live more effectively.
4. NBCC also shares a firm commitment with ACA toward legislative advocacy, promoting the value of counseling, professionalism, and public awareness of quality counseling.
5. All counseling organizations have a specific role in the development and maintenance of the professional identity of counselors. Working together for the benefit of professional counselors and the public will ultimately serve to enhance the image of professional counseling.
6. Our profession is still a young one, and it continues to grow and develop. As professionals, we also must learn to grow and develop our own professional identity

through a lifelong commitment. While there may continue to be many specialties within our profession, our professional identity is deeply rooted in our historical beginnings of being helpers. And regardless of our

specialty area within the counseling profession, our professional identity must remain strong in order to continue to develop, promote, and advocate for our profession.

REVIEW QUESTIONS

1. List the steps involved in defining a profession.
2. What is the primary mission of ACA?
3. How many divisions are part of ACA?
4. List five of ACA's divisions.
5. What is the body responsible for accrediting counseling programs?
6. What is the primary mission of CACREP?
7. What board oversees the certification of counselors?
8. Why are ethical codes important?
9. How can counselors engage in advocacy?

ADDITIONAL RESOURCES

- American Association of State Counseling Boards (http://www.aascb.org/)
- American Counseling Association (http://www.counseling.org/)
- American Counseling Association Ethics Code (http://www.counseling.org/Resources/CodeOfEthics/TP/Home/CT2.aspx)
- Council for the Accreditation of Counseling and Related Educational Programs (http://www.cacrep.org/)
- National Board for Certified Counselors (http://www.nbcc.org/)

REFERENCES

American Counseling Association. (2008, October 24). *Bylaws*. Retrieved May 1, 2009, from http://www.counseling.org/AboutUs/ByLaws/TP/Home/CT2.aspx.

American Counseling Association. (2009). *About us*. Retrieved from http://www.counseling.org/AboutUs/.

Goodman, J. (2009). Starfish, salmon, and whales: An introduction to the special section. *Journal of Counseling and Development, 87*, 259.

Klatt, L. (1967). The professionalization of everyone. *Personnel Journal, 46*, 508–509, 522.

Lewis, Arnold, House, & Toporek (2002). *The ACA advocacy competencies*. Retrieved July 6, 2009, from http://www.counseling.org/Resources/.

National Board for Certified Counselors (1993). *A work behavior analysis of professional counselors*. Muncie, IN: Accelerated Development, Inc.

National Board for Certified Counselors. (2009). *About us*. Retrieved May 1, 2009, from http://www.nbcc.org/whoWeAre/About.aspx.

National Career Development Association. (1997). *Career development competencies*. Retrieved July 6, 2009, from http://www.ncda.org/pdf/counselingcompetencies.pdf.

National Career Development Association. (2007). *Career convergence*. Retrieved July 6, 2009 from http://associationdatabase.com/aws/NCDA/pt/sp/career_convergence.

Skovholt, T. M. & Ronnestad, M. H. (1992). Themes in therapist and counselor development. *Journal of Counseling & Development, (70)*, 505–515.

Stauffer, M. D. & Kurpius, S. E. R. (2005). Ethics and the beginning counselor: Being ethical right from the start. In D. Capuzzi and D. R. Gross (Eds.), *Introduction to the counseling profession* (pp. 75–99). Boston, MA: Pearson Education, Inc.

Sue, D. W., Arredondo, P., & McDavis, R. J. (1992). Multicultural competencies and standards: A call to the profession. *Journal of Counseling & Development, 70*, 477–486.

CHAPTER 17

Integrating Technology and Counseling

LEARNING OBJECTIVES

After reading this chapter, you should be able to

- describe the current state of technology use in counseling;
- identify technology competencies for counselors established by the Association for Counseling and Supervision;
- discuss the use of various forms of technology in a counseling context;
- explain how to protect client confidentiality when using technology; and
- discuss ways to use technology for supervision and training.

CHAPTER OUTLINE

INTRODUCTION

According to *Wikipedia* ("Technology," n.d.), technology is defined as "a broad concept that deals with ... usage and knowledge of tools and crafts, and how it affects ... [one's] ability to control and adapt to ... [one's] environment" (¶ 1). While *Wikipedia*—an online encyclopedia everyone can contribute to—would not be considered a professional source for a course paper or presentation, it is useful in this context because it's a good example of how innovative technology is changing the way we gather and use information.

Active Learning Exercise **17.1**

How do you use technology? Take a few minutes to think about different activities you may have engaged in today. Did you buy a cup of coffee or gasoline using your debit card, check your e-mail, order a book online, or send a text message? Did you go on a social networking site like Facebook or MySpace to see what your friends have been up to? Did you review a digitally recorded counseling session, or use a CD or DVD that came with one of your textbooks? Did you search the Internet? All of these activities use various forms of technology.

All the activities you thought about in terms of the kinds of technology you've already used today (see Active Learning Exercise 17.1) require that you possess technological literacy, which Tyler and Sabella (2004) define as the "intellectual processes, abilities, and dispositions needed for counselors to understand the link among technology, themselves, their clients, and a diverse society ... to satisfy human needs and wants for themselves and others" (p. 5). Technologically literate counselors understand the role of technology in their lives. They understand how technology can be used effectively (including being able to assess the risks and benefits of using various forms of technology), are able to resolve ethical and legal dilemmas associated with the use of technology, and feel confident and comfortable using various forms of technology in all aspects of their lives (Tyler & Sabella, 2004). The challenge is that some counselors may not be well educated about how to use various technologies available to them and their clients.

Just in writing this chapter I used several types of technology, including a desktop and a laptop (both Macintosh computers), the spelling and proofreading features in Microsoft Word to help with editing, the Penn State library and the search engine Google to find online resources and research materials, the alarm feature on my Blackberry to remind me of appointments, and e-mail and online Scrabble when I wanted a diversion from writing. This is a small illustration of the ways we use technology on a daily basis to do our work, whether we are counselors, counselors-in-training, supervisors, or faculty. In addition to using technology, we need to be flexible in adapting to new forms of technology, especially if they can help us to be more efficient. I say this because even two years ago, I didn't use some of the technology

I just noted. As a result of the growing relevance of technology to the field of counseling, the purpose of this chapter is to provide an overview of the wide variety of technologies currently used in counseling, including guidelines for how to use them ethically and appropriately.

Active Learning Exercise **17.2**

Take a minute to think about the following questions, adapted from Peterson, Hautamaki, and Walton (2007):

- How much do you invite and use technology in your everyday activities?
- How comfortable are you with using different kinds of technology in general (this can be everything from using an electric toothbrush to using text messaging) and in counseling?
- How might your perspectives on technology affect your views of a client who wants you to provide online counseling, or a supervisor who wants to meet with you via videoconferencing?

There are no right or wrong answers to these questions but given the increasing use of technology in counseling settings, it's important that we're aware of our thoughts, feelings, and behaviors regarding technology.

COUNSELING AND TECHNOLOGY

Computer-assisted counseling, in the form of software used by counselors in session or as a part of the counseling process, was developed in the 1960s but it wasn't used on a larger scale until the 1980s when it was typically used to help clients rehearse new behaviors through simulated practice experiences, complete tests and assessments, and learn new and more effective ways to interact with other people (Peterson et al., 2007). And while the use of the World Wide Web (WWW) is now commonplace in most parts of the world, the first Web page was posted fewer than 20 years ago, on December 10, 1991 (Tyler & Guth, 2004).

Perspectives on the Use of Technology in Counseling

Counselors view the constantly expanding use of technology in counseling, including the use of Web-based information, online counseling, and video-based supervision, in different ways. Some counselors view using technology as an innovative and creative way to access information and to reach clients who may be too busy or too isolated to come in for face-to-face counseling. Other counselors view technology as both a blessing and a curse, in that some forms of technology can be used to enhance the counseling process while others may create more distance between clients and counselors. And some counselors experience *cyberphobia*, meaning they experience anxiety around the use of computers, although the anxiety is typically related to the reactions of others rather than a resistance to learning or an opposition to technology (Bloom & Walz, 2004). Remember in all instances that the technologies described are tools that can be used to help counselors work with their clients. They do not replace the need for effective, appropriate, and ethical counseling knowledge and skills.

The upside of using technology includes an increased ability to access information at faster speeds; increased independence because we can obtain information no matter where we are; the ability to streamline routine tasks; an increased sense of connectedness with others; and the ability to reach clients in rural or isolated areas, or clients who can't access counseling services during traditional nine-to-five, Monday-through-Friday hours. The downside of technology includes limited access for some people as a result of disability, technological illiteracy, or lack of financial resources; being inundated with more information than we have time to process; physical health problems related to the use of technology, such as repetitive stress injuries; increased anxiety as a result of feeling we have less free time because technology allows us to assess work 24 hours a day, seven days a week; and an increased sense of the need to multitask since technology permits us to do several tasks at one time. There can also be an increase in employer expectations that we can do more in less time because of computers and other kinds of technology (Casey, 2000). Finally, there exists the challenge of how to learn all the new technologies while maintaining a caseload and meeting the needs of clients and colleagues, even when the new technology can help reduce workloads once it is learned.

Technology Competencies and Counselor Training

Realizing the growing importance of technology in counseling, in the late 1990s a group of counselor educators developed a list of 12 technology-related competencies they believed counselors should possess (Tyler & Sabella, 2004). The latest version of these competencies, known as the *Technical Competencies for Counselor Education Students: Recommended Guidelines for Program Development* (ACES Technology Interest Network, 2007), can be found at http://www.acesonline.net/documents.asp. In general these competencies suggest that well-trained counselors are able to use a variety of software programs, like Microsoft Word or Excel, as well as audiovisual equipment; are able to access e-mail, as well as counseling-related Listservs and discussion groups; can use assessment software programs; and can use the Internet to gather and transmit information to others. As you go through your counseling training program, periodically review the list of competencies to ensure that you're learning the necessary technology skills so you can do your best work with clients. At the same time, look for new kinds of technology and new uses for existing technology that aren't addressed in the competencies.

Now think back to the technologically related activities you've already engaged in today. How did you learn to perform those tasks? How easy or difficult was it to learn them and how quickly did they become second nature to you? In what ways do you envision using technology in your work with clients this year, in 5 years, in 10 years, and how will you go about learning how to perform those activities? The answers to these questions will not only help you, but being aware of your own perspectives about and experiences with technology can help you educate and empathize with your clients and colleagues as they work with technology.

Cultural Diversity and Technology

One of the larger concerns about using technology in counseling is that not all people have access to technology, particularly computer-based technology. This may be the result of financial constraints, limited reading and writing skills, cyberphobia, lack of technological literacy, or not having the use of accessible technology, in the case of people with disabilities. This lack of access is often referred to as the digital or technological divide and can influence how we use technology with our clients. According to Remley and Herlihy (2007), a 2000 report from the United States Department of Commerce noted that 51 percent of the households they surveyed had a computer in the home, and 42 percent had access to the Internet. Of the people who had Internet access, 46 percent were White, 57 percent were Asian American, 24 percent were Hispanic, and 24 percent were African American. Of the people who had home access to the Internet, 86 percent had household incomes over $75,000 a year and only 13 percent had household incomes of less than $15,000 (Remley & Herlihy). In contrast, Cook and Doyle (2002) found equal representation across income levels, but they found that Whites, people with higher levels of education, and people living in urban areas were more likely to have home access to the Internet.

Peterson et al. (2007) note, "Socially responsible practitioners must make every effort to keep progressive technology in counseling equally accessible to all who need it, lest the technology itself becomes a vehicle of disenfranchisement rather than one of empowerment" (p. 194). As counselors, we have a responsibility to be aware of community resources, such as libraries and community centers, where clients can access free computer services. We also have a responsibility to help clients who have limited literacy or who do not have strong English reading and writing skills to access information and resources using technology, including helping them receive services so they can learn to use technology independently, if they so choose.

MAKING USE OF TECHNOLOGY IN COUNSELING

There are many ways to categorize how technology is used in counseling situations but to keep things clear and simple I'll discuss technology in four broad categories: (1) direct client services, (2) online counseling, (3) record keeping and documentation, and (4) counselor training and supervision. Each section will address relevant technologies including an explanation of the technology, how counselors might use it, and possible ethical and legal implications.

Direct Client Services

This category includes any technology that is used directly with clients, including telephones (both landline and cell phones) and answering services, fax machines, e-mail, the Internet and the WWW, computerized assessments, and counseling issues specific to computer technology. For example, computer technology can be used to gather or record information about clients during intake or throughout the counseling process. And some researchers have found that when asked about sensitive topics like criminal history, suicidal ideation, sexual concerns, and addiction history, clients disclose more when recording the information via computer than they do when talking with a counselor (Newman, 2004).

Telephones and Answering Services

There are several cautions to keep in mind when using telephones to communicate with clients or to discuss clients, some of which are directly addressed in standard B.3.e of the American Counseling Association's (ACA) *Code of Ethics* (2005). First, check to make sure you are actually talking with the client before you disclose confidential information. In the future we may all use videophones to talk with each other, but until then we need to find ways to verify the people we are talking with are our actual clients. And be conscious about discussing client information in a private area where other people can't hear what you're saying. Second, if discussing client information with another professional by phone, make sure you have a signed release of information from the client. Don't talk with anyone who says he or she has a release without seeing a copy of the signed document.

Third, be aware that using landline phones are the only way to ensure the conversation is confidential, since cell phone conversations can be intercepted. This is important for counselors but also for clients who may be talking with counselors on their cell phones. Even landline phones may be monitored, recorded, or intercepted without your knowledge (Remley & Herlihy, 2007). With regard to cell phones, if you contact clients, there is a record of their phone number and possibly their names in your phone, so make an effort to erase confidential information. Even if someone cannot tell the number is a client's number, they may call the number to see who you've been talking to and may inadvertently find out someone is your client. Fourth, do not make "off the record" comments since anything you say may be passed on to someone else. Only state information you feel comfortable having passed on to others.

Answering machines and answering services, voice mail systems, and pagers are other forms of technology that can be helpful during the counseling process but should be used carefully. In terms of voice mail and answering machines, Remley and Herlihy (2007) note two cautions: (1) leaving a message creates a voice record of information that exists until it's erased, and (2) there is no way to ensure that the person you leave the message for will be the only person to listen to the message. Protect client confidentiality when leaving and receiving messages since you don't know who may listen to a message. Leave only your name and content that will not disclose that the person is a client. Listen to your phone messages in a private area, and don't provide unnecessary people with access to your answering machine or your access code. You will also want to educate people who take messages for you about the importance of client confidentiality. Many phone systems now use password protected voice mail systems, but if your agency doesn't, work with your staff to ensure other people don't have access to your phone or to messages from clients.

Fax Machines

Facsimile or fax machines, whether sending a paper fax or "directly from a computer file" fax, are another form of technology used in counseling settings. Fax machines are often located in public spaces, so if you're sending or receiving information via fax, call the sender before transmitting the fax to make sure he or she knows it's coming and can be at the machine to receive the information. Use a cover sheet stating that the information is confidential and to whom it is directed, but keep in mind that the cover sheet does not protect confidential information from being intercepted by the wrong person. With that in mind, don't send sensitive client information such as session notes or assessment results by fax. You should also obtain a signed client release specific to sending information via faxes (Welfel, 2006).

Electronic Mail

E-mail is another form of technology used in counseling that has rapidly increased in recent years. While e-mail can be an easy and efficient way to contact clients and colleagues, keep in mind e-mail is not a confidential method of communication. Check with clients to see if they want you to contact them by e-mail, particularly since other people may have access to their e-mail account, and be sure you type the correct address when you send an e-mail. The same applies if you use the text message feature on your phone. If you do use e-mail with clients, it is best to use it for scheduling purposes or as between-sessions support (Tyler & Sabella, 2004) and not for counseling or consulting unless you are providing e-counseling (this topic will be addressed later in more detail). Even if you send an e-mail to one person, that e-mail can be forwarded to hundreds of people in a matter of seconds, so don't put information in an e-mail that you wouldn't want to have printed in the newspaper or read on the evening news.

Reread your e-mails before you hit the "send" key to make sure your content and grammar are correct, and use a profession tone in your writing (e.g., "Dear ..." rather then "Hey dude ..."). Even though we're used to using e-mail in an informal way, always present yourself in a professional manner just as you would in a formal letter or client report. Every e-mail can easily become a printed document, and you should consider either printing copies of e-mails and keeping them in client files, if you keep paper files, or using some form of computer backup system to save e-mail correspondence regarding clients. When you use your agency or program e-mail, your employer has the right to access any and all of your e-mails so don't use your work e-mail for personal correspondence. In addition, if you use major e-mail service providers like AOL or Hotmail, they may keep copies of all e-mails for one year after transmission on their server (Welfel, 2006). As with other forms of computer technology, keep in mind that deleting e-mail doesn't always mean the document is completely deleted. Finally, although the law might not support this view, all e-mails should be treated as copyrighted materials and should not be used unless they're cited as personal communication. When possible, you should obtain written permission prior to using an e-mail in a communication other than the format for which it was originally intended (Tyler & Sabella, 2004).

The Internet

Use of the Internet has increased greatly in the past decade, and should be used as another tool in the counseling process. This is not markedly different from counselors reviewing any printed documents, such as books or journals, they recommend to clients and colleagues to ensure the information provided is accurate and well documented. The difference is the exponential number of sites available to clients with just a few keystrokes. Because there are no restrictions or guidelines about what information can be posted on the Internet, counselors should review Web sites carefully before recommending them to clients or colleagues. When reviewing sites, (a) check the content to make sure it's current, accurate, and consistent with other well-documented information; (b) consider the source of the content; (c) assess who owns the Web site to determine if they have a vested interest in the view they promote on the site (e.g., a site that provides information about antidepressants is sponsored by a pharmaceutical company); (d) determine if the relevant links are active; and (e) decide who would benefit from viewing the site. As with e-mail, be aware that your employer can access your Internet search history.

Counselors can also create lists of Web sites to share with clients who want to learn specific information. For example, counselors who specialize in working with people with eating disorders can create a list of recovery sites that have been helpful to previous clients. Or a counselor working with a parent of an adolescent child with Asperger's syndrome can suggest the client go to YouTube to watch videos of people describing their experiences living with Asperger's. Another option is to work with clients to help them become good consumers of Web-based information independent of counseling. In this case, counselors can sit with clients as they search for information, assessing the clients' computer and critical thinking skills and providing guidance when necessary. Some sites may not be accessible to people with disabilities, people with low reading levels or low literacy, or people for whom English is not their first language. In these cases, clients can be encouraged to surf the Internet with family or friends who can help them interpret the information. Counselors can also encourage clients to bring the information they find into session for discussion (Tyler & Sabella, 2004).

Another option is for counselors to develop their own Web sites. This may occur for a variety of reasons, including advertising their counseling practice, educating clients about particular topics, and providing information to previous, current, and future clients. If you choose to create your own Web site, make sure you acknowledge your content sources and don't take information from a source without noting that on your site. Counselors should not only make sure the content is accurate and correctly attributed to the original author (i.e., don't present other people's Web site content as your own), but they should develop and maintain a Web site that is accessible to all people. While describing the elements needed to create a Web site is beyond the scope of this chapter, there are a variety of resources counselors can use. The Web Accessibility Initiative (WAI, 2008) Web site provides information and resources to develop a Web site that is accessible for people with disabilities. As the developers of the WAI note, the Internet is increasingly becoming an essential resource for people, and "it is essential that the Web be accessible in order to provide equal access and equal opportunity to people with disabilities. An accessible Web can also help people with disabilities more actively participate in society" (¶ 5).

Some of the technology that people with visual impairments use to access Web site content includes the JAWS screen reader program and computer programs that can translate computer text into Braille, enlarge the text on their computer screen, or read computer text aloud. People with physical disabilities can use programs that translate their speech into text on the screen, change the rate of speed on their keyboard, or use commands to create words or phrases out of a few keystrokes (e.g., typing the letters "sc" can become "school counselor"). There are a number of simple ways counselors can make their Web sites universally accessible, including using alternative tags (or alt-tags) for all photographs and audiovisual clips on their site, which provide text explaining the pictures for people with visual impairments and people who use older generation computers. In addition, use Web page layouts that allow screen readers, which translate text into speech, to access all the content on the page, and add closed-captioning (adding text for all the sounds and spoken words) for all audiovisual content for people with hearing impairments. Closed-captioning is also helpful for people with low literacy and people for whom English is a second language (Wheaton & Granello, 2004). Counselors who develop their own sites should also make sure there is adequate contrast between the text and the background (there's actually a whole science to this), and shouldn't rely solely on color to transmit information since some viewers may be color-blind. Fortunately, there are free and low-cost Web development programs that can help you create accessible and visually attractive Web sites.

Computerized Assessments

One of the earliest and still most common ways counselors use computer technology in their work with clients is through computer-assisted assessments, using computers to administer, score, and interpret a wide variety of career, personal, and cognitive assessments (Peterson et al., 2007). Computerized assessment refers to any test or assessment that is administered or interpreted using computer software, while Internet-based assessment refers to computerized assessments that use Internet servers for some part of the assessment process (Tyler & Sabella, 2004). Computer-assisted assessments can be computer based, which is essentially posting a paper-and-pencil test on a computer, or computer adaptive, where the test or assessment is customized to the client by "building into the test a decision making model that responds to the client's level of errors and adjusts the items administered based on this information" (Abney & Maddux, 2004, p. 4). When using computerized versions of tests and assessments, counselors should not use pirated software or assessments. For example, copies of the Myers-Briggs Type Indicator and the Beck Depression Inventory can easily be found on the WWW, but both are copyrighted instruments and should only be used with permission. Counselors also need to know and understand the psychometric properties (e.g., reliability, validity, norming groups) of the computerized version rather than assuming the psychometric properties are the same as for the paper and pencil version of the test. They should also determine whether the assessment has been extensively tested using a computer format (National Career Development Association [NCDA], 1997). Much the same as they would with a paper and pencil assessment, counselors should receive training and supervision before giving or reviewing the results of a computerized assessment.

There are numerous reasons why counselors use computerized tests and assessments. For example, computer-based assessments can be tailored to specific clients or situations, they often require less time then paper-and-pencil versions of the same assessments, and clients can receive immediate feedback as well as track their progress over time (Abney & Maddux, 2004). Computerized assessments are also effective at providing reliable, consistent, and repetitive information, for example, presenting instructions on how to complete an assessment. While computerized assessments are frequently used, counselors should take several precautions before using them as they would more traditional assessments. First, counselors should ensure that the computerized assessments are accessible to clients, particularly clients who have visual or physical disabilities. Second, counselors should assess clients' computer literacy and their comfort and confidence with using computerized testing. Third, when using technology to interpret assessment results, counselors need to review the content carefully and supplement the results when necessary (e.g., adding content about testing conditions, observed behaviors as the client completed the assessment) to ensure the findings are relevant and specific to the client (Peterson et al., 2007). As with all written word–based assessments, counselors should also determine clients' literacy level as well as their ability to read English. Finally, counselors should have a back-up plan in case problems develop with the technology.

Online Counseling

One of the most controversial issues with regard to technology in counseling is the use of online counseling in place of face-to-face counseling. At this point in time there are a number of names for online counseling, including Internet counseling, webcounseling, e-counseling, e-therapy, and cybercounseling. I will use the term *online counseling* to refer to any counseling interactions that occur using the Internet, e-mail, or a chat feature like IM (instant messaging) or meeting software (e.g., Go To Meeting) for communication that uses typed text rather than the spoken word. While the research in this area is still somewhat limited, some researchers have found that clients who engaged in online counseling were able to develop a "collaborative, bonding relationship" and found the experience to be a positive one (Cook & Doyle, as cited in Peterson et al., 2007). Day and Schneider (as cited in Peterson et al., 2007) also found that clients who engaged in online counseling increased their length of participation compared to clients engaged in face-to-face counseling. Some reasons given for making online counseling available to clients include lack of access to counseling services (e.g., clients in rural areas); disability-related limitations that require accommodations that don't fit into a 50-minute counseling session (e.g., a client who uses augmentative communication methods); clients with schedules that prohibit attending counseling on a nine-to-five, Monday-through-Friday schedule; and people who prefer expressing themselves through written communication rather than the spoken word (Remley & Herlihy, 2007).

Concerns have been raised, however, about using online counseling. These concerns include the lack of visual and auditory clues that exist when using online counseling, the possibility of breaches of confidentiality related to Internet security, how to assess and intervene with clients who may be considering harming themselves or others, how to effectively build a counseling alliance or relationship when the clients and the counselors don't share the same physical space (Remley & Herlihy, 2007), and whether counselors will have the time and the energy, as well as the training, to work with what could potentially be increased contacts with clients, especially given that the Internet can be accessed 24 hours a day, seven days a week.

Given the reality that counselors are providing online counseling services, a number of professional organizations have created guidelines to ensure counselors are providing the most effective and ethical services possible for their clients. These guidelines include the *The Practice of Internet Counseling* (National Board for Certified Counselors [NBCC], n.d.) and *NCDA Guidelines for the Use of the Internet for Provision of Career Information and Planning Services* (NCDA, 1997). In addition, the Center for Credentialing and Education, an affiliate of NBCC, recently developed a certification for counselors providing online counseling called the Distance Credentialed Counselor.

NCDA (1997) raises a number of questions and concerns to consider when using online counseling. First, how will you ensure that client information is kept confidential when using an online format for contact? Second, what will you do if you have a client in crisis? Because you may be counseling clients in a different state or even a different country, you need to have a plan for how to intervene if a client expresses suicidal or homicidal ideation, as well as for how you'll learn about resources in your client's home community. Third, how valid will your counseling credentials be in your client's area of the country, or the world? Counselors need to be aware of and honestly relay information about which licenses and certifications will be applicable to potential clients. For example, a counselor who is a Licensed Professional Counselor (LPC) in Pennsylvania cannot say she is an LPC when providing online counseling services to a client in Hawaii, since counselor licensure is not reciprocal across states.

Fourth, what steps will you take to ensure that your client is really who he or she says? Client identity, especially for clients who may be underage, is a concern with online counseling since the counselor can neither see nor hear the client. Fifth, how will you market and present yourself and your qualifications to potential clients? Counselors need to be explicit about their qualifications and training to provide online counseling, and someone who has expertise in online counseling should, at least initially, supervise them. Counselors should also be clear in their promotion materials about what kinds of counseling issues can benefit from online counseling, which requires counselors to stay current on the latest research about the efficacy of online counseling, much as they would with the efficacy of face-to-face counseling. Counselors should be clear about when and how often clients can expect to hear from them, and they should also be prepared to help clients access referrals to face-to-face counselors where the client lives if online counseling is not appropriate (NCDA, 1997). NBCC (n.d.) also has a comprehensive list of recommendations for counselors providing online counseling.

Counselors using online counseling need to be explicit about their fees, ensuring their fees are comparable to other online counseling providers (e.g., flat rate per e-mail, fee per minute of e-mail response, no fee), as well as how clients will pay for services (Peterson et al., 2007). If using insurance, clients need to be informed up front which services would be covered by their insurance. Finally, counselors need to provide clients with detailed information about what kinds of technology they need to have access to in order to effectively receive online counseling services, as well as developing a back-up plan to contact each other in case the client or counselor has problems with technology. Guidelines should also be developed about how to communicate with the counselor off-line, when necessary (Tyler & Sabella, 2004).

One way to make sure you address all of these issues is to develop a written contract that can be faxed to the client or downloaded off the Internet. The contract functions the same as an informed consent document for any type of counseling (e.g., counselor's credentials, costs and billing options, where to report unethical behavior) but in addition includes information about the counselor's expertise delivering online or computer-based counseling services, agreed upon goals for counseling using a computer-based method, a statement about the degree of confidentiality one can expect using computer-based services, how client data will be collected and stored and for how long, a statement about the need for clients to be in a private environment when they communicate with the counselor, and emergency contact information (NCDA, 1997).

Mallen, Vogel, and Rochlen (2005) recommend that counselors providing online services have clients provide basic contact information and discuss what steps the counselor would take in case of a danger of harm to self or others. Relevant demographic information would include home address and telephone numbers, as well as physician and emergency contact names and numbers. They also provide guidance on how counselors should market themselves for online counseling (e.g., credentials, areas of expertise). Additional helpful information for clients includes content to help them decide whether online counseling is the best option for them, possible limits of online counseling, fees, and scope of services. Once they're providing online counseling, counselors should check in with clients regularly to ensure that empathic statements are coming across to the clients. For example, counselors can type out their emotional reactions to client content (e.g., "I felt sad when I read about your fight with your son"), use emoticons, and even write about their nonverbal reactions to client content since clients can't see the counselor's nonverbal responses (Mallen et al., 2005).

Record Keeping and Documentation

As noted in the *ACA Code of Ethics* (2005), counselors are responsible for protecting and maintaining confidential client information, including information stored using a variety of electronic means. Section B.3.e defines electronic media as "computers, electronic mail, facsimile machines, telephones, voicemail, answering machines, and other electronic or computer technology" (ACA, p. 8). Protecting client records transmitted through electronic means is also mandated under the Health Information Portability and Accountability Act (HIPAA; Peterson et al., 2007). This section will address how to use various forms of technology for record keeping purposes, including computer disks, flash drives, and computers, but first we'll begin with an overview of HIPAA.

Designed to create uniform standards and increase the efficiency by which protected health information (PHI) is transferred from one health professional to another or to an insurance company, HIPAA was signed into law in 1996. HIPAA consists of three main rules. The Electronic Transaction Rule addresses protecting the confidentiality of any PHI transmitted using electronic means from the counselor to an insurance carrier. The Privacy Rule requires all counselors who could potentially transfer records using electronic means (e.g., fax, e-mail attachments) to inform clients in writing of the steps they will take to safeguard the clients' PHI. The Security Rule addresses how to appropriately store and manage PHI using electronic means (Peterson et al., 2007; Welfel, 2006).

One aspect of maintaining confidential client records is being aware of who has access to your office and when it has been accessed. Your supervisor, colleagues, maintenance staff, and janitorial staff are examples of people who might have access to your office. It is important to not only keep client records in the form of printed documents and paper files secured when you're away from your desk, but you should password protect your computer and any methods used to store data (e.g., CDs, DVDs, flash drives) so they cannot be accessed by others. Train the office staff you work with about password security. If other people need to access your computer files, an administrative assistant for example, select a shared password that is not the same password you use for other files that only you have access to. When sharing a password, be sure the password itself is kept in a secure location. I've seen situations where passwords are posted on computer screens, which defeats the purpose of having a password.

Computer storage is another way that technology is changing how we provide services to our clients. As technology advances, we're able to store information about clients in more compact ways. The good side of this is that we can now save large volumes of information in ways that are transportable, don't take up a lot of space, and are easier to access locally and from a distance (e.g., being able to access a client's file from an Internet-based site while on a home visit). The bad side is that we need to take new precautions to protect client records. Computer storage includes online storage and back-up systems, where the information is stored in cyberspace rather than on a disk or in a paper file, and computer disks, CDs, DVDs, and jump or flash drives, which can hold tremendous amounts of information and are easy to transport (and potentially easy to lose). Labeling these forms of technology is the most effective way to know what is stored where. To protect clients, use codes rather than client names on labels, and keep the list that connects client names with codes in a secure place. Whether you're archiving client records or accessing them on a regular basis, make regular backup copies of files and keep them in a secure but separate location. And be sure to update your virus protection on a regular basis. Many programs allow users to set a consistent time where the computer will search for and update virus protection software.

When using printed client records, keep them in locked file cabinets when you are not using them. No matter how rigorous your agency policies on client confidentiality, leaving a file unattended even for a few minutes provides an opportunity for someone to have access to confidential client information. A final word on computer storage has to do with deleted documents. Computer technicians can retrieve most deleted files, so check your agency policy about how to dispose of disks and other pieces of technology (Remley & Herlihy, 2007). If there is no policy, work with your technology staff to develop a policy for safely disposing of technology that may contain information about clients.

Another potential use for technology is software developed to help counselors maintain their counseling practice. Software programs have been developed that can assist with everything from managing case records (including how to format and organize case notes to using voice-to-text software), to generating treatment plans, to managing billing, to creating presentations for community education and outreach, to creating a Web site to advertise services to potential clients (Tyler & Sabella, 2004). A community mental health counselor, for example, could develop a Web site of local resources in several languages that could be used by refugee clients who could come to the office or go to the local library for computer access. Newer technologies include programs that help counselors develop podcasts and DVDs that can be used for client education, community outreach, professional development, and training of allied professionals. For example, a school counselor could develop a podcast about living with and managing obsessive-compulsive disorder (OCD) that could be used to educate students with OCD, as well as their friends, families, and teachers.

The advent of computers has created new opportunities and new challenges for counselors. While computers allow counselors to create their own documents and manage their case files in their offices and out in the field, there are potential ethical concerns. Many counselors use laptops they take with them when they visit clients so they can access client files and the Internet. If you're using a laptop in a public space, keep the screen turned away from other people's view. Whether the computer is portable or not, using password protections is the most effective way to protect client records. If counselors share a computer to type client notes, they should store all confidential client records on a disk rather than the hard drive, and the disks should be kept in a locked cabinet or desk when not in the counselors' possession. Client files should not be kept on a network or shared server, unless it is designed specifically to protect client records, since other people could inadvertently or intentionally access those records (Peterson et al., 2007). In addition, if counselors share a printer, they should retrieve documents immediately to ensure confidential information is protected.

Counselor Training and Supervision

A final way that technology has changed counseling is the area of computer-assisted consultation, supervision, and distance learning, which is defined as any activity where learning takes place using some form of electronic means (e.g., computer, videotaped materials viewed on a television) between the student and teacher in different locations (Tyler & Sabella, 2004). Counselor educators and supervisors are beginning to use technology to provide training and supervision from a distance, including videoconferencing, digital recording of sessions, online lectures, and discussion groups using e-mail or other text-based formats conducted in real time, like IM, or in asynchronous time.

While limited research exists to show whether supervision and consultation using distance technology is as effective as face-to-face interactions, there are some guidelines we can follow to get the most out of these experiences. When using technology to provide supervision, consultation, or education, first determine the level of training and comfort people have with using technology in this way. Using distance formats may create barriers to mentoring and modeling of professional behaviors, since the people can't see each other unless they're using video technology like iChat (Peterson et al., 2007). When using technology for supervision or consultation, first talk about whether you want to use a video- or audio-based format or if the content will be presented in a reading and writing format, since that decision can affect when and how information is transmitted. Also check for compatibility of technology (e.g., Web access, Mac/PC interfacing). If the selected format includes video or audio content, make sure everyone present is cleared to have access to confidential information. Set clear goals of who is responsible for what activities and when you'll communicate with each other (e.g., time changes, frequency of contact). Finally, have a back-up plan in case technology problems arise, including how to access technology support.

Distance learning is another emerging area in counselor training. Some of the positive reasons for using distance learning formats include the flexibility it offers in that students can go to school when it fits their schedule, rather than only when the courses are offered like in a traditional face-to-face course. Distance learning also works well for non-traditional students and students who live in remote areas or work full-time and cannot make the commitment to full-time study. In terms of continuing education, distance learning can be less costly than attending a conference or workshop and can be completed when and where the counselor chooses. For online courses that are frequently updated, students can also learn the most current information, and participants can select the instructor they want to work with based on their reputation or the training topic (Tyler & Sabella, 2004).

Possible downsides of distance learning include lack of in-person access to faculty since most or all contact will occur online, faculty and students who may be ill-prepared to teach and learn using distance technology, and problems with technology like the Web site "crashing" or having computer technology that is not compatible with the course technology. People considering using distance learning should investigate the course or program closely to ensure these concerns don't become a reality. Many online programs include a mandatory orientation course students must complete that educates them about how to use distance learning programs to their best advantage. Potential students should also check to see if the distance learning course or workshop they want to take will be accepted by their licensing or certification boards or by a university since not all distance learning programs have been approved by these organizations. Finally, at this time the majority of the learning in a distance learning course occurs through reading and writing, including the use of discussion groups and chat rooms, so if people don't like to read then distance learning may not be a good format for them. Students must also be organized, have good time management skills, and be well disciplined to successfully complete online courses, given their autonomous and independent nature (Tyler & Sabella, 2004). Faculty who are interested in teaching an online or distance learning course can find a variety of Web sites and even online courses that will help them learn how to design a Web-based course or training program.

COUNSELING ISSUES SPECIFIC TO CLIENT USE OF THE INTERNET

There are a number of counseling issues that can arise specific to clients using computer technology. I will give a brief description of these issues, and you are encouraged to seek out other resources to learn more about each issue and possible treatment options.

Internet abuse/addiction relates to clients who either can't control or can't stop their online behavior, and common addictions are to viewing online pornography, engaging in Internet gambling, and compulsive or excessive online shopping. Counseling services are often offered online as a way to teach clients how to use the Internet in a healthy and productive way, since many people can't just stop using computers altogether as they would if they were addicted to alcohol or heroin.

Computer-related identity theft is another emerging counseling concern that can have serious implications for people whose identities are stolen. Counselors can help people work through their feelings of being victimized as well as developing plans to handle the stress involved with the often years of work it takes to clear their names and credit histories as a result of the identity theft (Rollins, 2008).

With the growing popularity of social networking sites like MySpace and Facebook, cyberbullying is on the increase, especially among adolescents. Cyberbullying refers to actions taken to cause harm to another person through any electronic means, like a computer or cell phone or through the Internet, and can lead to dire consequences, including suicide, on the part of people who are being victimized. The increase in online sexual predators also has counseling implications in terms of providing services for people who have been victimized as well as for perpetrators (Rollins, 2008). Kennedy (2008) provides a list of guidelines counselors can use to educate parents and children about how to access the Internet safely. A related issue is whether counselors want to "friend" clients and students on social networking sites.

If counselors do choose to make their Facebook, LinkedIn, or MySpace pages available to clients, they should review the content to ensure it presents them in a professional and positive light (Thompson, 2008). Counselors who friend their clients—which is not recommended but may be OK in some settings, like a secondary school or college—need to consider how they will handle related ethical issues, including inadvertent self-disclosure as result of content they place of their pages, boundary issues, and what they will do if they learn information from a client's social networking page that leads the counselor to believe the client is at risk of harming him- or herself or others. The same is true when counselors write blogs or develop personal Web sites.

A final computer-related counseling issue is the easy access people with eating disorders have to information about how to maintain and hide their disease from others. For example, Web sites exist, often referred to as "pro-ana communities," that argue that anorexia is a lifestyle rather than an illness, and they provide support and suggestions for maintaining and increasing weight loss.

CONCLUSION

In closing, I have a few suggestions that can help you use technology more effectively and efficiently while you're in school and once you begin working full time as a counselor. First, as the use of technology in counseling increases, it's imperative that we learn to manage technology so that it works for us, and not vice versa. Jencius (2008) calls this *lifehacking*, which he describes as "the practice of finding simple and elegant solutions to solve life's common problems, often using technology" (p. 28). It's really about finding ways to manage the technology we use, from cell phones to e-mail to online calendars, so that we are more productive in less time and with less effort. For example, e-mail is an important communication tool but it can also be a big distraction. Instead of leaving your e-mail on all day so you're frequently disrupted by the "you have mail" tone, check your e-mail two to three times a day at set times for a set period of time. That way you are not constantly interrupting yourself by reading and possibly responding to e-mails throughout the day. Instead, you'll be responding to e-mails when you know you have the time to do so with your full attention. It is also most effective to respond to e-mails as you read them, rather than reading through all of your e-mails first and then going back and answering them. In addition, there are Web sites that provide suggestions for how to manage e-mail, Web site bookmarks, computer folders, and other forms of online technology. Two good sources are David Allen's Getting Things Done Web site (http://www.davidco.com/index.php) and Merlin Mann's Web site (www.43folders.com).

Second, making the time to learn how to use a word processing program, a presentation program (like PowerPoint or Keynote), and spreadsheet (Excel, Lotus) and statistical software (SPSS, SAS) can help you in school and beyond. All of these programs have shortcuts that make them that much more efficient to use. For example, you can create a word processing template so that all of your papers begin with one-inch margins and are double-spaced without having to set those parameters each time you begin a writing assignment. Some students also benefit from programs that store reference information, like Endnote, or programs that create papers using the American Psychological Association publication format. When using programs such as these, be sure to carefully check your final product since the program may not have recorded all the information accurately. Counselors can also benefit from learning how to create PDF (portable document format) files using Adobe systems to ensure the documents they send to others cannot be altered by the receiver (Tyler & Sabella, 2004).

Third, decide whether computer and technology upgrades will actually enhance your work productivity. Because a new upgrade or a new product exists doesn't mean you have to have it. Technical support staff can be a great resource in determining what upgrades you really need, as well as how to use technology most effectively. Fourth, create your own boundaries around when and how you'll make use of technology. Just because you can access your e-mail, voice mail, and the Internet 24 hours a day doesn't mean you have to. You can decide when and where you'll use technology in your life and your work. As Casey (2000) notes, "Technology is a tool, not a lifestyle" (p. 26). Finally, expect the unexpected. Always have a back-up plan in case something happens to your technology, be sure to back-up your documents, have extra print cartridges and paper on hand, and allow yourself adequate time when using technology.

CHAPTER REVIEW

1. The use of technology in counseling has evolved from computerized tests and assessments developed in the 1960s to Web sites that address specific counseling issues, podcasts that provide practicing counselors with continuing education, and online support groups.
2. The most effective way to work through anxiety related to the use of technology (for both clients and counselors) is through education, consultation, and support.
3. Staying current with how technology is addressed in counseling codes of ethics is essential to providing ethical and responsible services to our clients.
4. Types of technology that counselors use include computers, electronic and Internet-based calendars, fax machines, smart phones, CDs and DVDs to store client files, the Internet and the WWW for continuing education, and videoconferencing and e-mail for supervision and consultation. As technology continues to evolve and expand, counselors will need to learn how to use new forms of technology ethically and responsibly.
5. Counselors can feel pressure to learn the latest technology and to be accessible 24 hours a day. It is important that counselors learn how to manage technology as a tool to help them be productive, including knowing when to disconnect, so that the technology works for them and not vice versa.

REVIEW QUESTIONS

1. How has the use of technology changed in the past three decades?
2. What are three ways counselors can use the Internet and the WWW to help them in their job?
3. Describe five ways counselors can maintain their clients' confidentiality when using technology.
4. How can you use technology to help you be successful as a student and as a counselor?
5. What are three things counselors can do to manage technology so they don't feel like it is managing them?

ADDITIONAL RESOURCES

- Association for Counselor Education and Supervision: Technical Competencies for Counselor Education: Recommended Guidelines for Program Development (http://www.acesonline.net/documents.asp)
- Journal of Technology in Counseling (http://jtc.colstate.edu/)
- National Board for Certified Counselors: *The Practice of Internet Counseling* (http://www. nbcc.org/ethics/Default.aspx)
- NCDA *Guidelines for the Use of the Internet for Provision of Career Information and Planning Services* (http://www.ncda.org)
- Web Accessibility Initiative (http://www. w3.org/WAI/)

REFERENCES

Abney, P. C., & Maddux, C. D. (2004). Counseling and technology: Some thoughts about the controversy. *Journal of Technology in Human Services, 23*(3), 1–24.

ACES Technology Interest Network. (2007). *Technical competencies for counselor education: Recommended guidelines for program development.* Retrieved June 15, 2008, from http://www.acesonline.net/documents.asp.

American Counseling Association. (2005). *ACA code of ethics.* Alexandria, VA: Author.

Bloom, J. W., & Walz, G. R. (Eds.). (2004). *Cybercounseling cyberlearning: An encore.* Alexandria, VA: American Counseling Association.

Casey, J. A. (2000). Managing technology wisely: New counselor competency. In J. W. Bloom & G. R. Walz (Eds.), *Cybercounseling and cyberlearning: Strategies and resources for the millennium* (pp. 17–28). Alexandria, VA: American Counseling Association.

Cook, J. E., & Doyle, C. (2002). Working alliance in online therapy as compared to face-to-face therapy: Preliminary results. *Cyberpsychology and Behavior, 5,* 95–105.

Jencius, M. (2008). Hacking your life. *Counseling Today, 51*(1), 28–29.

Kennedy, A. (2008). Plugged in, turned on and wired up. *Counseling Today, 51*(2), 34–38.

Mallen, M. J., Vogel, D. L., & Rochlen, A. B. (2005). The practical aspects of online counseling: Ethics, training, technology, and competency. *The Counseling Psychologist, 33,* 776–818.

National Board for Certified Counselors. (n.d.). *The practice of Internet counseling.* Retrieved October 24, 2007, from http://www.nbcc.org/ethics/Default.aspx.

National Career Development Association. (1997). *NCDA guidelines for the use of the Internet for provision of career information and planning services.* Retrieved October 24, 2007, from http://www.ncda.org.

Newman, M. (2004). Technology in psychotherapy: An introduction. *JCLP/In Session, 60,* 141–145.

Peterson, D. B., Hautamaki, J. B., & Walton, J. L. (2007). Ethics and technology. In R. R. Cottone & V. M. Tarvydas, *Counseling ethics and decision making* (3rd ed., 184–211). New York: Prentice Hall.

Remley, T. P., Jr., & Herlihy, B. (2007). *Ethical, legal, and professional issues in counseling* (Updated 2nd ed.). Upper Saddle River, NJ: Pearson.

Rollins, J. (2008, July). Emerging client issues. *Counseling Today, 51*(1), 28–29.

Technology. (n.d.). *Wikipedia*. Retrieved August 21, 2008, from http://en.wikipedia.org/wiki/Technology.

Thompson, A. (2008). Counselors' right to privacy: Potential boundary crossings through membership in online communities. *Counseling Today, 51*(2), 44–45.

Tyler, J. M., & Guth, L. J. (2004). Understanding online counseling services through a review of definitions and elements necessary for change. In J. W. Bloom & G. R. Walz (Eds.), *Cybercounseling and cyberlearning: An encore* (pp. 133–150). Alexandria, VA: American Counseling Association.

Tyler, J. M., & Sabella, R. A. (2004). *Using technology to improve counseling practice: A primer for the 21st century*. Alexandria, VA: American Counseling Association.

Web Accessibility Initiative. (1994–2008). *WAI resources on introducing Web accessibility*. Retrieved June 18, 2008, from http://www.w3.org/WAI/.

Welfel, E. R. (2006). *Ethics in counseling and psychotherapy: Standards, research, and emerging issues* (3rd ed.). Pacific Grove, CA: Brooks/Cole.

Wheaton, J. E., & Granello, P. F. (2004). In J. W. Bloom & G. R. Walz (Eds.), *Cybercounseling and cyberlearning: An encore* (pp. 3–17). Alexandria, VA: American Counseling Association.

INDEX